W0112804

Omics Approaches in Veterinary Parasitology

Omics Approaches in Veterinary Parasitology: Diagnosis, Biomarkers, and Drug Development explores applications of omics approaches for diagnosis, biomarker discovery, and drug development against parasites of veterinary importance. It presents the fundamental principles of parasite biology and their complex physiological processes. The chapters review key aspects such as parasite life cycles, host–parasite interactions, and the molecular mechanisms that underlie parasitic diseases. The subsequent chapters delve into the principles and applications of genomics, transcriptomics, proteomics, and metabolomics in understanding parasites at a molecular level. The use of next-generation sequencing, PCR-based assays, and metagenomics in identifying and characterizing parasites for accurate and efficient diagnosis are also covered in detail. Toward the end, the book focuses on target identification, drug repurposing, and the optimization of drug efficacy while minimizing drug resistance using omics data. The book is useful for researchers, students, and professionals in the field of veterinary parasitology.

Omics Approaches in Veterinary Parasitology

Diagnosis, Biomarkers, and Drug Development

Edited by
Muhammad Sohail Sajid and
Hafiz Muhammad Rizwan

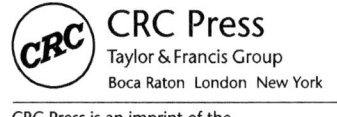

CRC Press
Taylor & Francis Group
Boca Raton London New York

CRC Press is an imprint of the
Taylor & Francis Group, an **informa** business

Designed cover image: ShutterStock Images

First edition published 2025
by CRC Press
2385 NW Executive Center Drive, Suite 320, Boca Raton FL 33431

and by CRC Press
4 Park Square, Milton Park, Abingdon, Oxon, OX14 4RN

CRC Press is an imprint of Taylor & Francis Group, LLC

© 2025 selection and editorial matter, Muhammad Sohail Sajid and Hafiz Muhammad Rizwan; individual chapters, the contributors

Reasonable efforts have been made to publish reliable data and information, but the author and publisher cannot assume responsibility for the validity of all materials or the consequences of their use. The authors and publishers have attempted to trace the copyright holders of all material reproduced in this publication and apologize to copyright holders if permission to publish in this form has not been obtained. If any copyright material has not been acknowledged please write and let us know so we may rectify in any future reprint.

Except as permitted under U.S. Copyright Law, no part of this book may be reprinted, reproduced, transmitted, or utilized in any form by any electronic, mechanical, or other means, now known or hereafter invented, including photocopying, microfilming, and recording, or in any information storage or retrieval system, without written permission from the publishers.

For permission to photocopy or use material electronically from this work, access www.copyright.com or contact the Copyright Clearance Center, Inc. (CCC), 222 Rosewood Drive, Danvers, MA 01923, 978-750-8400. For works that are not available on CCC please contact mpkbookspermissions@tandf.co.uk

Trademark notice: Product or corporate names may be trademarks or registered trademarks and are used only for identification and explanation without intent to infringe.

Library of Congress Cataloging-in-Publication Data

Names: Sajid, Muhammad Sohail, editor. | Rizwan, Hafiz Muhammad, editor.
Title: Omics approaches in veterinary parasitology : diagnosis, biomarkers, and drug development / edited by Muhammad Sohail Sajid, Hafiz Muhammad Rizwan
Description: First edition | Boca Raton, FL : CRC Press, 2025 | Includes bibliographical references and index
Identifiers: LCCN 2024023200 (print) | LCCN 2024023201 (ebook) | ISBN 9781032644455 (hardback) | ISBN 9781032644455 (paperback) | ISBN 9781032651071 (ebook)
Subjects: LCSH: Veterinary parasitology. | Domestic animals--Parasites.
Classification: LCC SF810.A3 O65 2025 (print) | LCC SF810.A3 (ebook) | DDC 636.089/696--dc23/eng/20240703
LC record available at https://lccn.loc.gov/2024023200
LC ebook record available at https://lccn.loc.gov/2024023201

ISBN: 9781032644455 (hbk)
ISBN: 9781032651064 (pbk)
ISBN: 9781032651071 (ebk)

DOI: 10.1201/9781032651071

Typeset in Nemilov
by Deanta Global Publishing Services, Chennai, India

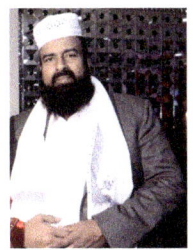

I, Dr. Hafiz Muhammad Rizwan, am honored to present this book titled "Omics Approaches in Veterinary Parasitology; Diagnosis, Biomarkers, and Drug Development." *With heartfelt reverence and deep respect, I dedicate this book to my late father, Mr. Mashooq Ali. His unwavering support, boundless wisdom, and relentless encouragement have been the guiding force behind my academic and professional journey. Though he is no longer with us, his memory continues to inspire and motivate me in every endeavor. May Allah grant my father the highest place in Jannah and shower his soul with eternal peace and blessings. His legacy of kindness, integrity, and dedication to family and community remains a beacon of light for all who knew him. I pray that his soul finds comfort and that he is rewarded abundantly for all the goodness he brought into this world. Ameen.*

Dr. Hafiz Muhammad Rizwan

Contents

Preface

As students and researchers delve deeper into the intricate world of biotechnology, biochemistry, and genetic engineering, the need for comprehensive resources becomes increasingly evident. With this in mind, *Omics Approaches in Veterinary Parasitology: Diagnosis, Biomarkers, and Drug Development* aims to provide a valuable foundation for those navigating the fields of veterinary science, health science, medicine, and related disciplines. This book serves as a gateway to understanding the fundamental principles of various omics technologies in the context of veterinary and medical parasitology. Designed to cater to students, researchers, and professionals alike, it offers a comprehensive overview of genomics, transcriptomics, proteomics, and metabolomics—collectively referred to as "omics." By elucidating the applications of these technologies in parasitic diagnosis and research, this book equips readers with essential knowledge to address the challenges posed by parasitic diseases. We believe that this book fills a crucial gap in parasitology literature, particularly at the molecular and genome levels. With a focus on applicable outcomes, including diagnostics, therapeutics, prevention, and control measures, it provides valuable insights into combating veterinary and medically important parasites worldwide. For students preparing to enter the healthcare field, a solid understanding of disease aetiology, diagnosis, and management is paramount. This book not only offers a comprehensive review of foundational concepts but also explores the cutting-edge applications of omics technologies in parasitic research. In an era of rapidly evolving scientific information, educational resources that are concise yet informative play a pivotal role in facilitating learning and skill development. We hope that *Omics Approaches in Veterinary Parasitology* serves as a valuable resource for students, researchers, and practitioners alike, guiding them through the complexities of parasitic diseases and empowering them to make meaningful contributions to the field. It is our sincere belief that this book will inspire curiosity, foster learning, and ultimately contribute to the advancement of veterinary and medical parasitology.

About the Editors

Muhammad Sohail Sajid got his early education from Kamalia and Khanewal and higher secondary education from Govt. Emerson College, Multan, Punjab, Pakistan. He secured a silver medal in his Doctor of Veterinary Medicine (DVM) degree from the University of Agriculture, Faisalabad (UAF), Pakistan, in 2002. Since then, he started his professional career as a lecturer in the Department of Parasitology, UAF while continuing in MSc (Hons) and PhD in Parasitology. He served as Assistant Professor, Associate Professor, Chairman, and Member, Climate Change Chair of the US–Pakistan Center for Advanced Studies in Agriculture and Food Security, established through the USAID, in the UAF, Pakistan, and finally as tenured Professor. His thematic research area is molecular epidemiology and control of arthropods and arthropod-borne diseases of one health significance. His competitive successes include PhD fellowship sponsored by the Higher Education Commission (HEC), Islamabad, Pakistan, HEC-funded post-doc fellowship from the University of Southern Mississippi (USM), Hattiesburg, MS, USA, USAID-funded project through the HEC Pak-US S&T Cooperation Program (Phase IV), and the Fulbright Post-Doc fellowship at UC Davis, USA. So far, he has been awarded 10 grants as PI/Co-PI and mentored more than 50 M.Phil and 12 PhD graduate students as Chairman/Co-supervisor/Member. The Ministry of Science and Technology, Islamabad, Pakistan, has awarded him competitive Research Productivity Awards consecutively for 6 years (2010 to 2015). To date, he has published approximately 90 research papers in ISI indexed journals having an IF of ~100, presented at various national and international conferences, authored one textbook, two chapters in an international book, and 150 abstracts in proceedings. He has served as "Section Editor" of the UAF's Official Journal *PJAS* (IF-0.785) for more than a decade and has edited books published by CABI, Oxfordshire, UK. He is the co-author of the first guidelines for the "Institutional Animal Care and Use" at UAF. His hard work and commitment enabled him to achieve the top-ranked academic position of Tenured Professor of Parasitology in the Department of Parasitology, UAF, Pakistan.

Hafiz Muhammad Rizwan is an accomplished researcher and academician in the field of Parasitology. He has made significant contributions to the understanding and management of parasitic diseases through his research and publications. Dr Rizwan's expertise lies in the areas of molecular parasitology, host–parasite interactions, omics-based approaches for diagnosing and managing parasitic diseases, and parasitic control strategies. Dr Rizwan is currently affiliated with the University of Veterinary and Animal Sciences (UVAS), Narowal Campus, Pakistan, where he serves as an Assistant Professor of Parasitology in the Department of Pathobiology. He is actively involved in teaching and mentoring students, sharing his knowledge and passion for the subject. With a strong academic background, Dr. Rizwan holds a PhD in Parasitology. He has published numerous research articles in reputable journals, contributing to the scientific literature on parasitic infections. Dr Rizwan's dedication and commitment to his field have earned him recognition and respect from his peers. He continues to make valuable contributions to the field of parasitology through his research, teaching, and academic endeavours.

Contributors

Haider Abbas
Section of Parasitology
Department of Pathobiology
KBCMA College of Veterinary and
    Animal Sciences, Narowal
Sub-campus University of Veterinary
    and Animal Sciences
Lahore, Pakistan

Sumra Wajid Abbasi
Department of Biological Sciences
National University of Medical
    Sciences
Rawalpindi, Pakistan

Haroon Ahmad
Department of Parasitology
Faculty of Veterinary Sciences
University of Agriculture
Faisalabad, Pakistan

Qurat Ul Ain
Department of Forensic Science
Faculty of Medicine and Allied Health
    Sciences
The Islamia University of Bahawalpur
Bahawalpur, Punjab, Pakistan
and
Center for Advanced Interdisciplinary
    Science and Biomedicine of IHM
Division of Life Sciences and
    Medicine
University of Science and Technology
    of China
Hefei, Anhui, China

Rana Muhammad Athar Ali
Department of Clinical Medicine and
    Surgery
University of Agriculture
Faisalabad, Pakistan

Mughees Aizaz Alvi
Department of Clinical Medicine and
    Surgery
University of Agriculture
Faisalabad, Pakistan

Nimra Anwar
Department of Pharmacology and
    Toxicology
Faculty of Bio-Sciences
University of Veterinary and Animal
    Sciences
Lahore, Pakistan

Muhammad Waqar Arshad
Departments of Urology and
    Biochemistry and Molecular
    Genetics
Northwestern University
Feinberg School of Medicine
Chicago, Illinois USA

Syed Awais Attique
School of Interdisciplinary Engineering
    & Science (SINES)
National University of Sciences &
    Technology (NUST)
Islamabad, Pakistan

Muhammad Haziq Bajwa
Faculty of Veterinary Sciences
KBCMA College of Veterinary and
    Animal Sciences
Lahore, Pakistan

**Shameeran Salman Ismael
Bamarni**
Head of Medical Laboratory Sciences
    Department
University Of Duhok
College Of Health Science
Duhok, Iraq

Amina Basheer
Department of Biological Sciences
National University of Medical
    Sciences
Rawalpindi, Pakistan

Usman Elahi
Faculty of Agriculture and Veterinary
    Sciences
Superior University
Lahore, Pakistan

Sadia Ghazanfer
Department of Parasitology
Faculty of Veterinary Science
University of Agriculture
Faisalabad, Pakistan

Syed Soban Hassan
Faculty of Veterinary Sciences
KBCMA College of Veterinary and
    Animal Sciences, Narowal
Sub-campus University of Veterinary
    and Animal Sciences
Lahore, Pakistan

Muhammad Faisal Hayat
Department of Zoology, Wildlife and
    Fisheries
University of Agriculture
Faisalabad, Pakistan

Muhammad Umar Ijaz
Department of Zoology, Wildlife and
    Fisheries
University of Agriculture
Faisalabad, Pakistan

Syed Babar Jamal
Department of Biological Sciences
National University of Medical Sciences
Rawalpindi, Pakistan

Muhammad Usman Mazhar
Senior Scientist, Animal Sciences Division
National Institute of Animal
    Biotechnology
Faisalabad, Pakistan

Mahvish Maqbool
Department of Parasitology
University of Agriculture
Faculty of Veterinary Science
Faisalabad, Pakistan
and
College of Agricultural and Life
    Sciences
Virginia Tech
Blacksburg, Virginia, USA

Hizqeel Ahmed Muzaffar
Faculty of Veterinary Sciences
KBCMA College of Veterinary and
    Animal Sciences, Narowal
Sub-campus University of Veterinary
    and Animal Sciences
Lahore, Pakistan

Shumaila Naz
Department of Biological Sciences
National University of Medical
    Sciences
Rawalpindi, Pakistan

Nadia Nazish
Department of Zoology
University of Sialkot
Sialkot, Pakistan

HazratUllah Raheemi
Department of Health and Biological
    Sciences
Faculty of Life Sciences
Abasyn University
Peshawar, Pakistan

Hafiz Muhammad Rizwan
Section of Parasitology
Department of Pathobiology
KBCMA College of Veterinary and
    Animal Sciences, Narowal
Sub-campus University of Veterinary
    and Animal Sciences
Lahore, Pakistan

Mourad Ben Said
Laboratory of Microbiology
National School of Veterinary Medicine
    of Sidi Thabet
University of Manouba
Manouba, Tunisia
and
Department of Basic Sciences
Higher Institute of Biotechnology of
    Sidi Thabet
University of Manouba,
Manouba, Tunisia

Muhammad Sohail Sajid
Department of Parasitology
Faculty of Veterinary Sciences
University of Agriculture
Faisalabad, Pakistan

Muhammad Nadeem Saleem
Section of Animal Breeding and
    Genetics Section
Department of Animal Sciences
KBCMA College of Veterinary and
    Animal Sciences, Narowal
Sub-campus University of Veterinary
    and Animal Sciences
Lahore, Pakistan

Muhammad Saqib
Department of Clinical Medicine and
    Surgery
Faculty of Veterinary Science
University of Agriculture
Faisalabad, Pakistan

Raja Adil Sarfraz
Department of Chemistry
Faculty of Science
University of Agriculture
Faisalabad, Pakistan

Muhammad Shafeeq
Department of Clinical Medicine and
    Surgery
University of Agriculture
Faisalabad, Pakistan

Asim Shamim
Department of Veterinary Parasitology
Faculty of Veterinary and Animal
    Sciences
University of the Poonch Rawalakot
Azad Kashmir, Pakistan.

Muhammad Sulman Ali Taseer
Section of Pathology
Department of Pathobiology
KBCMA College of Veterinary and
    Animal Science, Narowal
Sub-campus University of Veterinary
    and Animal Sciences
Lahore, Pakistan

Muhammad Younus
Section of Pathology
Department of Pathobiology
KBCMA College of Veterinary and
    Animal Sciences, Narowal
Sub-campus University of Veterinary
    and Animal Sciences
Lahore, Pakistan

Muhammad Zeeshan
Department of Parasitology
Faculty of Veterinary Science
University of Agriculture
Faisalabad, Pakistan

Saadiya Zia
Department of Biochemistry
University of Agriculture
Faisalabad, Pakistan

1 Molecular Biology and Physiology of Parasites

Muhammad Faisal Hayat[1],
Rana Muhammad Athar Ali[2],
Muhammad Umar Ijaz[1]*, Mughees Aizaz Alvi[2]*, and
Muhammad Shafeeq[2]

[1]Department of Zoology, Wildlife and Fisheries,
University of Agriculture, Faisalabad, Pakistan

[2]Department of Clinical Medicine and Surgery,
University of Agriculture, Faisalabad, Pakistan

*Corresponding Authors

1.1 INTRODUCTION

Parasites (protozoa, helminths, and arthropods) belong to several taxonomic families and are responsible for significant veterinary and public health issues all over the world. Each of these numerous parasites has a biological life cycle that differs significantly from the others, and their tissue tropism also varies greatly (Gazzinelli-Guimaraes and Nutman, 2018). The clinical outcomes of parasitic infections exhibit variations that correspond to these distinctions. The majority of infections produce pathologic effects that correlate with the number of parasites and the duration of the underlying infection (Zvinorova et al., 2016).

Although there are species-specific variations, it is revealed that parasites collectively influence and control the immune reaction of the host to themselves (parasite-specific immunoregulation) (Maizels and McSorley, 2016). However, these parasites can change the immunological reaction to allergens, vaccinations, and vaccinations as well as antigens (Metenou et al., 2012; Babu and Nutman, 2016). Extensive research has delved into understanding the molecular processes responsible for parasite-induced immune modulation. Parasites possess the capability to manipulate the host immune system, a phenomenon partially reversible through drug therapy (Robinson et al., 2009). The focus has largely been on parasite-generated substances, which hold potential applications in vaccines, medicines, diagnostic testing, and as treatments for autoimmune and inflammatory conditions (Gazzinelli-Guimaraes and Nutman, 2018).

Research on parasite biology has progressed with developments in genome sequencing and proteome characterisation tools. The genomes of parasites are

DOI: 10.1201/9781032651071-1

extremely complex, with up to 18,000 protein-coding genes and genomic sizes ranging from 42 to over 1000 Mb (International Helminth Genome Consortium, 2019). The quick introduction of new sequencing platforms has allowed for a 1000-fold improvement in output over Sanger's sequencing and enabled the subsequent reporting of more parasite genomes. Examples of these platforms are the Roche 454 sequencing platforms and the Illumina sequencing system (Sotillo et al., 2019). The growth of transgenesis and genome-editing research has been supported by the accessibility of these "omics" data, which provides important insights into the molecular biophysiology of parasites (Yoo et al., 2011). In this chapter, we highlight the biology and physiology of parasites at the molecular levels under various conditions, as well as applications and potential future challenges to livestock animals and researchers.

1.2   MOLECULAR MECHANISMS OF PARASITIC INFECTIONS

Parasitic life cycles are intricate, involving multiple phases of development. Each phase exhibits a unique antigenic repertoire and often targets specific organ systems. For instance, *Ascaris* targets the gastrointestinal tract (GIT), *Onchocerca* targets the lungs, and *Schistosoma* targets the hepatic system. Moreover, brain and muscle infections with *Taenia* create a challenge when attempting to draw broad conclusions about parasites as a unified species (Nutman, 2015).

Immune reactions are often governed differently based on the resident tissues or parasites' duration of life, as these developmental transformations and migrations take place over time. Both individuals, as well as experimentally infected rodents, experience a localised inflammatory reaction in their lungs as a result of migratory Ascarid larvae, which results in a condition resembling Löffler's disease (Dold and Holland, 2011). It has been determined that the inflammation in mice is a Type 2 reaction, with interleukin (IL)-4, IL-13, and some IL-5 predominating. Increases in IL-1 beta (β) and tumour necrosis factor-alpha (TNF-α) have also been identified in the pulmonary tissues caused by the larval movements. In extensive Ascarid larval movements, there is a significant IL-6 production that is assumed to be connected to the significant neutrophil infiltration (Gazzinelli-Guimarães et al., 2013).

Both eosinophils and macrophages substitute the neutrophil infiltrate in the pulmonary system when the larvae begin to migrate from the connective tissue in the lungs to the digestive tract to finish their life cycle. These macrophages are important for remodelling tissues and preventing reinfection (Nogueira et al., 2016). After returning to the GIT, the immature forms develop into adult worms and cause an infection that lasts a long time owing to the markedly reduced parasite-specific response (Midttun et al., 2018).

1.3   PARASITIC FUNCTIONAL GENOMICS

Parasitic genomics are associated with parasitic diversity and adaptation to diversified habitats and hosts. The most comprehensive source of knowledge is genome analysis, which offers nearly full details on an organism's capability for producing different compounds and carrying out chemical processes (Kochneva et al., 2023). The antigen-presenting cells (APCs) are the first stages in the adaptive immune reaction to infection. They take up, process, and present antigens to the T-cells. Later on, APCs enhance the production of extracellular ligands and soluble chemicals that activate T-lymphocytes associated with antigens. Additionally, this interaction may influence the response's qualitative characteristics by favouring a dominant Th1 or Th2 mode (Moser and Murphy, 2000).

Numerous parasite products have the ability to obstruct this pathway, causing a delay in the development of an immune response. When cultivated with *Schistosoma* soluble egg antigen, human or mouse dendritic cells (DCs) can trigger Th2 events *in vitro* or upon transfer to a naïve host in a way that is independent of both MyD88 and IL-4 (Jankovic et al., 2004). However, they do not undergo the conventional maturation of co-stimulatory ligand production. Even when lipopolysaccharide (LPS), a potent pro-inflammatory stimulus, is integrated with parasite antigen-pulsed DCs, the Th2-triggering effects of parasite products remain predominant (Everts et al., 2009). For example, helminth products from *Heligmosomoides polygyrus*, *Echinococcus granulosus*, *Fasciola hepatica*, *E. multilocularis*, and *Taenia crassiceps* commonly decrease the inflammatory (Th1) pathway (Massacand et al., 2009).

The CD4+ T-cells are responsible for orchestrating adaptive immune reactions. Numerous studies have examined the immune-modulating impact of helminth products on T-cells, which is mediated through various mechanisms (Aranzamendi et al., 2012).

1.4 PARASITIC TRANSCRIPTOMICS

A transcriptome analysis that unravels the gene expression in parasites e.g. of *Angiostrongylus (A.) vasorum* that is a dog parasite, was conducted by Ansell et al. (2013). A vast range of enzymes and compounds involved in anabolic or catabolic processes or signalling were encoded by the transcript contigs that the study compiled. Later, Yu et al. (2017) conducted a transcriptomic analysis of *A. cantonensis*, correlating adult females with L4 larvae at the time of brain invasion by the parasite.

Dictyocaulus (D.) filaria and *D. viviparus* are the two most significant ruminant lungworms. For *D. viviparus*, McNulty et al. (2016) assembled the genome and examined the difference in transcriptome over the whole life cycle. According to the research, in self-sustaining L1s–L3s, there were many transcripts linked to chemotaxis/signalling, transcriptional control, and oxygen transportation. The L4 and pre-adult stages of *D. viviparus* had similar transcriptomes; however, a thorough investigation revealed that the latter had increased levels of lipid metabolism, proteolysis, and several transcription elements. Additional *Dictyocaulus* transcriptome investigations comprise evaluations of male and female adults and L3s based on 454 (Cantacessi et al., 2011), as well as comparisons of mixed adult *Dictyocaulus* and *Dictyofilaria* based on Illumina (Mangiola et al., 2014).

Schwarz et al. (2015) presented the most comprehensive transcriptome analysis of an ancylostomatoid (also known as a "hookworm") of veterinary significance to date. They not only characterised the draft *Ancylostoma (An.) ceylanicum* genome but also observed changes in transcript abundance from infectious L3s until maturity. Transcriptomic investigations of *Oesophagostomum (O.) dentatum* involved tracking them during the larval stage (L2 to L4) and maturity in pigs (Gasser et al., 2007). The transformation from L3s to L4s in the swine gut was indicated by the increase of serine and metallo- and excretory cysteine enzymes, and protease inhibitors to subtilisin and aprotinin. These were observed as typical alterations in nematode parasitism following host infection and persisted at high throughout adulthood (Tyagi et al., 2015).

Haemonchus (H.) contortus genome draft assemblies were reported in separate MHco3(ISE) investigations. The MHco3(ISE) line is a *H. contortus* strain, susceptible to all the major anthelmintic classes (Laing et al., 2013; Schwarz et al., 2013). Laing et al. (2013) ascertained RNA-seq evidence for a total of 17,483 coding genes, out of which 11,295 exhibited differential transcription across the whole lifespan. Increased transcription linked to fat and glucose metabolism, cuticle formation, protein synthesis, and growth was noted following the moult to L4 and the start of blood-feeding. Additionally, investigating the transcriptome in the *H. contortus* gut found an overexpression of peptidase inhibitors and cysteine-type peptidases, which have their role in blood-feeding. Similar findings were reported by Schwarz et al. (2013), who also observed an elevation of class A and SR-type G-protein-coupled receptors in L1 stages (usually linked to proprioception, chemosensation, mechanosensation, and osmosensation in *Caenorhabditis* worms).

1.5 PARASITIC FUNCTIONAL PROTEOMICS

Functional proteomics, as the name implies, investigates the expression and function of proteins in parasites. The most useful application for proteomics lies in characterising the different aspects of metabolism that are truly active at a given moment. Proteomic studies not only offer insights into the end products of genetic information deployment, but also enable the determination of individual protein levels within a cell, the identification of significant and minor components of the proteome, the assessment of post-translational modifications in proteins, and the detailed investigation of the isozyme profile of specific amino acid groups (Cui et al., 2013). Additionally, proteome analysis can greatly enhance the outcomes of molecular genetic techniques in animals whose genomes have not yet been fully mapped (Cho, 2007).

With a quick look at UniProt, one of the biggest databases (DBs) containing recognised protein molecules, we can determine that around 95% of the protein sequences of parasitic worms that have been discovered were produced by genome translation (The UniProt Consortium, 2017). When considering the preservation of a parasitic lifestyle, several protein categories are particularly intriguing (Tritten et al., 2021). These include proteins that negatively affect other species, storage proteins essential for accumulating absorbed substances, excreted proteins potentially involved in signalling to the host and creating the worm's microenvironment, proteins related to germ cell development, signalling proteins potentially controlling host metabolism, and protective proteins against toxins (Kochneva et al., 2023).

Muscle proteins are an essential part of the proteome of adult phases in parasites and are involved in locomotor activity. The most prevalent ones are myosin chains and actin (Liu et al., 2006). Glycolytic enzymes are well recognised as being among the proteins involved in metabolising energy in adult parasites. Moreover, finding species-specific antigens for the creation of a vaccination against parasitic infections is made possible by the identification of the main proteins found in the adult stages of parasitic worms (Chen et al., 2012). Consequently, it has been demonstrated that enolase from parasites may be used as an antigen in the creation of vaccinations (Arce-Fonseca et al., 2018).

1.6 PARASITIC METABOLOMICS

Metabolic pathways in parasitic organisms are profiled using metabolomics. A comprehensive investigation of the transcriptome and genome of parasites, as reported in the analytical review by Carey et al. (2022), presents important insights regarding the unique metabolic organisation of parasites in relation to their specific niche as obligatory parasites (Carey et al., 2022). The provided data on metabolomics revealed that parasites lack the ability to oxidising steroids and xenobiotics but possess a huge potential for reduction reactions and release of hydrophobic compounds, which ultimately help in anti-parasitic drug metabolism (Tsai et al., 2013).

Through a variety of metabolic activities, parasites release a large number of biologically active substances into the surrounding environment. These chemical compounds are crucial in decreasing the immune response, aiding in the parasites' invasion into the host tissues, and even helping to restructure the metabolism of host tissues to meet their own demands (Robinson et al., 2009). Calcium-binding proteins associated with metabolic control are examples of housekeeping proteins that are often found in the proteomes of parasites (Boukli et al., 2011; Sotillo et al., 2012).

1.7 EPIGENETICS IN PARASITES

According to Bozdech et al. (2003), during the life cycles of parasites, various sorts of environmental as well as genetic alterations occur. Studying any heritable or environmental alterations in gene expressions which are not attributed to underlying DNA is called epigenetics. These alterations involve loss of imprinting, disruptions in chromatin, and DNA methylation (Hamilton, 2011). Epigenetics is one of the simplest justifications for elucidating how cells and organisms with similar DNA have different phenotypes (Jirtle and Skinner, 2007). Epigenetics plays a significant role in the development of host–parasite interactions. It is found that the normal architecture of chromatin is essential in the epigenetic regulation of various protozoans' genes. Epigenetic gene regulation depends upon cellular control, differentiation, and the virulence of parasites. Recent investigations demonstrated the role of various genes in regulating the expression of regulatory genes in protozoans by different chemical modifications of constituent nucleosomes (Croken et al., 2012). For example, malarial parasites are well-known owing to their higher rates of infections, which can be estimated from the fact that approximately 200 million infected cases are documented every year due to various parasites of malaria (WHO, 2018). The genomic sequence of malaria revealed that it consists of 23 million base pairs per haploid (1n) genome, which are sequenced on 14 chromosomes (Gardner et al., 2002). Furthermore, 80% of the malarial genome is composed of AT base pairs, which makes it the most AT-rich genome among eukaryotic genomes to date.

It is reported that alterations in histone proteins play a crucial role in gene regulation in *Plasmodium (P.) falciparum*. This is particularly true for various virulent genes (*var* genes) involved in immune evasion. In *P. falciparum*, the *var* genes are responsible for encoding variants of erythrocyte membrane proteins (PfEMP1). This protein transfers to the outer surface of infectious erythrocytes and plays an essential role in cyto-adherence and immune evasion within the host (Miller et al., 1994). It is documented that the *P. falciparum* genome comprises approximately 60 *var* genes, and only one *var* gene is expressed at a specific time, facilitating various antigenic variations that allow the parasite to evade the host's immune system (Scherf et al., 2008). A plethora of *in vitro* investigations elucidated that the expression of these *var* genes is controlled by various epigenetic factors (Abel and Le-Roch, 2019).

Furthermore, it has been revealed that 59 silenced *var* genes are marked by repressive histone modifications such as *P. falciparum* heterochromatin protein 1 (PfHP1) and histone 3 lysine 9 trimethylation (H3K9me3) (Lopez-Rubio et al., 2009; Flueck et al., 2009). The PfHP1 binds with H3K9me3 and ensures the regulation of repressive heterochromatin. It is found that the unavailability of PfHP1 results in the uncontrolled expression of approximately all *var* genes, which arrests the cellular cycle during the asexual developmental stages of the parasite. Additionally, another gene called PfAP2-G is present on chromosome 12, which is crucial for regulating gametocyte stages in malarial parasites (Brancucci et al., 2014). When a parasite is in its regular growth stage, PfAP2-G remains silent owing to the existence of H3K9me3 and PfHP1. It was revealed that when PfHP1 was eliminated, PfAP2-G initiates the expression of other genes involved in gametocytogenesis, thereby producing a huge number of gametocytes (Lopez-Rubio et al., 2009). In another investigation, the gametocyte development 1 gene (GDV1) was identified as playing an essential role in the sexual differentiation of malarial parasites. However, various investigations have found that different environmental factors are responsible for the activation of gametocytogenesis in parasites, which regulate the expression of the aforementioned genes (Filarsky et al., 2018).

1.8 MOLECULAR INSIGHTS OF THE HOST–PARASITE INTERACTIONS

Hosts and parasites interact with each other through various sorts of communications at molecular levels. One of the most prominent communication channels involves the utilisation of microRNA vesicles to stimulate the immune system of hosts by parasites. It is reported that *Schistosoma (S.) mansoni* (flatworm) secretes microRNA-10, which affects the fate of T-cells of the host's immune system by the manipulation of the nuclear factor kappa B (NF-κB) pathway (Hamway et al., 2022). This species of flatworm is responsible for the development as well as progression of schisto-somiasis, which affects millions of animals and humans globally. These parasites persist for years and establish a complicated association between host and parasite. These interactions involve: (a) utilisation of host components for development, (b) modulation of the host's immune system of host, and (c) utilisation of microRNAs in extracellular vesicles (Ofir-Birin and Regev-Rudzki, 2019; Angeles et al., 2020).

It is documented that *S. mansoni* possesses several miRNAs in its genome, but interestingly sma-miR-10-5p, sma-miR-125a-5p, and sma-miR-bantam-3p enter the T-cells of the host. These miRNAs are involved in triggering immune responses of hosts, particularly the Th2 immune response (Amoil et al., 2018; Liu et al., 2019). Furthermore, it is observed that sma-miR-10 targets the expression of MAP37K and reduces the activity of NF-κB. The NF-κB controls the expression of *jubn* as well as *gata3*, which play significant role in mediating the Th2 immune response by escalat-ing the expression of *il4* (Katagiri et al., 2021).

1.9   IMMUNE EVASION STRATEGIES OF PARASITES

Immune evasion refers to the strategies used by various pathogenic bacteria, para-sites, & viruses to avoid detection & destruction by the immune system of a particular host (Sorci et al., 2013). Different parasites, including malarial parasites, demon-strate different strategies to prevent interacting with the host defence system. Risco-Castillo et al. (2015) elucidated that a single bite of an infected mosquito roughly transmits 200 sporozoites into the dermal layer, and despite a strong immune system, very low numbers of these sporozoites are still able to develop an infection. The dermal surface, or skin is considered the first and foremost barrier against patho-genic encounters in vertebrates (Cirimotich et al., 2010). These sporozoites cross this hurdle by using various strategies such as cell traversal and motility (Tavares et al., 2013). It is reported that sporozoites contain special proteins which aid them in suc-cessfully passing through the skin (Patarroyo et al., 2011). Sporozoites traverse the immune cells, which ultimately inactivate the immune cell defences thereby opening a gateway for their penetration (Sinnis and Zavala, 2012). It is reported that a protein called "TRAP" contributes to enhancing the motility of sporozoites during pen-etration. TRAP assists the parasite in communicating with the surface of host mol-ecules, thereby improving gliding motility to pass through the dermis. Furthermore, in hepatic tissues, TRAP binds with sulfated glycoconjugate motifs, which allows recognition as well as entry to hepatic cells (Müller et al., 1993).

Despite a strong immune system, parasites evade the immune response and initi-ate the development as well as progression of successful infection at the erythrocytic stage (Singh et al., 2010). After crossing all the cellular barriers, sporozoites reach the blood and then the lymphatic system of the body (Crompton et al., 2014). In the circulatory system, sporozoites quickly attack the sinusoid cavity of the hepatic region and the infection phases are described as the "exoerythrocytic stage." This stage is asymptomatic as the liver is an immune-privileged organ which is highly safeguarded against various pathogens (Liehl et al., 2015). However, various reports revealed that hepatic immune cells remain active during the initial phases of infections in rodent malaria models. It is reported that *Plasmodium* RNA activates the "Type I interferon" pathway in our body through Melanoma Differentiation-Associated protein 5 (MDA5) receptors (Liehl et al., 2014). Type I interferons are highly potent inflammatory cytokines which could inhibit the growth of malarial parasites inside the host body (Hisaeda et al., 2005). It is found that different cells such as Natural Killer (NK)-T, γ δT as well as NK cells inhibit the growth of parasites through the secretion of interferons like IFN-γ and Type I interferon (Risco-Castillo et al., 2015). Many other molecules such as hepcidin are also involved in the inhibition of parasites at the exoerythrocytic phase (Spottiswoode et al., 2014).

In order to invade the hepatic cells, sporozoites must cross the phagocytic immune cells called Kupffer cells (KCs) (Tavares et al., 2013). To establish a successful infection, these sporozoites interact with KCs at the infection site (Meslin et al., 2007). When they reach the liver, they interact with different sulfated molecules that are present on KCs and endothelial cells (ECs). The interaction between KCs and sporozoites is mediated by heparan sulfate proteoglycans (HSPGs) as well as circumsporozoite protein (CSP) at the surface of host immune cells. Similarly, P39 and CD38 are also reported in this process. Various microscopic studies revealed that sporozoites prefer the KCs pathways instead of ECs (Cha et al., 2015). It is documented that sporozoites manipulate various pathways at the same time to cross the sinusoidal barrier. In some cases, sporozoites pass through the gaps between ECs and KCs instead of any interaction (Meis et al., 1983). However, it is still unclear why KCs do not destroy parasites during early stages of infection despite their immense immune strength against other microorganisms in hepatic tissues (Sinnis and Zavala, 2012). It is revealed that sporozoites modulate the cytokine profile of KCs, which ultimately lowers the Th1 cytokines (TNF-α, IL-6, and MCP-1) and upregulates the Th2 cytokines (IL-10) to ensure their safe passage (Klotz and Frevert, 2008). Furthermore, CSP present on the outer region of KCs interacts with lipoproteins having low-density receptor-related proteins, which escalated cAMP/EPAC levels, thereby preventing the generation of reactive oxygen species, a natural byproduct during external stresses that can evade the parasites (Ikarashi et al., 2013). However, in some cases, parasites trigger apoptotic pathways and force the KCs into programmed cell death (Steers et al., 2005). Evasion strategies of parasites to cross the skin barrier are outlined in Figure 1.1.

1.10   SIGNALLING PATHWAYS IN PARASITE PHYSIOLOGY AND DEVELOPMENT

Various pathogenic parasites, including flatworms, are considered as significant health threats to both humans and animals worldwide. It is estimated that approximately 1 billion individuals are infected by parasites such as hookworms, common roundworms, and whipworm (Jourdan et al., 2018). Recent investigations in the fields of genomics, proteomics, transcriptomics, and metabolomics have established various pathways to understand the genetics, physiology, biochemistry, and neurology of these worms (Howe et al., 2017). Parasitic worms generally develop from an

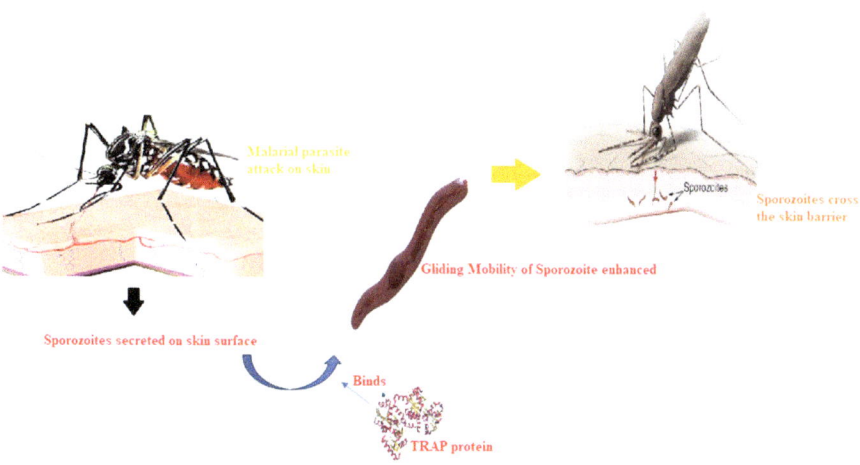

Malarial parasite
attack on skin

Sporozoites

Sporozoites cross
the skin barrier

Gliding Mobility of Sporozoite enhanced

Sporozoites secreted on skin surface

Binds

TRAP protein

FIGURE 1.1 Evasion strategies of parasites to cross the skin barrier.

embryonic egg to an adult through a series of physical and physiological transitions such as feeding, moulting, and metabolism (Rougvie and Moss, 2013). It is reported that nematodes change their physiological states in response to environmental conditions (Lutzelschwab et al., 2005).

In recent decades, investigators have delved into the molecular and cellular pathways to understand the physiology and development of parasites, including *Caenorhabditis (C.) elegans* (Faunes and Larraín, 2016). It is documented that transforming growth factor β (TGF-β), cyclic guanosine monophosphate (cGMP), hormones, and insulin-like peptides (INS) play a significant role as a signalling molecules for the development of *C. elegans* in response to environmental conditions (Butcher et al., 2007). Researchers have identified approximately 150 specific signalling molecules called "ascarosides" in nematodes (von Reuss et al., 2012). These ascarosides interact with other messengers to ensure growth and behavioural development in parasites (Ludewig and Schroeder, 2013). Some of these ascarosides, such as ascr#2, ascr#3, and ascr#5, are well studied. It is revealed that these ascarosides interact with special proteins called G protein-coupled receptors (GPCRs) such as SRBC-64 and SRG-36. These interactions play a significant role in a process called "dauer formation" in *C. elegans* (Butcher, 2017). Furthermore, the interactions between ascarosides and GPCRs produce various other messengers such as cGMP, TGF-β and INS (Ludewig and Schroeder, 2013). cGMP is a primary signalling molecule which ensures the transmission of information between nerve cells of *C. elegans* (Figure 1.2). It activates specific channels in nerve cells which help the nematodes to sense their surroundings (Bargmann, 2006).

When the production of cGMP reduces in *C. elegans*, it triggers the dauer formation, which is known as a developmental pause in nematodes. It is revealed that any substitute for cGMP can fill this gap and activate the developmental stages (Birnby et al., 2000). Similarly, TGF-β acts as a traffic directors of cellular activities. It is

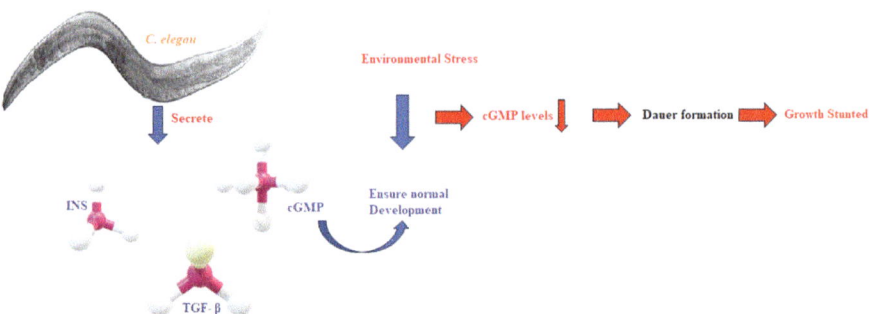

FIGURE 1.2   Mechanistic approaches in the development of *Caenorhabditis elegans.*

documented that there are five different genes that produce TFG-β molecules in *C. elegans*. Furthermore, the DAF-7 gene plays a significant role in the regulation of the "dauer" process (Gumienny and Savage-Dunn, 2013). Interestingly, the aforementioned TGF-β genes and their homologous receptors are reported to be involved in activating infective larvae in parasitic nematodes (He et al., 2018).

Insulin-like peptides (INS) are special types of proteins that are similar to human insulin, and they are secreted by *C. elegans*. It is elucidated that there is only one receptor called "DAF-2" for these INS. These INS play a significant role in the early growth of *C. elegans*. Recent investigations revealed that DAF-28, INS-4, and INS-6 interact with the IGF-1 signalling molecule which mediates the growth of worms, while INS-1, INS-17, and INS-18 work antagonistically to INS-4 and INS-6, thereby retarding the normal development of *C. elegans* (Murphy and Hu, 2013). Moreover, Kaplan et al. (2019) demonstrated that INS maintains the developmental stages of worms, which are controlled by positive and negative feedback systems. In conclusion, the signalling molecules (cGMP, TGF-β, and INS) serve as agonists as well as antagonists for the development and neural transmission in *C. elegans* (Table 1.1). These signalling molecules and their associated receptors trigger various intercellular or intracellular signalling pathways which ultimately regulate growth and development in worms.

1.11   DRUG TARGETS AND RESISTANCE MECHANISMS IN PARASITES

Since decades, novel anti-infective agents (drugs) have gained currency owing to the emergence of novel and/or previously neglected infectious diseases (Cassell and Mekalanos, 2001). This does not only account for viral or bacterial diseases but also includes various parasitic infectious diseases (Egan and Kaschula, 2007). Currently, a wide range of anti-parasitic drugs are available in the market, and in case of resistance, there are substantial alternatives. *Giardia (G.) lamblia* is responsible for millions of diarrhoeal cases worldwide, which are commonly treated with "metronidazole" (Gardner and Hill, 2001).

TABLE 1.1

Various Regulators in Physiology and Development of *C. elegans*

Regulators	Physiological Role in *C. elegans*	References
Cyclic guanosine monophosphate (cGMP)	Cell signalling during development	(Butcher et al., 2007)
Hormones and insulin-like peptides (INS)	Acts as growth regulators	(Jeong et al., 2005)
Transforming growth factor β (TGF-β)	Direct cellular trafficking	(Gumienny and Savage-Dunn, 2013)
G protein-coupled receptors (GPCRs)	Interacts with ascarosides to enhance cellular growth	(Ludewig and Schroeder, 2013)
Circumsporozoite protein (CSP)	Assist in immune evasion	(Cha et al., 2015)

There are numerous approaches used to combat parasitic infections, including direct targeting of DNA. Quinacrine was the first drug used to fight against giardiasis and malaria. It is documented that quinacrine directly interacts with the DNA of host and retards the processes of replication, transcription, and translation (Ciak and Hahn, 1967). Quinacrine serves as an intercalating agent, similar to other acridine-based compounds. Furthermore, it has been revealed that quinacrine inserts itself between adenine and thymine-rich regions of DNA base pairs to disrupt the normal processes of the central dogma. Similarly, ethidium bromide is another well-known intercalating agent used to fight against *Trypanosoma* parasites in African cattle since the 1950s (Chowdhury et al., 2010).

Since DNA is a ubiquitous target, the effectiveness of DNA-intercalating drugs is closely associated with targeting parasites as well as host cells. The specificity of these drugs depends on their uptake as well as metabolism in parasites. For instance, the *G. lamblia* strain shows resistance to quinacrine due to different uptakes (Upcroft et al., 1996). However, some parasites have special structures, such as kinetoplasts in trypanosomes (Shapiro and Englund, 1990) and apicoplasts in apicomplexans. These organelles may render these parasites more susceptible to intercalating drugs (Dahl and Rosenthal, 2008). Additionally, intercalating drugs not only interact with DNA but also engage with DNA-modifying enzymes. This dual nature of intercalating agents escalates their specificity, making them more selective in targeting microorganisms; for example, pentamidines bind to trypanosome DNA and trigger DNA cleavage in a pattern that resembles the action of topoisomerase II inhibitors (Shapiro and Englund, 1990).

The integrity of the cytoskeleton is crucial for the survival and infection-causing ability of protozoa and helminths. It is elucidated that the cytoskeleton, particularly a protein called tubulin, can be a promising target to combat these parasites (Werbovetz, 2002). Albendazole is one of the renowned antimicrobial drugs, which disrupts the integrity of the cytoskeleton in parasites. Various investigations have compared the susceptibility and resistance to albendazole among different parasites, including nematodes and flatworms (Hemphill and Müller, 2009). These studies have demonstrated a strong correlation between susceptibility or resistance to albendazole and the presence of specific alleles of β-tubulin genes. For example, a change in single codon of genetic code (phenylalanine to tyrosine) at position 200 is sufficient to shift an organism from susceptible to resistant against benzimidazole drugs (Kwa et al., 1995). Moreover, molecular modelling of albendazole-binding sites in albendazole-resistant *Acanthamoeba* exhibits 13 different residues from tubulin-susceptible organisms (Henriquez et al., 2008).

1.12 APPLICATION OF SYSTEMS BIOLOGY IN VETERINARY PARASITOLOGY

Recent advancements in proteomics, metabolomics, transcriptomics, as well as genome sequencing, have opened a gateway for the early detection of parasites and the determination of their target drugs (Kumar et al., 2021). The use of molecular biology tools is increasing drastically, advancing our understanding of veterinary parasitology. Over the last three decades, these tools have played a pivotal role in the early diagnosis and control of infections, which is attributed to growing accessibility to the genomics and proteomics of parasites through various databases such as HelmCop, EuPathDB, and GeneDB (Aurrecoechea et al., 2017). The polymerase chain reaction (PCR) is an advancement in systems biology which is extensively used to detect and recognise different parasites in veterinary investigations. Various variants of PCR such as RAPD, qPCR, Race PCR, nested PCR, and LAMP show different levels of accuracy and sensitivity in parasite detection. It is reported that ITS-1 and TBR primer-based PCR can detect incredibly small pieces (0.1 nanogrammes) of DNA in samples (Sharma et al., 2012). Besides DNA probes, DNA microarrays have proven valuable in screening huge numbers of parasite genotypes in different epidemiological studies related to veterinary parasites (Kumar et al., 2021).

Parasites are emerging day by day owing to their highly modified genome; thereby a plethora of investigations have been carried out to assess their presence and mode of action against different hosts. These investigations have led to the discovery of novel pharmaceutical drugs. For instance, phylum Apicomplexa is reported to cause toxoplasmosis, malaria, cryptosporidiosis, and coccidiosis in humans and animals. However, the integration of systems biology, including omics and CRISPR/Cas9 tools, has revolutionised the study of apicomplexans. These technologies develop a holistic approach to the development of vaccines by identifying novel antigens and their underlying mechanistic strategies (Tomazic et al., 2022). Another investigation was designed to assess the potential biomarkers for resistance in nematode infections of sheep. Various techniques, such as gene expression, gene co-expression network analysis, and quantitative genetic analysis, were employed. These techniques revealed specific genes associated with the infections, which offer a valuable insight for the development of novel therapeutic interventions against gastrointestinal infection resistance in animals (Kadarmideen et al., 2011).

1.13 FUTURE PROSPECTS AND CHALLENGES IN MOLECULAR BIOLOGY OF PARASITES

Despite the fact that molecular biology opens a wide range of gateways for the discovery of novel drugs as well as the diagnosis of different infections, owing to high rate of genomic variations among parasites, it still it needs to be explored further. It is found that a multi-omics approach has the potential to enhance future research in parasitology, particularly in the study of helminth biology. This approach includes the understanding of host–parasite interactions, underlying molecular mechanisms, as well as disease pathogenesis (Smith et al., 2003). Ma et al. (2019) elucidated intriguing models for bile acid-like signalling as well as dauer-like signalling pathways that may demonstrate a high degree of conservation between parasitic nematodes. The concept of dauer-like signalling pathways produces new avenues for understanding the mechanistic approaches of parasitic nematodes to infect and survive in their hosts. Moreover, it offers significant insight into the evolutionary strategies employed by parasites, which is pivotal for advancing disease management strategies and their control measures (Smith et al., 2020).

Aside from these, there are numerous other developmental pauses in parasites such as (i) hypobiosis, in which parasites such as *Haemonchus*, *Ostertagia*, *Cooperia,* and *Teladorsagia* pause their fourth developmental stage in their hosts (Gibbs, 1986) and (ii) larvae of *Bacylisascaris*, *Ancylostome*, and *Toxocara* arrest their development when passing through the host tissues (Strube et al., 2013). It is revealed that different hormonal signalling pathways might play a pivotal role in activating the arrested state of parasites in response to host conditions (Ogawa et al., 2009). Therefore, understanding the nature and signalling approach of hormones can help to understand how helminths and other parasites detect chemicals during their journey from tissues to body organs. For example, the larval stage of different parasites such as *Toxocara*, *Baylisascaris*, and *Angiostrongylus* migrate through the paratenic hosts and target the central nervous system. Interestingly, it was reported that this intriguing behaviour of larval species was influenced by different hormones (Strube et al., 2013; Janecek et al., 2014).

Although significant advancements have been made in helminth biology at genomics, proteomics, and transcriptomics levels (Jex et al., 2019) but many molecular components (genes, lipids, proteins, and carbohydrates) in parasites remain unidentified or need comprehensive studies. The availability of transcriptomes and draft genomes provides a baseline for biomedical research, comprehensive definition, and identification of these components, but there are still difficulties in defining all proteins and lipids using present bioinformatics and mass-spectrometry-based approaches. For instance, various molecules have low expression, abundance, or transcription levels and fall below the detection thresholds of currently available techniques (Luck et al., 2015).

1.14 CONCLUSION

Molecular biology comprehensively elucidates a plethora of insights and challenges in parasitology. Epigenetics plays a pivotal role in host–parasite interactions as well as development, with major focus on their regulatory mechanisms, as exemplified in malarial species. Various signalling molecules such as TGF-β, cGMP, and insulin-like peptides, emerge as key players in the physiology and development of different parasitic species. The diverse applications of systems biology revolutionised veterinary parasitology to detect and control pathogenic parasites. However, development is indispensable in molecular biology for the early detection, diagnosis, and treatment of parasitic infection.

REFERENCES

Abel, S., and K. G. Le-Roch. 2019. The role of epigenetics and chromatin structure in transcriptional regulation in malaria parasites. *Briefings in Functional Genomics* 18:302–313.

Amoil, V., M. Dagenais, V. Ganapathy, J. Aldridge, A. Glebov, A. Jardim, and P. Ribeiro. 2018. Vesicle-based secretion in schistosomes: Analysis of protein and microRNA (miRNA) content of exosome-like vesicles derived from *Schistosoma mansoni*. *Scientific Report* 8:3286

Angeles, J. M. M., V. J. P. Mercado, and P. T. Rivera. 2020. Behind enemy lines: Immunomodulatory armamentarium of the schistosome parasite. *Frontiers in Immunology* 11:1018.

Ansell, B. R., M. Schnyder, P. Deplazes, P. K. Korhonen, N. D. Young, R.S. Hall, S. Mangiola, P. R. Boag, A. Hofmann, P. W. Sternberg, and A. R. Jex. 2013. Insights into the immuno-molecular biology of *Angiostrongylus vasorum* through transcriptomics – pros- pects for new interventions. *Biotechnology Advances* 31:1486–1500.

Aranzamendi, C., F. Fransen, M. Langelaar, F. Franssen, P. van der Ley, J. P. van Putten, V. Rutten, and E. Pinelli. 2012. *Trichinella spiralis*-secreted products modulate DC functionality and expand regulatory T cells in vitro. *Parasite Immunology* 34:210–223.

Arce-Fonseca, M., M. C. González-Vázquez, O. Rodríguez-Morales, V. Graullera-Rivera, A. Aranda-Fraustro, P. A. Reyes, A. Carabarin-Lima, and J. L. Rosales-Encina. 2018. Recombinant enolase of *Trypanosoma cruzi* as a novel vaccine candidate against chagas disease in a mouse model of acute infection. *Journal of Immunology Research* 2018:8964085.

Aurrecoechea C, A. Barreto, E. Y. Basenko, J. Brestelli, B. P. Brunk, S. Cade, K. Crouch, R. Doherty, D. Falke, S. Fischer, and B. Gajria. 2017. EuPathDB: The eukaryotic pathogen genomics database resource. *Nucleic Acids Research* 45:581–D591.

Babu, S., and T. B. Nutman. 2016. Helminth-Tuberculosis Co-infection: An Immunologic Perspective. *Trends in Immunology* 37:597–607.

Bargmann, C. I. 2006. Chemosensation in *C. elegans*. *WormBook* 25:1–29.

Birnby, D. A., E. M. Link, J. J. Vowels, H. Tian, P. L. Colacurcio, and J. H. Thomas. 2000. A transmembrane guanylyl cyclase (DAF-11) and Hsp90 (DAF-21) regulate a common set of chemosensory behaviors in *Caenorhabditis elegans*. *Genetics* 155:85–104.

Boukli, N. M., B. Delgado, M. Ricaurte, and A. M. Espino. 2011. *Fasciola hepatica* and *Schistosoma mansoni*: Identification of common proteins by comparative proteomic analysis. *Journal of Parasitology* 97:852–861.

Bozdech, Z., M. Llinás, B. L. Pulliam, E. D. Wong, J. Zhu, and J. L. DeRisi. 2003. The transcriptome of the intraerythrocytic developmental cycle of *Plasmodium falciparum*. *PLoS Biology* 1:e5.

Brancucci, N. M., N. L. Bertschi, L. Zhu, I. Niederwieser, W. H. Chin, R. Wampfler, C. Freymond, M. Rottmann, I. Felger, Z. Bozdech, and T. S. Voss. 2014. Heterochromatin protein 1 secures survival and transmission of malaria parasites. *Cell Host Microbe* 16:165–176.

Butcher, R. A. 2017. Small-molecule pheromones and hormones controlling nematode development. *Nature Chemical Biology* 13:577–586.

Butcher, R. A., M. Fujita, F. C. Schroeder, and J. Clardy. 2007. Small-molecule pheromones that control dauer development in *Caenorhabditis elegans. Nature Chemical Biology* 3:420–422.

Cantacessi, C., R. B. Gasser, C. Strube, T. Schnieder, A. R. Jex, R. S. Hall, B. E. Campbell, N. D. Young, S. Ranganathan, P. W. Sternberg, and M. Mitreva. 2011. Deep insights into *Dictyocaulus viviparus* transcriptomes provides unique prospects for new drug tar- gets and disease intervention. *Biotechnology Advances* 29:261–271.

Carey, M. A., G. L. Medlock, M. Stolarczyk, W. A. Petri Jr, J. L. Guler, and J. A. Papin. 2022. Comparative analyses of parasites with a comprehensive database of genome-scale metabolic models. *PLoS Computational Biology* 18(2):e1009870.

Cassell, G. H., and J. Mekalanos. 2001. Development of antimicrobial agents in the era of new and reemerging infectious diseases and increasing antibiotic resistance. *JAMA* 285:601–605.

Cha, S. J., K. Park, P. Srinivasan, C. W. Schindler, N. Van Rooijen, M. Stins, and M. Jacobs-Lorena. 2015. CD68 acts as a major gateway for malaria sporozoite liver infection. *Journal of Experimental Medicine* 212:1391–1403.

Chen, N., Z. G. Yuan, M. J. Xu, D. H. Zhou, X. X. Zhang, Y. Z. Zhang, X. W. Wang, C. Yan, R. Q. Lin, and X. Q. Zhu. 2012. *Ascaris suum* enolase is a potential vaccine candidate against ascariasis. *Vaccine* 30:3478–3482.

Cho, W. C. 2007. Proteomics technologies and challenges. *Genomics Proteomics Bioinformatics* 5(2):77–85.

Chowdhury, A. R., R. Bakshi, J. Wang, G. Yildirir, B. Liu, V. Pappas-Brown, G. Tolun, J. D. Griffith, T. A. Shapiro, R. E. Jensen, and P. T. Englund. 2010. The killing of African trypanosomes by ethidium bromide. *PLoS Pathogen* 6:e1001226.

Ciak, J., and F. E. Hahn. 1967. Quinacrine (atebrin): Mode of action. *Science* 156:655–656.

Cirimotich, C. M., Y. Dong, L. S. Garver, S. Sim, and G. Dimopoulous. 2010. Mosquito immune defenses against Plasmodium infection. *Developmental & Comparative Immunology* 34:387–395.

Croken, M. M., S. C. Nardelli, and K. Kim. 2012. Chromatin modifications, epigenetics, and how protozoan parasites regulate their lives. *Trends in Parasitology* 28:202–213.

Crompton, P. D., J. Moebius, S. Portugal, M. Waisberg, G. Hart, L. S. Garver, L. H. Miller, C. Barillas-Mury, and S. K. Pierce. 2014. Malaria immunity in man and mosquito: insights into unsolved mysteries of a deadly infectious disease. *Annual Review of Immunology* 32:157–187.

Cui, S. J., L. L. Xu, T. Zhang, M. Xu, J. Yao, C. Y. Fang, Z. Feng, P. Y. Yang, W. Hu, and F. Liu. 2013. Proteomic characterization of larval and adult developmental stages in *Echinococcus granulosus* reveals novel insight into host-parasite interactions. *Journal of Proteomics* 84:158–175.

Dahl, E. L., and P. J. Rosenthal. 2008. Apicoplast translation, transcription and genome replication: Targets for antimalarial antibiotics. *Trends in Parasitology* 24:279–284.

Dold, C., and C. V. Holland. 2011. *Ascaris* and ascariasis. *Microbes and Infection* 13(7):632–637.

Egan, T. J., and C. H. Kaschula. 2007. Strategies to reverse drug resistance in malaria. *Current Opinion in Infectious Diseases* 20:598–604.

Everts, B., G. Perona-Wright, H. H. Smits, C. H. Hokke, A. J. van der Ham, C. M. Fitzsimmons, M. J. Doenhoff, J. van der Bosch, K. Mohrs, H. Haas, M. Mohrs, M. Yazdanbakhsh, and G. Schramm. 2009. Omega-1, a glycoprotein secreted by *Schistosoma mansoni* eggs, drives Th2 responses. *Journal of Experimental Medicine* 206:1673–1680.

Faunes, F., and J. Larraı́n. 2016. Conservation in the involvement of heterochronic genes and hormones during developmental transitions. *Developmental Biology* 416:3–17.

Filarsky, M., S. A. Fraschka, I. Niederwieser, N. M. Brancucci, E. Carrington, E. Carrió, S. Moes, P. Jenoe, R. Bártfai, and T. S. Voss. 2018. GDV1 induces sexual commitment of malaria parasites by antagonizing HP1-dependent gene silencing. *Science* 359:1259–1263.

Flueck, C., R. Bartfai, J. Volz, I. Niederwieser, A. M. Salcedo-Amaya, B. T. Alako, F. Ehlgen, S. A. Ralph, A. F. Cowman, Z. Bozdech, and H. G. Stunnenberg. 2009. *Plasmodium falciparum* heterochromatin protein 1 marks genomic loci linked to phenotypic variation of exported virulence factors. *PLoS Pathogens* 5:e1000569.

Gardner, M. J., N. Hall, E. Fung, O. White, M. Berriman, R. W. Hyman, J. M. Carlton, A. Pain, K. E. Nelson, S. Bowman, and I. T. Paulsen. 2002. Genome sequence of the human malaria parasite *Plasmodium falciparum*. *Nature* 419:498–511.

Gardner, T. B., and D. R. Hill. 2001. Treatment of giardiasis. *Clinical Microbiology Reviews* 14:114–128.

Gasser, R. B., P. Cottee, A. J. Nisbet, B. Ruttkowski, S. Ranganathan, and A. Joachim. 2007. *Oesophagostomum dentatum*: potential as a model for genomic studies of strongylid nematodes, with biotechnological prospects. *Biotechnology Advances* 25:281–293.

Gazzinelli-Guimaraes, P. H., and T. B. Nutman. 2018. *Helminth parasites and immune regulation*. F1000Research, 7: F1000 Faculty Rev-1685.

Gazzinelli-Guimarães, P. H., A. C. Gazzinelli-Guimarães, F. N. Silva, V. L. T. Mati, L. de Carvalho Dhom-Lemos, F. S. Barbosa, L. S. A. Passos, S. Gaze, C. M. Carneiro, D. C. Bartholomeu, and L. L. Bueno. 2013. Parasitological and immunological aspects of early *Ascaris* spp. Infection in mice. *International Journal of Parasitology* 43:697–706.

Gibbs, H. C. 1986. Hypobiosis in parasitic nematodes—an update. *Advances in Parasitology* 25:129–174.

Gumienny, T. L., and C. Savage-Dunn. 2013. TGF-β signaling in *C. elegans*. *WormBook* 1:1–34.

Hamilton, J. P. 2011. Epigenetics: principles and practice. *Digestive Diseases* 29:130–135.

Hamway, Y., K. Zimmermann, M. J. Blommers, M. V. Sousa, C. Haberli, S. Kulkarni, S. Skalicky, M. Hackl, M. Gotte, J. Keiser, and C. P. da Costa. 2022. Modulation of host–parasite interactions with small molecules targeting *Schistosoma mansoni* microRNAs. *ACS Infectious Diseases* 8:2028–2034.

He, L., R. B. Gasser, P. K. Korhonen, W. Di, F. Li, H. Zhang, F. Li, Y. Zhou, R. Fang, J. Zhao, M. Hu. 2018. A TGF-β type I receptor-like molecule with a key functional role in *Haemonchus contortus* development. *International Journal of Parasitology* 48:1023–1033.

Hemphill, A., and J. Müller. 2009. Alveolar and cystic echinococcosis: towards novel chemotherapeutical treatment options. *Journal of Helminthology* 83:99–111.

Henriquez, F. L., P. R. Ingram, S. P. Muench, D. W. Rice, and C. W. Roberts. 2008. Molecular basis for resistance of *Acanthamoeba tubulins* to all major classes of antitubulin compounds. *Antimicrobial Agents and Chemotherapy* 52:1133–1135.

Hisaeda H., K. Yasutomo, and K. Himeno. 2005. Malaria: Immune evasion by parasites. *International Journal of Biochemistry & Cell Biology* 37:700–706.

Howe, K. L., B. J. Bolt, M. Shafie, P. Kersey, and M. Berriman, 2017. WormBase ParaSite—a comprehensive resource for helminth genomics. *Molecular and Biochemical Parasitology* 215:2–10.

Ikarashi, M., H. Nakashima, M. Kinoshita, A. Sato, M. Nakashima, H. Miyazaki, K. Nishiyama, J. Yamamoto, and S. Seki. 2013. Distinct development and functions of resident and recruited liver Kupffer cells/macrophages. *Journal of Leukocyte Biology* 94:1325–1336.

International Helminth Genome Consortium. 2019. Comparative genomics of the major parasitic worms. *Nature Genetics* 51:163–174.

Janecek, E., A. Beineke, T. Schnieder, and C. Strube. 2014. Neurotoxocarosis: Marked preference of *Toxocara canis* for the cerebrum and *T. cati* for the cerebellum in the paratenic model host mouse. *Parasites & Vectors* 7:1–13.

Jankovic, D., M. C. Kullberg, P. Caspar, and A. Sher. 2004. Parasite-induced Th2 polarization is associated with down-regulated dendritic cell responsiveness to Th1 stimuli and a transient delay in T lymphocyte cycling. *Journal of Immunology* 173:2419–2427.

Jeong, P. Y., M. Jung, Y. H. Yim, H. Kim, M. Park, E. Hong, W. Lee, Y. H. Kim, K. Kim, and Y. K. Paik. 2005. Chemical structure and biological activity of the *Caenorhabditis elegans* dauer-inducing pheromone. *Nature* 433:541–545.

Jex, A. R., R. B. Gasser, and E. M. Schwarz. 2019. Transcriptomic resources for parasitic nematodes of veterinary importance. *Trends in Parasitology* 35:72–84.

Jirtle, R. L., and M. K. Skinner. 2007. Environmental epigenomics and disease susceptibility. *Nature Reviews Genetics* 8:253–262.

Jourdan, P. M., P. H. L. Lamberton, A. Fenwick, and D. G. Addiss. 2018. Soil-transmitted helminth infections. *Lancet* 391:252–265.

Kadarmideen, H. N., N. S. Watson-Haigh, and N. M. Andronicos. 2011. Systems biology of ovine intestinal parasite resistance: Disease gene modules and biomarkers. *Molecular Biosystems* 7:235–246.

Kaplan, R. E. W., C. S. Maxwell, N. K. Codd, and L. R. Baugh. 2019. Pervasive positive and negative feedback regulation of insulin-like signaling in *Caenorhabditis elegans*. *Genetics* 211:349–361.

Katagiri, T., H. Kameda, N. H. Akano, and Y. S. Amazake. 2021. Regulation of T cell differentiation by the AP-1 transcription factor JunB. *Immunological Medicine* 44:197–203.

Klotz C., and U. Frevert. 2008. *Plasmodium yoelii* sporozoites modulate cytokine profile and induce apoptosis in murine Kupffer cells. *International Journal of Parasitology* 38:1639–1650.

Kochneva, A. A., E. V. Borvinskaya, D. S. Bedulina, L. P. Smirnov, and I. V. Sukhovskaya. 2023. Proteomics research on features of life activity of parasitic worms. *Biology Bulletin Reviews* 13:S155–S171.

Kumar, S., S. Gupta, A. Mohmad, A. Fular, B. C. Parthasarathi, and A. K. Chaubey. 2021. Molecular tools-advances, opportunities and prospects for the control of parasites of veterinary importance. *International Journal of Tropical Insect Science* 41:33–42.

Kwa, M. S., J. G. Veenstra, M. Van Dijk, and M. H. Roos. 1995. Beta-tubulin genes from the parasitic nematode *Haemonchus contortus* modulate drug resistance in *Caenorhabditis elegans*. *Journal of Molecular Biology* 246:500–516.

Laing, R., T. Kikuchi, A. Martinelli, I. J. Tsai, R. N. Beech, E. Redman, N. Holroyd, D. J. Bartley, H. Beasley, C. Britton, and D. Curran. 2013. The genome and transcriptome of *Haemonchus contortus*, a key model parasite for drug and vaccine discovery. *Genome Biology* 14:R88

Liehl, P., P. Meireles, I. S. Albuquerque, M. Pinkevych, F. Baptista, M. M. Mota, M. P. Davenport, and M. Prudêncio. 2015. Innate immunity induced by *Plasmodium* liver infection inhibits malaria reinfections. *Infection and Immunity* 83:1172–1180.

Liehl, P., V. Zuzarte-Luís, J. Chan, T. Zillinger, F. Baptista, D. Carapau, M. Konert, K. K. Hanson, C. Carret, C. Lassnig, and M. Müller. 2014. Host-cell sensors for *Plasmodium* activate innate immunity against liver-stage infection. *Nature Medicine* 20:47–53.

Liu, F., J. Lu, W. Hu, S. Y. Wang, S. J. Cui, M. Chi, Q. Yan, X. R. Wang, H. D. Song, X. N. Xu, J. J. Wang, X. L. Zhang, X. Zhang, Z. Q. Wang, C. L. Xue, P. J. Brindley, D. P. McManus, P. Y. Yang, Z. Feng, Z. Chen, and Z. G. Han. 2006. New perspectives on hostparasite interplay by comparative transcriptomic and proteomic analyses of *Schistosoma japonicum*. *PLoS Pathogens* 2:268–281.

Liu, J., Z. L. hu, J. Wang, Q. L. Iu, Y. Chen, R. E. Davis, and G. Cheng. 2019. *Schistosoma japonicum* extracellular vesicle miRNA cargo regulates host macrophage functions facilitating parasitism. *PLoS Pathogens* 15:e1007817

Lopez-Rubio, J.J., L. Mancio-Silvaand, and A. Scherf. 2009. Genome-wide analysis of heterochromatin associates clonally variant gene regulation with perinuclear repressive centers in malaria parasites. *Cell Host Microbe* 5:179–190.

Luck, A. N., K. G. Anderson, C. M. McClung, N. C. VerBerkmoes, J. M. Foster, M. L. Michalski, and B. E. Slatko. 2015. Tissue-specific transcriptomics and proteomics of a filarial nematode and its Wolbachia endosymbiont. *BMC Genomics* 16:1–17.

Ludewig, A. H., and F. C. Schroeder. 2013. Ascaroside signaling in *C. elegans*. *WormBook*, 1–22.

Lutzelschwab, C. M., C. A. Fiel, S. I. Pedonesse, R. Najle, E. Rodrı́guez, P. E. Steffan, C. Saumell, L. Fuse, and L. Iglesias. 2005. Arrested development of *Ostertagia ostertagi*: Effect of the exposure of infective larvae to natural spring conditions of the humid pampa (Argentina). *Veterinary Parasitology* 127:253–262.

Ma, G., T. Wang, P. K. Korhonen, S. Nie, G. E. Reid, A. J. Stroehlein, A. V. Koehler, B. C. H. Chang, A. Hofmann, N. D. Young, R. B. Gasser. 2019. Comparative bioinformatic analysis suggests that specific dauer-like signalling pathway components regulate *Toxocara canis* development and migration in the mammalian host. *Parasite & Vectors* 12:32.

Maizels R. M., and H. J. McSorley. 2016. Regulation of the host immune system by helminth parasites. *Journal of Allergy and Clinical Immunology* 138:666–675.

Mangiola, S., N. D. Young, P. W. Sternberg, C. Strube, P. K. Korhonen, M. Mitreva, J. P. Scheerlinck, A. Hofmann, A. R. Jex, and R. B. Gasser. 2014. Analysis of the transcriptome of adult *Dictyocaulus filaria* and comparison with *Dictyocaulus viviparus*, with a focus on molecules involved in host–parasite interactions. *International Journal of Parasitology* 44:251–261

Massacand, J. C., R. C. Stettler, R. Meier, N. E. Humphreys, R. K. Grencis, B. J. Marsland, and N. L. Harris. 2009. Helminth products bypass the need for TSLP in Th2 immune responses by directly modulating dendritic cell function. *Proceedings of National Academy of Science of United States of America* 106:13968–13973.

McNulty, S. N., C. Strübe, B. A. Rosa, J. C. Martin, R. Tyagi, Y. J. Choi, Q. Wang, K. Hallsworth Pepin, X. Zhang, P. Ozersky, and R. K. Wilson. 2016. *Dictyocaulus viviparus* genome, variome and transcriptome elucidate lungworm biology and support future intervention. *Scientific Reports* 6:20316.

Meis J. F., J. P. Verhave, P. H. Jap, and J. H. Meuwissen. 1983. An ultrastructural study on the role of Kupffer cells in the process of infection by *Plasmodium berghei* sporozoites in rats. *Parasitology* 86:231–242.

Meslin, B., C. Barnadas, V. Boni, C. Latour, F. De Monbrison, K. Kaiser, and S. Picot. 2007. Features of apoptosis in *Plasmodium falciparum* erythrocytic stage through a putative role of PfMCA1 metacaspase-like protein. *The Journal of Infectious Diseases* 195:1852–1859.

Metenou, S., M. Kovacs, B. Dembele, Y. I. Coulibaly, A. D. Klion, and T. B. Nutman. 2012. Interferon regulatory factor modulation underlies the bystander suppression of malaria antigen-driven IL-12 and IFN-γ in filaria-malaria co-infection. *European Journal of Immunology* 42:641–650.

Midttun, H. L., N. Acevedo, P. Skallerup, S. Almeida, K. Skovgaard, L. Andresen, S. Skov, L. Caraballo, I. Van DIe, C.B. Jørgensen, and M. Fredholm. 2018. *Ascaris suum* infection downregulates inflammatory pathways in the pig intestine *in vivo* and in human dendritic cells *in vitro. Journal of Infectious Diseases* 217:310–319.

Miller, L. H., M. F. Good, and G. Milon. 1994. Malaria pathogenesis. *Science* 264:1878–1883.

Moser, M., and K. M. Murphy. 2000. Dendritic cell regulation of TH1–TH2 development. *Nature Immunology* 1:199–205.

Müller H. M., I. Reckmann, M. R. Hollingdale, H. Bujard, K. J. Robson, and A. Crisanti. 1993. Thrombospondin related anonymous protein (TRAP) of *Plasmodium falciparum* binds specifically to sulfated glycoconjugates and to HepG2 hepatoma cells suggesting a role for this molecule in sporozoite invasion of hepatocytes. *EMBO Journal* 12:2881–2889.

Murphy, C. T., and P. J. Hu. 2013. Insulin/insulin-like growth factor signaling in *C. elegans. WormBook* 1:1–43.

Nogueira, D. S., P. H. Gazzinelli-Guimarães, F. S. Barbosa, N. M. Resende, C. C. Silva, L. M. de Oliveira, C. C. O. Amorim, F. M. S. Oliveira, M. S. Mattos, L. R. Kraemer, and M. V. Caliari. 2016. Multiple exposures to *Ascaris suum* induce tissue injury and mixed Th2/Th17 immune response in mice. *PLoS Neglected Tropical Diseases* 10:e0004382.

Nutman, T.B. 2015. Looking beyond the induction of Th2 responses to explain immunomodulation by helminths. *Parasite Immunology* 37:304–313.

Ofir-Birin, Y., and N. Regev-Rudzki. 2019. Extracellular vesicles in parasite survival. *Science* 363:817–818.

Ogawa, A., A. Streit, A. Antebi, and R. J. Sommer. 2009. A conserved endocrine mechanism controls the formation of dauer and infective larvae in nematodes. *Current Biology* 19:67–71.

Patarroyo, M. E., M. P. Alba, and H. Curtidor. 2011. Biological and structural characteristics of the binding peptides from the sporozoite proteins essential for cell traversal (SPECT)-1 and -2. *Peptides* 32:154–160.

Risco-Castillo, V., S. Topçu, C. Marinach, G. Manzoni, A. E. Bigorgne, S. Briquet, X. Baudin, M. Lebrun, J. F. Dubremetz, and O. Silvie. 2015. Malaria sporozoites traverse host cells within transient vacuoles. *Cell Host Microbe* 18:593–603.

Robinson, M. W., R. Menon, S. M. Donnelly, J. P. Dalton, and S. Ranganathan. 2009. An integrated transcriptomics and proteomics analysis of the secretome of the helminth pathogen *Fasciola hepatica*: Proteins associated with invasion and infection of the mammalian host. *Molecular and Cellular Proteomics* 8:1891–1907.

Rougvie, A. E., and E. G. Moss. 2013. Developmental transitions in C. elegans larval stages. *Current Topics in Developmental Biology* 105:153–180.

Scherf, A., J. J. Lopez-Rubio, and L. Riviere. 2008. Antigenic variation in *Plasmodium falciparum. Annual Review of Microbiology* 62:445–470.

Schwarz, E. M., Y. Hu, I. Antoshechkin, M. M. Miller, P. W. Sternberg, and R. V. Aroian. 2015. The genome and transcriptome of the zoonotic hookworm *Ancylostoma ceylanicum* identify infection- specific gene families. *Nature Genetics* 47:416–422.

Schwarz, E. M., P. K. Korhonen, B. E. Campbell, N. D. Young, A. R. Jex, A. Jabbar, R. S. Hall, A. Mondal, A. C. Howe, J. Pell, and A. Hofmann. 2013. The genome and developmental transcriptome of the strongylid nematode *Haemonchus contortus. Genome Biology* 14:R89

Shapiro, T. A., and P. T. Englund. 1990. Selective cleavage of kinetoplast DNA minicircles promoted by antitrypanosomal drugs. *Proceedings of National Academy of Science of United States of America* 87:950–954.

Sharma P, P. D. Juyal, L. D. Singla, D. Chachra, and H. Pawar. 2012. Comparative evaluation of real time PCR assay with conventional parasitological techniques for diagnosis of Trypanosoma evansi in cattle and buffaloes. *Veterinary Parasitology* 190:375–382.

Singh S., M. M. Alam, I. Pal-Bhowmick, J. A. Brzostowski, C. E. Chitnis. 2010. Distinct external signals trigger sequential release of apical organelles during erythrocyte invasion by malaria parasites. *PLoS Pathogens* 6:e1000746.

Sinnis, P., and F. Zavala. 2012. The skin: where malaria infection and the host immune response begin. *Seminars in Immunopathology* 34:787–792.

Smith, L. M., F. C. Motta, G. Chopra, J. K. Moch, R. R. Nerem, B. Cummins, K. E. Roche, C. M. Kelliher, A. R. Leman, J. Harer, and T. Gedeon. 2020. An intrinsic oscillator drives the blood stage cycle of the malaria parasite *Plasmodium falciparum*. *Science* 368:754–759.

Smith, W. D., G. F. Newlands, S. K. Smith, D. Pettit, and P. J. Skuce. 2003. Metalloendopeptidases from the intestinal brush border of *Haemonchus contortus* as protective antigens for sheep. *Parasite Immunology* 25:313–323.

Sorci, G., S. Cornet, and B. Faivre. 2013. Immune evasion, immunopathology and the regulation of the immune system. *Pathogens* 2:71–91.

Sotillo, J., M. S. Pearson, and A. Loukas. 2019. Trematode genomics and proteomics. *Digenetic Trematodes* 1154:411–436.

Sotillo, J., M. Trelis, A. Cortés, M. L. Valero, M. S. del Pino, J. Guillermo Esteban, A. Marcilla, and R. Toledo. 2012. Proteomic analysis of the pinworm *Syphacia muris* (Nematoda: Oxyuridae), a parasite of laboratory rats, *Parasitology International* 61:561–564.

Spottiswoode N., P. E. Duffy, and H. Drakesmith. 2014. Iron, anemia and hepcidin in malaria. *Frontiers in Pharmacology* 5:125.

Steers N., R. Schwenk, D. J. Bacon, D. Berenzon, J. Williams, and U. Krzych. 2005. The immune status of Kupffer cells profoundly influences their responses to infectious *Plasmodium berghei* sporozoites. *European Journal of Immunology* 35:2335–2346.

Strube, C., L. Heuer, and E. Janecek. 2013. *Toxocara* spp. infections in paratenic hosts. *Veterinary Parasitology* 193:375–389.

Tavares, J., P. Formaglio, S. Thiberge, E. Mordelet, N. Van Rooijen, A. Medvinsky, R. Ménard, and R. Amino. 2013. Role of host cell traversal by the malaria sporozoite during liver infection. *Journal of Experimental Medicine* 210:905–915.

Tomazic, M. L., V. Marugan-Hernandez, and A. E. Rodriguez. 2022. Next-generation technologies and systems biology for the design of novel vaccines against apicomplexan parasites. *Frontiers in Veterinary Science* 8:800361.

Tritten, L., C. Ballesteros, R. Beech, T. G. Geary, and Y. Moreno. 2021. Mining nematode protein secretomes to explain lifestyle and host specificity. *PLoS Neglected Tropical Diseases* 15(9):e0009828.

Tsai, I. J., M. Zarowiecki, N. Holroyd, A. Gasciarrubio, A. Sanchez-Flores, K. L. Brooks, A. Tracey, R. J. Bobes, G. Fragoso, E. Sciutto, M. Aslett, H. Beasley, H. M. Bennett, X. Cai, F. Camicia, R. Clark, M. Cucher, N. De Silva, T. A. Day, P. Deplazes, K. Estrada, C. Fernandez, P. W. H. Holland, J. Hou, S. Hu, T. Huckvale, S. S. Hung, L. Kamenetzky, J. A. Keane, F. Kiss, U. Koziol, O. Lambert, K. Liu, X. Luo, Y. Luo, N. Macchiaroli, S. Nichol, J. Paps, J. Parkinson, N. Pouchkina-Stantcheva, N. Riddiford, M. Rosenzvit, G. Salinas, J. D. Wasmuth, M. Zamanian, and Y. Zheng. 2013. The genomes of four tapeworm species reveal adaptations to parasitism. *Nature* 496:57–63.

Tyagi, R., A. Joachim, B. Ruttkowski, B. A. Rosa, Martin J. C., K. Hallsworth-Pepin, X. Zhang, P. Ozersky, R. K. Wilson, S. Ranganathan, and P. W. Sternberg. 2015. Cracking the nodule worm code advances knowledge of parasite biology and biotechnology to tackle major diseases of livestock. *Biotechnological Advances* 33:980–991.

UniProt Consortium. 2017. UniProt: the universal protein knowledgebase. *Nucleic Acids Research* 45(D1):D158–D169.

Upcroft, J. A., R. W. Campbell, and P. Upcroft. 1996. Quinacrine-resistant *Giardia duodenalis*. *Parasitology* 112:309–313.

von Reuss, S. H., N. Bose, J. Srinivasan, J. J. Yim, J. C. Judkins, P. W. Sternberg, and F. C. Schroeder. 2012. Comparative metabolomics reveals biogenesis of ascarosides, a modular library of small-molecule signals in *C. elegans*. *Journal of American Chemical Society* 134:1817–1824.

Werbovetz, K. A. 2002. Tubulin as an antiprotozoal drug target. *Mini Reviews in Medicinal Chemistry* 2:519–529.

WHO. 2018. *World Health Organization WHO: The world Malaria report 2018*. WHO.

Yoo, W. G., D.W. Kim, J. W. Ju, P. Y. Cho, T. I. Kim, S. H. Cho, S. H. Choi, H. S. Park, T. S. Kim and S. J. Hong. 2011. Developmental transcriptomic features of the carcinogenic liver fluke, *Clonorchis sinensis*. *PLoS Neglected Tropical Diseases* 5:e1208.

Yu, L., B. Cao, Y. Long, M. Tukayo, C. Feng, W. Fang, and D. Luo. 2017. Comparative transcriptomic analysis of two important life stages of *Angiostrongylus cantonensis*: fifth-stage larvae and female adults. *Genetics and Molecular Biology* 40:540–549.

Zvinorova, P. I., T. E. Halimani, F. C. Muchadeyi, O. Matika, V. Riggio, and K. Dzama. 2016. Prevalence and risk factors of gastrointestinal parasitic infections in goats in low-input low-output farming systems in Zimbabwe. *Small Ruminant Research* 143:75–83.

2 Introduction to Omics Technologies

Muhammad Sohail Sajid[1], Sadia Ghazanfer[1],
Hafiz Muhammad Rizwan[2],
Muhammad Haziq Bajwa[3],
Nimra Anwar[4], and Muhammad Saqib[5]

[1]Department of Parasitology, Faculty of Veterinary Sciences, University of Agriculture, Faisalabad, Pakistan

[2]Section of Parasitology, Department of Pathobiology, KBCMA College of Veterinary and Animal Sciences, Narowal, Sub-campus University of Veterinary and Animal Sciences, Lahore, Pakistan

[3]Faculty of Veterinary Sciences, KBCMA College of Veterinary and Animal Sciences, Lahore, Pakistan

[4]Department of Pharmacology and Toxicology, Faculty of Bio-Sciences, University of Veterinary and Animal Sciences, Lahore, Pakistan

[5]Department of Clinical Medicine and Surgery, Faculty of Veterinary Science, University of Agriculture, Faisalabad, Pakistan

2.1 INTRODUCTION

The Greek word *ome* and the word *omics* are the sources of the suffix -ome, which denotes "whole," "all," or "complete." Cellular molecules such as genes, transcripts, proteins, and metabolites can be referred to as genomes, transcriptomes, proteomes, and metabolomes, respectively, when the suffix "-ome" is added. Systems biology and omics technologies represent the cutting edge of molecular medicine (Yadav and Shukla, 2007). Genomics, transcriptomics, proteomics, and lipidomics are high-throughput analyses. These analyses are integrated using systems biology, computational tools, and bioinformatics. They study the interactions, mechanisms, and functions of organs, tissues, cell populations, and entire organisms. This is done at the molecular level in a non-biased and non-targeted manner. This field is known as omics (Carlos et al., 2012; Lavelle and Sokol, 2018). The systematic study of an organism's whole genome is known as genomics (Horgan and Kenny, 2011).

The human genome comprises approximately 3 billion base pairs of nucleotides, consisting of adenine, guanine, cytosine, and thymine. Within DNA lie the genetic

DOI: 10.1201/9781032651071-2

instructions essential for cellular construction and maintenance (Hartl, 2014). Genes, specific units of DNA, encode the blueprints necessary for generating functional proteins. The sequence of nucleotides within DNA dictates the information it holds (Schmidt, 2022). The advent of high-throughput sequencing technologies, like next-generation sequencing (NGS), facilitates the examination of genetic variations among individuals (Lohmann and Klein, 2014).

The study of transcriptomics focuses on the transcriptome, which is the totality of RNA sequences in a cell known as transcripts (Pang et al., 2023). RNA is divided into two categories: i) Coding RNAs, or mRNAs, which are translated into protein sequences; ii) non-coding RNA is divided into two subgroups: long non-coding RNA and short non-coding RNA, which includes microRNA. Gene regulation involves non-coding RNA (Dinger et al., 2008). Advanced RNA sequencing technologies enable a comprehensive comprehension of gene expression and variation among different types of RNA molecules (Han et al., 2015).

The study of proteomics focuses on the proteome, encompassing all expressed proteins, along with the intricate network of protein families and metabolic pathways found within cells, tissues, or organisms. While the exact number of proteins remains uncertain, estimates suggest several hundred thousand (Müller et al., 2020). Metabolomics, on the other hand, explores the metabolome present in biofluids, cells, organisms, or tissues (Figure 2.1). The metabolome comprises small molecules and their interactions within biological systems, influenced by genetic, dietary, and environmental factors (Wishart, 2019). As the downstream product of gene and protein expression, the metabolome is chemically and physically intricate, reflecting changes and interactions shaped by the environment. Among various omics techniques, metabolomics closely resembles the phenotypic characteristics of organisms (Belhaj et al., 2021). The molecular phenotype of health and illness is most effectively modulated and represented by metabolomics (Guijas et al., 2018). It is an excellent source of disease-associated biomarkers in this sense. A helpful

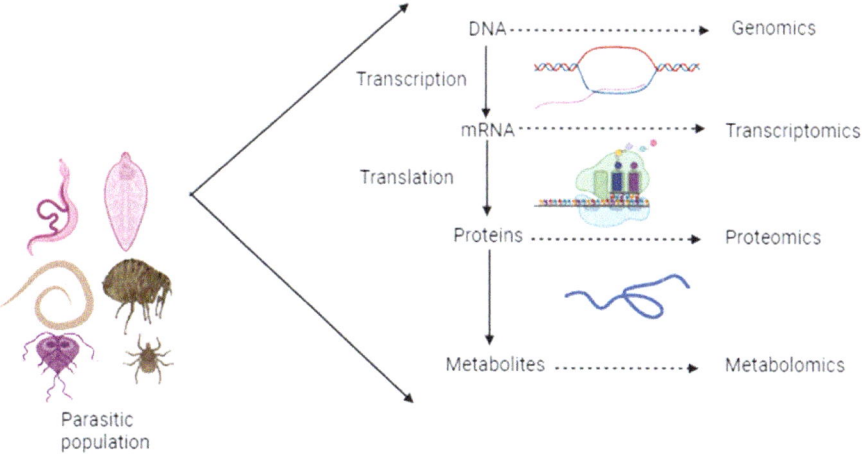

FIGURE 2.1 Overview of omics in parasitic research.

method for classifying disease- or treatment-associated molecular patterns derived from metabolites, as well as for identifying disease-related metabolites in biofluids, is mass spectrometry-based metabolomics. It also distinguishes between various disease severity types (Gowda et al., 2008).

2.2   EVOLUTIONARY DEVELOPMENT AND TYPES OF OMICS

Numerous seminal moments in the history of genomics have profoundly influenced our understanding of genetics and provided the foundational framework for modern genomics research. The terminology "genomics," signifying the thorough examination of entire genomes, including analysis of structural and functional aspects, was introduced during the latter part of the 20th century (Dwivedi et al., 2017). Undoubtedly, one of the most transformative events in the realm of genomics occurred with the groundbreaking discovery by James Watson and Francis Crick in 1953. Their elucidation of the double-helix structure of DNA stands as an iconic moment in scientific history. This monumental breakthrough established the fundamental framework that has allowed us to grasp how genetic information is encoded, stored, and transmitted within living organisms (Klug, 2004).

In 1977, another significant milestone was reached when researchers sequenced the complete genome of a virus, Phi X 174. This achievement was closely followed by sequencing the bacteriophage MS2 (Sanger and Coulson, 1975). These accomplishments represented a pivotal advancement in the field of genomics. They not only showcased the viability of sequencing entire genomes but also played a crucial role in paving the path for more ambitious genome sequencing endeavours that followed. These pivotal moments in the history of genomics not only enriched our understanding of genetics but also acted as catalysts for the evolution of genomics research. They laid the foundation for in-depth exploration of genomes in all their intricate complexity, ushering in a new era of scientific discovery (Heather and Chain, 2016). The evolution of omics techniques is shown in Figure 2.2.

The Human Genome Project (HGP), started in 1990 and completed in 2003, was a huge worldwide undertaking to sequence the whole human genome (Lander et al., 2001). The introduction of next-generation sequencing (NGS) technology in the early 21st century revolutionised genomics research by enabling faster and more cost-effective sequencing of complete genomes (Metzker, 2010). This led to the study of RNA and the transcriptomics revolution began in the 21st century with the introduction of RNA-seq technology. It permits high-throughput sequencing of RNA molecules, making it possible to measure gene expression (Wang et al., 2009). Microarray technology, which enabled researchers to simultaneously analyse the expression of thousands of genes, played a significant role in transcriptomics prior to RNA-seq (Schena et al., 1995).

Protein separation and purification were made possible by early methods such as electrophoresis and chromatography (Lee, 2017). Two-Dimensional Polyacrylamide Gel Electrophoresis (2D-PAGE) became an efficient technique for protein separation and quantification in the 1970s (O'Farrell, 1975). The Human Proteome Project (HPP), similar to the Human Genome Project, was started in the 21st century to

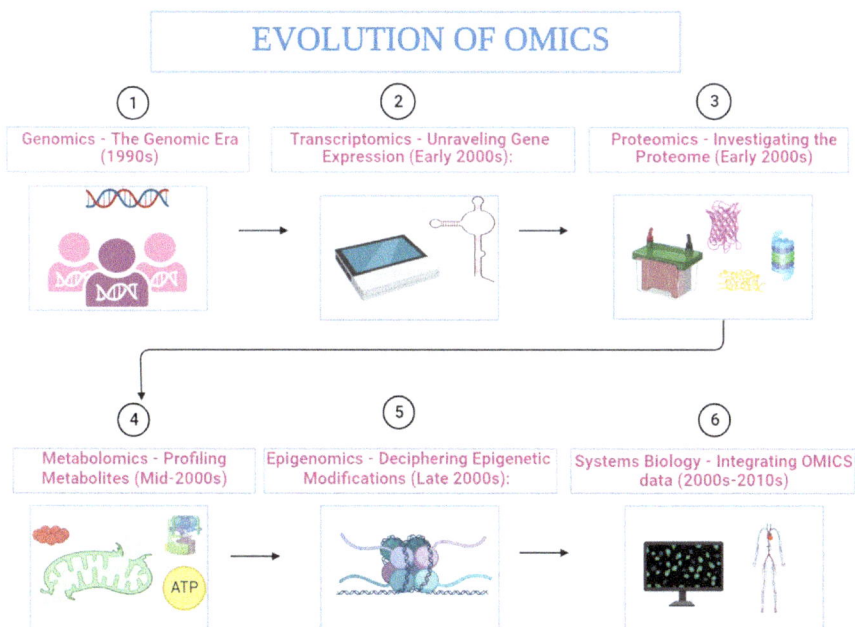

FIGURE 2.2 The timeline of omics development over time.

map the whole human proteome, giving rise to proteomics (Consden et al., 1947). The development of mass spectrometry also provided the analytical tools necessary for comprehensive lipid analysis (Aebersold and Mann, 2003). The high-throughput lipid profiling methods of liquid chromatography-mass spectrometry (LC-MS) and gas chromatography-mass spectrometry (GC-MS) enabled the identification and quantification of numerous lipid species, hence developing lipidomics (Han and Gross, 2003).

In the mid-20th century, researchers began identifying glycoproteins and glyco-lipids, molecules consisting of proteins or lipids linked to carbohydrates (Varki, 2017). The field of glycomics emerged in the late 20th century, with the development of techniques for studying complex carbohydrates and glycoconjugates (Harvey, 2012). The latest branch of omics called epigenomics, gained prominence after the invention of high-throughput sequencing techniques, such as ChIP-seq (chromatin immunoprecipitation followed by bisulfite sequencing), which enabled genome-wide profiling of epigenetic marks (Kim et al., 2017). Further details of different omics techniques and their applications are given in Table 2.1.

2.3 GENOMICS AND ITS SIGNIFICANCE IN PARASITIC RESEARCH

In the eukaryotic tree of life, parasites are classified as eukaryotic organisms. Parasitic worms that cause widespread diseases are significant for humans and animals (Loker and Hofkin, 2022). For over a decade, genome sequencing has both

TABLE 2.1
The Different Omics Techniques and Their Applications

Fields of Omics	Definition	Applications
Genomics	The study of an organism's whole genome, including how genes are arranged, used, and interact with one another (Lander et al., 2001).	Genetic variations connected to diseases have been discovered through the application of genomics (Manolio et al., 2009).
Transcriptomics	The study that involves analysing the patterns of gene expression and activity levels of genes in a biological sample (Wang et al., 2009).	Transcriptomics has enabled the identification of disease-specific gene expression profiles, which has aided in the development of personalised medicines (Subramanian et al., 2005).
Proteomics	The study of all the proteins (proteome) in a cell, tissue, or organism. It includes the detection and quantification of proteins, as well as their interactions and post-translational changes (Aebersold and Mann, 2003).	Proteomics is crucial in biomarker discovery and understanding disease mechanisms at the protein level (Mertins et al., 2016).
Metabolomics	The study of metabolites, small molecules involved in biological activities. It offers an understanding of metabolic pathways and how diseases result from their disruption (Fiehn, 2002).	Metabolomics has been used to identify biomarkers for various diseases, such as diabetes and cancer (Patti et al., 2012).
Lipidomics	The study of lipid molecules to understand their function in biological systems and disorders (Han and Gross, 2003).	Lipidomics has contributed to understanding lipid-related disorders and has helped study drug development targeting lipid metabolism (Ecker and Liebisch, 2014).
Glycomics	The study of carbohydrates (glycans) and their functions that are involved in various biological processes (Varki et al., 2009).	Glycomics has proved to be useful in cancer research, immunology, and infectious diseases (Ohtsubo and Marth, 2006). By understanding glycan structures and interactions, glycan-based drugs can be developed.
Epigenomics	The study that deals with the process of gene regulation by observing modifications to DNA and histones (Feinberg and Vogelstein, 1983).	Epigenomics plays a crucial role in understanding the epigenetic basis of diseases and developing epigenetic drugs (Feinberg et al., 2006; Dawson and Kouzarides, 2012).

redefined relationships among eukaryotic organisms and set fresh challenges, especially in the case of parasites, which have complex life cycles and thrive in impoverished environments. With few exceptions, the inner workings of parasites have been largely obscure (Martin, 2002). However, due to the burgeoning number of parasite genomes obtained mostly from field isolates, this is no longer the case. Sequencing projects, both individual and what can be referred to as "statistical," by large sequencing facilities have led to hundreds of parasite genomes being sequenced (Broder and Venter, 2000). The "sequencing tsunami" of genomic information has provided answers to long-held questions about genetic diversity of parasites, molecular evolution under the immunological pressure of hosts, population genetics of organisms of ancient pedigree, and mutable epidemiological and infection characteristics (Hupalo et al., 2015). Here we discuss the current state of parasitic protist genomics, innovative sequencing approaches driven by unique genomes, and how NGS transforms our understanding of disease control and parasite population genomics.

Before the widespread availability of rapid and cost-effective NGS, the limited data on parasite genome sequences constrained population studies to a few genetic loci. These initial investigations identified loci suitable for classifying patient isolates and provided insights into genetic diversity, local and global population structures, and gene flow among different parasite species (Kanai et al., 2022). These studies typically relied on a small number of microsatellite markers spread across chromosomes and single nucleotide polymorphisms (SNPs) in single-copy genes. Such genotyping methods have proven valuable for epidemiological investigations and disease classification (Boité et al., 2012). Furthermore, single-locus analyses have been instrumental in identifying genetic changes associated with parasite traits such as drug resistance and virulence (Su et al., 2002).

Recently, advancements in whole-genome sequencing have enabled the study of parasite populations, including naturally occurring isolates from patients and laboratory-modified strains. This has enhanced our understanding of important population genetic characteristics (Garçon et al., 2007). The NGS data are proving influential in shaping population genetic studies of parasites (Conway, 2007). The ability of an organism to carry out sexual recombination directly impacts the distribution of crucial genes related to virulence or treatment resistance, underscoring the importance of considering recombination as a key population genetic characteristic in parasites (Dapper and Payseur, 2017).

Population genetic studies on various parasite species have indicated recent or potential genetic exchange events in their evolutionary histories. The first reference genome analysis of the intestinal pathogen *Entamoeba (E.) histolytica* revealed the presence of genes necessary for meiosis, indicating the possibility of sexual reproduction in wild populations (Stanley, 2005). Subsequent analysis of lab-cultured lines from Mexico and Bangladesh using NGS techniques provided more robust evidence of sexual reassortment and meiotic recombination, suggesting that *E. histolytica* may indeed reproduce sexually (Weedall et al., 2012). Further research by Gilchrist et al. (2012) utilised genotyping of 84 samples and identified specific loci associated with clinical symptoms, indicating a linkage between genotype and virulence. These studies underscore the substantial diversity within *E. histolytica* populations and suggest frequent and recent recombination events.

The NGS data have significantly impacted population genetic studies of species within the monkey malaria clade, as demonstrated by Gilchrist et al. (2012). This paper involved sequencing of *Plasmodium (P.) vivax* isolates adapted to monkeys and strains of closely related *P. cynomolgi* isolated from macaques (Neafsey et al., 2012). The NGS has improved the ability to identify lineage-specific changes in loci that were previously unnoticed. For example, NGS facilitated the creation and enhancement of reference genomes for *Leishmania* species, aiding in the detection of chromosomal and gene copy number variations (Downing et al., 2011). Studies revealed diverse chromosome copy numbers, with up to nine supernumerary chromosomes per individual, but only a few lineage-specific genes showed significant differences between species. A recent study examined genomic sequences of *Leishmania donovani* clinical isolates with varying treatment susceptibilities. Notably, genomics has contributed to identifying a locus linked to artemisinin resistance (Rogers et al., 2011).

The malaria community has been alarmed by the discovery of widespread resistance of *P. falciparum* to all available antimalarial drugs. Clinical resistance to artemisinin and its derivatives has emerged in patients from Cambodia, Vietnam, and Thailand (Amato et al., 2018). Cheeseman et al. (2012) conducted genotyping experiments on 91 clones from Laos, Cambodia, and Thailand, revealing a region on chromosome 13 under strong selection and significant population differentiation. Further screening of 715 isolates with additional genetic markers identified a 35 kb area within a selective sweep containing numerous potential resistance genes. Concurrently, Takala-Harrison et al. (2013) identified several genomic regions associated with artemisinin resistance phenotypes—including a region on chromosome 13—through population genetic analysis of SNP array data from approximately 330 patient isolates in Southeast Asia. Miotto et al. (2013) utilised a population genomics approach to analyse 414 West African and 411 Southeast Asian *P. falciparum* genomes, aiming to establish a "population-level genetic framework" for defining molecular markers and investigating the biological origins of resistance.

The discovery of numerous distinct but sympatric parasite subpopulations revealed significant genetic differentiation among Cambodian parasites in whole-genome data, indicating founder effects and recent population expansion (Hupalo et al., 2015). The acquisition of artemisinin resistance appears to depend on inheriting a limited number of genetic loci from resistant ancestors, as no association was observed between admixture proportions and parasite artemisinin resistance testing (Miotto et al., 2020). Understanding the genetic structure and evolutionary patterns of parasite populations is crucial for designing effective control measures against diseases (Cable et al., 2017). Population genomic data, particularly in the *Plasmodium* genus, have illuminated the evolutionary dynamics of infections and provide a solid foundation for further research on other understudied parasites. As sequencing costs decline and bioinformatics techniques advance, both large and small laboratories will have the capability to address population genetic issues related to parasitic diseases (Selbach et al., 2019).

2.4 PROTEOMICS AND ITS SIGNIFICANCE IN PARASITIC RESEARCH AND DIAGNOSIS

Parasites are challenging to identify using traditional methods due to their complex life cycles and redundant molecules in infectious activities. Changes in host metabolic processes due to parasite diseases can be detected through metabolic fingerprint methods, providing potential biomarkers for diagnosis (Balog et al., 2011). Contemporary -omic technologies, aided by advanced bioinformatic tools, offer high-throughput approaches for investigating complex systems biology (Wang et al., 2015). Differential protein profiling of hosts or parasitic compounds can help develop biomarkers for parasitic infections, relying on peptide degradations and post-translational modifications (Cantacessi et al., 2012). Human and animal tissues, as well as biofluids, may contain molecular information about the organism's physiological and pathological status due to the transit and destination points for parasites and their secretions. Proximal biofluid proteomic characterisation may provide valuable data for prognostic, predictive, and diagnostic biomarkers (Skrjabin et al., 1967). Identifying widely distributed proteins in rare quantities remains challenging. Biomarkers offer higher downstream information content compared to nucleic acids, which can be crucial for early diagnosis (Blaxter et al., 1998).

Mass spectrometry (MS) is a highly sensitive and versatile analytical technique used to quantify and identify protein variations, splice isoforms, metabolites, and disease-specific substances accurately and efficiently. It enables the detection of post-translational changes in bodily fluids, tissues, or cell cultures (Ciocan-Cartita et al., 2019). The MS-based proteomics methods, including high-throughput systems, are valuable tools for discovering novel biomarkers due to their ability to detect subtle protein changes, even at the population level (Angel et al., 2012). These methods can be employed alone or in combination with traditional biochemical and proteomic techniques to identify biomarkers for parasite detection. For example, they have been used to discover potential malaria markers in patient serum and species-specific proteins in infected individuals (Olsen, 1986). The MS-based technologies such as SELDI-TOF-MS and surface-enhanced laser desorption/ionisation time-of-flight MS are particularly useful for examining protein-based biomarkers in parasitic diseases (Sánchez-Ovejero et al., 2016). The SELDI-TOF, for instance, can detect specific protein profiles in biofluids, including low molecular weight compounds, and has been used to identify host proteins altered in response to *Trypanosoma cruzi* infection with high sensitivity and specificity (Sommerville, 1957).

The MALDI-TOF has emerged as a valuable diagnostic method for distinguishing between infections caused by *Entamoeba* spp. and *Babesia canis canis* (Rogers and Sommerville, 1968). It is also becoming a compact bioanalytical tool for protein identification and classification in complex biological samples. MALDI-MS is utilised in various fields, including pathogen identification, biomarker discovery, and lipid-based biomarker sensing. It enables precise identification of vectors such as mosquitoes, which is crucial for understanding their role in disease transmission (Waller, 1997). Additionally, MALDI-TOF facilitates rapid identification of diseases and vectors in a single analysis, streamlining dual identification processes (Barker,

1975). Recent studies have highlighted the efficacy of MS in identifying indicators of parasite infections in biofluids and tissues, but its widespread adoption in research and clinical diagnosis is still needed (Baker et al., 2016). To maximise protein identifications using highly reproducible assays, careful consideration of pre-analytical processes during parasite sample preparation is essential (Fernandez-Becerra et al., 2023).

Several MS-based methods hold promise for advancing diagnostic parasitology (Waller, 1997): (i) MS imaging provides spatial distribution and relative abundance data of tissue-specific biomolecules, with potential applications in understanding disease pathogenesis and differentiating between diseases with similar histological features (Balic et al., 2000). (ii) PCR-electrospray ionisation mass spectrometry is a versatile technology for identifying tick-borne pathogens and characterising different strains and species (Loukas and Prociv, 2001). (iii) Multiple reaction monitoring mass spectrometric assays enable quantification of protein isoforms, specific proteins, or modified peptides, requiring enriched samples for accurate analysis of biomolecules relevant to parasites (Gause et al., 2003). (iv) Metabolomics techniques allow direct detection of substances originating from parasite physiology or metabolism within hosts, offering a means of detecting parasites through metabolic markers in bodily fluids, tissues, or cells (Maizels et al., 2004). Capillary electrophoresis MS and gas chromatography MS provide discriminatory power for identifying and interpreting metabolites derived from hosts or parasites, including medication metabolites during treatment of parasitic illnesses (Patel et al., 2009).

The integration of nanotechnologies and proteomics has led to the emergence of nanoproteomics, a new discipline focused on quick diagnostic screening at the nanoscale. Nanotechnology helps address complexities and protein modifications associated with proteomic technologies, offering detection benefits and enabling novel methodologies like multiplexing (Liu et al., 2010). Multiplexing, essential for analysing multiple factors simultaneously, is facilitated by techniques such as bead arrays, 3D printing, and protein and glycan microarrays in on-demand diagnostics platforms (Allen and Maizels, 2011). Micron-based dynamic sensing arrays and nano-sized beads applied in microfluidic systems enhance the level of multiplexing, contributing to advancements in immunoassays (Wu et al., 2022).

Protein microarrays are miniature immunoassays arranged in arrays, enabling simultaneous analysis of hundreds of proteins. They offer a high-throughput method for discovering novel biomarkers of infectious and parasitic disorders globally (Maxwell et al., 1987). Peptide chips serve as valuable tools for epitope characterisation and identification of immunodominant antigens (Miller and Horohov, 2006). Biochips with immuno-like polymer membranes are intriguing for point-of-care protein detection in serum samples. Novel single-domain antibodies, such as scFvs and nanobodies, offer advantages over monoclonal antibodies when used in conjunction with these techniques (Joachim et al., 1999). Glycan microarrays are effective for biomarker discovery, although advancements in synthesis, separation, and characterisation of glycans are necessary. These microarrays have the potential to identify carbohydrate antigens and improve the serodiagnosis of many parasitic illnesses

(Pearson et al., 2012). The diagnostic importance of glycans is evident in parasites like *Schistosoma*, *Leishmania*, and *Trichinella* (Nyame et al., 2004).

In diagnostic research, analysing specific isolated cellular compartments is increasingly crucial. Extracellular vesicles, particularly exosomes, play a vital role in intercellular communication and various biological processes (Gurunathan et al., 2019). With sizes ranging from 40 to 100 nm, exosomes carry a lipid coat and abundant surface protein concentrations, making them potential sources of circulating biomarker cargo (Mitchell et al., 2022). Exosomal protein markers displayed differently can serve as promising targets for diagnosis. Exosome-MS protein libraries, derived from whole exosome material or surface protein markers, offer optimal peptide libraries for GC-MS/MS analysis (Zhang et al., 2019). Intercommunicating extracellular vesicles released during parasitic infections play a critical role in the parasite's infectious life cycle (Holden-Dye and Walker, 2014). In diagnosing parasitic disorders, understanding and interpreting the cargo of parasite- or host-secreted biomarker-enriched microvesicles is crucial (Robertson et al., 2010). These microvesicles, including exosomes, hold potential for diagnosing long-term, complex diseases like cystic echinococcosis and vector-transmitted infections such as leishmaniasis (Keiser and Utzinger, 2008). MicroRNAs within exosome cargo show promise for diagnosing parasite illnesses (Ozturk and Caner, 2022). Lipids are another class of analytes worth investigating in exosomes for diagnostic purposes (Tenchov et al., 2022). Further research into the use of parasite-derived exosomes as diagnostic targets is warranted.

2.5 METABOLOMICS AND ITS SIGNIFICANCE IN PARASITIC RESEARCH AND DIAGNOSIS

Understanding the intricate interactions among genes, transcripts, proteins, and metabolites is a current challenge in biological research (Oliver et al., 1998). The metabolome, comprising all metabolites, closely reflects the phenotype and directly correlates with an organism's condition (Hu et al., 2020). Changes in both endogenous and environmental factors can impact the metabolome, serving as a vital link between the environment and biological systems (Lin et al., 2006). Despite numerous interactions among organisms, only a small fraction leads to dysregulation and subsequent illness (DiStefano, 2018). With infectious diseases ranking among the top causes of death, improved patient management is imperative. Unfortunately, some diagnostic techniques are cumbersome, slow, and lack sensitivity and specificity (Jain, 2010).

Metabolomics analysis offers potential in identifying metabolic biomarkers with novel characteristics (Figure 2.3) such as personalised treatment assessment, dynamic disease evaluation, non-invasive sampling, and improved diagnosis (Mayeux, 2004). A biomarker is a biological molecule capable of categorising individuals into specific groups, such as healthy or diseased, with sufficient sensitivity and specificity. However, this work is technically challenging (Xia et al., 2013). Scientists employ a comprehensive analytical process to discover and validate biomarkers, focusing

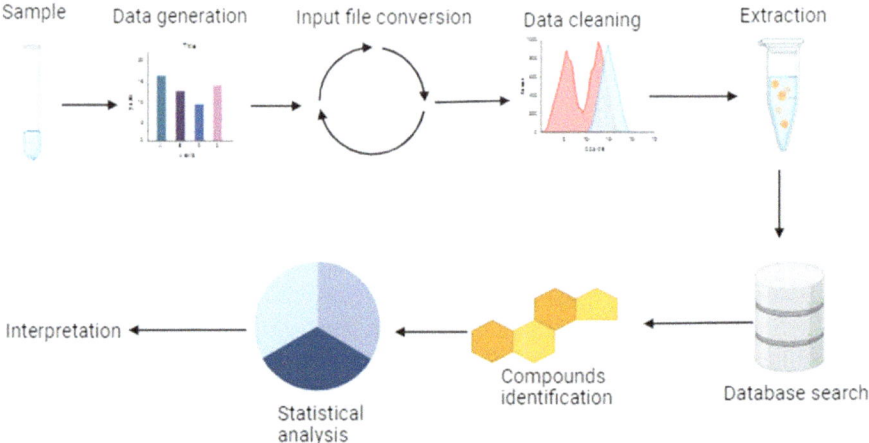

FIGURE 2.3 Workflow of metabolomics in parasitic research.

on data analysis, analytical platforms, sample preparation, and experimental design (Nakayasu et al., 2021). Metabolomics, strictly speaking, involves non-target analysis or global profiling, where the entire metabolome is examined without prior hypotheses, making it ideal for biomarker identification (Fiehn, 2002). However, biomarkers must undergo confirmation through traditional target analysis before being utilised in clinical settings. Nuclear magnetic resonance (NMR) and MS are the primary analytical platforms used in metabolomics fingerprinting, with NMR offering a non-destructive method for *in vivo* metabolism assessment (Letertre et al., 2021).

Gas chromatography (GC) separates metabolites based on their different vapour pressures and affinity for the column's stationary phase. Gas chromatography/mass spectrometry (GC-MS) typically uses small-bore capillary columns, with wall-coated open-tubular columns being the recommended kind (Mirnaghi and Caudy, 2014). The most commonly used stationary phases in metabolomics are DB-5 and DB-50, which represent (5%-phenyl)-methylpolysiloxane and (50%-phenyl)-methylpolysiloxane, respectively (Rojo, 2014). In liquid chromatography (LC), MS-linked system samples are injected into a packed column containing a stationary phase, allowing metabolites to be separated based on differing partition coefficients between the stationary phase and the eluotropic mobile phase (Bhattacharya, 2018). The LC procedures include normal-phase, hydrophilic interaction liquid chromatography (HILIC), and reverse-phase LC (such as C18, C8), each employing different stationary phases (Erkmen et al., 2021). Capillary zone electrophoresis, a type of capillary electrophoresis (CE), is a widely used technique in metabolomics, employing high voltages applied to two electrodes connected by a capillary to separate metabolites in a buffer solution (Zhang et al., 2017).

Parasites encompass a diverse array of organisms, including helminths and protozoa, which cause diseases like malaria, babesiosis, toxoplasmosis, and cryptosporidiosis (Akoolo et al., 2022). While extensive metabolomics studies have been conducted on *Plasmodium* spp., research on *Toxoplasma gondii* and *Cryptosporidium parvum* is limited (Bisanz et al., 2006; Sonawat and Sharma, 2012; Ramakrishnan et al., 2012). The genus *Plasmodium* comprises several obligatory intracellular parasites, including *P. falciparum*, *P. malariae*, *P. vivax*, *P. ovale*, and *P. knowlesi*, responsible for causing malaria (Autino et al., 2012). These parasites infect erythrocytes and hepatocytes, leading to varying degrees of illness severity and infection duration (Hänscheid, 2003). Severe malaria, commonly caused by *P. falciparum*, can result in life-threatening complications such as multiple organ dysfunction and respiratory distress. The gold standard for malaria diagnosis involves direct observation of parasites in blood smears, but this method has limitations (Njuguna and Newton, 2004). Lakshmanan et al. (2012) conducted LC-MS analysis of plasma samples from both *P. falciparum*-infected and non-infected patients and found significant group clustering in Partial Least-Squares Discriminant Analysis (PLS-DA). They identified substantial differences between the two groups in metabolites such as lipids, amino acids, and traumatin, a plant-like metabolite, suggesting the potential of alternative diagnostic biomarkers.

Other studies have focused on identifying biomarkers for the prognosis and differential diagnosis of malaria, particularly cerebral malaria (CM) or cerebral malaria with multiple organ dysfunction (CMMOD), which are severe forms of the disease affecting the central nervous system (Hellani, 2022). Surowiec et al. (2015) conducted a GC-MS study comparing plasma profiles of paediatric patients with mild and severe malaria and healthy controls. They found altered metabolites in binary comparisons of disease groups, enabling the creation of orthogonal partial least-squares-discriminant analysis (OPLS-DA) models with computed receiver operating characteristic (ROC) curves. These models successfully distinguished patients with moderate and severe malaria from healthy controls and from each other. Notably, urea, glucuronic acid, histidine, β-hydroxybutyric acid, cysteine, tryptophan, palmitoleic acid, and octadecatrienoic acid were among the most significantly altered metabolites identified in the investigation (Fernández-García et al., 2018).

Sengupta et al. (2016) conducted a 1H-NMR experiment assessing plasma profiles of patients infected with *P. falciparum*, presenting various clinical conditions including sepsis, viral encephalitis, moderate malaria, severe non-cerebral malaria, CM, and CMMOD. Principal component analysis (PCA) and OPLS-DA score plots showed partial segregation across all patient groups and controls, with important metabolites distinguishing malaria patients from controls, including lactate, glycoproteins, and lipoproteins (LDL/VLDL). Lactic acid, isoleucine, and LDL/VLDL distinguished patients with sepsis/encephalitis from those with *P. falciparum* infection. The CM and CMMOD patients exhibited lower levels of glycoproteins compared to other malaria patients, suggesting potential diagnostic biomarkers for CM. Pappa et al. (2015) investigated the plasma metabolic profile of children with CM, finding that brain volume was a strong predictor of disease prognosis. A multiplatform investigation utilising GC-MS and LC-MS identified a correlation between brain volume and several metabolites. Certain metabolites such as glucose, glutamine, alanine, ornithine, hippurate, and phenylalanine, along with N-butyrate and acetate, have been proposed as potential biomarkers for differentiating fever caused by viral CNS affectation from malaria. Additionally, a longitudinal 1H-NMR study by the same researchers analysed urine samples from patients with viral encephalitis and *P. vivax* infection to identify biomarkers related to therapy response and diagnosis (Sengupta et al., 2015).

2.6 OTHER OMICS TECHNIQUES

Metataxonomics offers a rapid and cost-effective approach to assess microbial community diversity and obtain semi-quantitative taxonomic abundance data (Carlos et al., 2012). It remains the primary method for profiling mucosally-adherent pathogens in tissues like the colon, especially in low-biomass environments. However, the technique is hindered by challenges associated with short-read sequencing based on PCR, including GC bias, sequencing errors, and limitations in assessing operational taxonomic units (OTUs) (Janda and Abbott, 2007).

Metagenomics, also known as shotgun metagenomics, involves randomly sequencing the entire DNA population of an environment (Escobar-Zepeda et al., 2015). This approach is commonly used to analyse the taxonomic composition and functional potential of diverse microbial populations, such as those found in stool samples (Zhernakova et al., 2016). Unlike metataxonomics, which focusses on amplifying a single marker gene, metagenomics shears all DNA from a sample into small fragments, which are then sequenced independently after barcoding (Quince et al., 2017). The resulting DNA sequences, or reads, are then matched to databases to provide precise quantitative taxonomic and functional characterisation, allowing researchers to identify the members of a parasitic community and understand their potential functions simultaneously (Galen et al., 2020).

When combined with metagenomics, the dynamic metatranscriptome provides insight into pathogen functional activity within the host phenotype, shedding light on molecular pathways influencing gut health and disease (Lavelle and Sokol, 2018). It moves beyond descriptive knowledge of the gut microbiome, offering a deeper understanding of host-microbial causal pathways in health and disease (Sun and Chang, 2014). In metatranscriptome studies, total RNA is isolated from tissue samples such as faeces or colon biopsies, with host mRNA often depleted to focus on microbial RNA. This depletion of host and pathogen ribosomal RNA is a critical step in metatranscriptome experiments (Reck et al., 2015). Metaproteomics involves analysing the complete protein profile of pathogens in a sample, offering direct insight into their functional activity and interactions (Jin et al., 2017). Unlike sequencing-based approaches, metaproteomics provides detailed information about protein content, abundances, and changes (Zhang and Figeys, 2019). Techniques used in proteomic investigations include nuclear magnetic resonance, mass spectrometry, gel-based and gel-free methods, and microarray-based technologies (Ruiz-Romero and Blanco, 2010).

Metabolomics involves quantitatively assessing the dynamic metabolic response of a living system to pathogenic stressors or genetic changes (Yan et al., 2018). On the other hand, metabonomics focuses on measuring the metabolic responses of individuals or populations to interventions like drug treatments over time (Holmes et al., 2008). While the terms are often used interchangeably, metabolomics primarily examines metabolic profiles at the cellular or organ level, whereas metabonomics incorporates environmental factors such as diet, toxins, medications, and gut microbiota (Kosmides et al., 2013). Integrated systems biology approaches are essential in metabonomics to comprehensively understand an organism's metabolic state (Fernie et al., 2004).

2.7 INTEGRATIVE OMICS APPROACHES IN PARASITIC RESEARCH

Integrative omics has uncovered a plethora of proteins crucial for the survival and growth of Tritryps, encompassing *Trypanosoma brucei*, *Trypanosoma cruzi*, and *Leishmania* spp. These proteins serve diverse functions, including roles in oxidative stress response and virulence. Identified through genomic and omics-based approaches, these proteins hold promise as potential targets for drug discovery (Rivara-Espasandín et al., 2023). The forward genetics IVIEWGA method stands out as a highly effective approach for pinpointing numerous specific targets for potential small drugs (Dziekan et al., 2020). As omics techniques become more accessible and affordable, they have revolutionised the study of protozoan pathogens, shedding light on novel therapeutic targets and enhancing our understanding of parasite biology (Vayssier-Taussat et al., 2014). Given the escalating threat of drug resistance, the development of innovative treatments for these critical infections is imperative (Cowell and Winzeler, 2019).

The integration of omics, coupled with bioinformatics tools, offers a systematic approach to pinpoint specific proteins within the comprehensive proteome of trematodes, paving the way for potential vaccine development (Heinson et al., 2015). Omics methodologies are poised to provide valuable insights into the biological characteristics of parasites and aid in the development of novel anti-trematode strategies, including helminth-based treatments for autoimmune diseases (Morales-Montor et al., 2022). Efficient methodologies for identifying proteins within the trematode proteome are crucial for maximising the benefits of omics research. Past successes in omics-based studies across various fields suggest promising prospects for translating research findings into effective trematode infection treatments (Haçarız and Sayers, 2016). Integrative omics has been instrumental in uncovering driver genes and molecular signatures associated with diseases, enabling prognostic insights and targeted therapies (Karczewski and Snyder, 2018). Leveraging unique datasets from omics research is expected to enhance our understanding of rare parasites and their interactions with hosts, aligning with global efforts to eliminate filarial infections (Hopkins, 2016).

2.8 OMICS-BASED DRUG DISCOVERY AND DEVELOPMENT FOR PARASITIC INFECTIONS

The shift towards cell-based phenotypic screening marks a pivotal advancement in antimalarial drug discovery, enabling screening for compounds targeting various malaria stages (Lage et al., 2018). *In vitro* development of compound-resistant parasites is crucial for identifying therapeutic targets in *P. falciparum* (Cowell and Winzeler, 2018). Promising drug targets like eEF2 and PheRS have been identified through this strategy, underscoring the importance of high-throughput integrative omics datasets for target identification (Cowell and Winzeler, 2019). The medical potential of metal complexes is a significant focus in bioinorganic chemistry, where omics approaches offer insights into the mechanisms of action for new metal-based medications. The pursuit of metallodrugs against *Trypanosoma cruzi* is a rapidly advancing field (Navarro et al., 2010).

The integration of metallomics, proteomics, and transcriptomics offers insights into molecular targets and metabolic pathways affected by potential anti-parasitic drugs like vanadium (V), platinum (Pt), and palladium (Pd). Studies suggest that Pt is more readily absorbed by parasites than Pd, with both accumulating similarly in parasite DNA. Surprisingly, vanadium does not appear to interact with DNA (Scalese et al., 2022). This combined approach of genomics, transcriptomics, and proteomics presents a cost-effective and time-efficient strategy for identifying potential target proteins in parasites. Ligands predicted to bind are currently under investigation for their efficacy in acanthocephalan control (Schmidt et al., 2022).

Limited options in existing anthelmintics have led to widespread multidrug resistance in helminths, necessitating the development of new drugs (Shalaby, 2013). Molecular and genomic data on helminths were previously scarce but have increased with the advent of NGS. This data, combined with chemogenomic screening and high-throughput techniques, allows for large-scale searches for novel drug targets and the experimental testing of associated compounds. Such multiomics, data-driven approaches offer promise in identifying effective treatments for helminth infections (Tyagi et al., 2019).

2.9 LIMITATIONS AND FUTURE DIRECTIONS IN OMICS-BASED PARASITIC RESEARCH

Advancements in technology have shifted the focus towards data analysis rather than data collection (Tomescu et al., 2014). The abundance of data from transcriptomics, proteomics, and metabolomics studies presents new challenges in integrating analytical approaches (Mitreva, 2022). Many parasite genomes remain in draft form, posing difficulties in analysis and interpretation due to gene fragmentation and model errors (Korhonen et al., 2016). Challenges arise in integrating large omics datasets, even if they lack the four Vs—velocity, variety, volume, and veracity—associated with big data (McCue and McCoy, 2017). The "curse of dimensionality" further complicates analysis, particularly in high-dimensional datasets with numerous variables (Ronan et al., 2016).

To deepen our understanding of health and disease complexities, we must leverage advanced technologies to integrate data from various sources, including sequenced genomes, functional genomics, protein profiling, metabolomics, and bioinformatics, ensuring comprehensive systems-based analysis (Matthews et al., 2016). Omics approaches are expected to play a crucial role in unravelling the biological characteristics of parasites and aiding in the development of innovative strategies to combat parasites, potentially offering therapeutic solutions for autoimmune diseases (Kumar et al., 2023). The development of efficient methods to select target proteins from the parasite proteome will be essential in maximising the benefits of omic technologies (Sánchez-Ovejero et al., 2016). Given the success of omics-based studies in other fields, it's anticipated that findings from relevant research will translate into practical interventions to prevent parasite diseases in the near future (Haçarız and Sayers, 2016).

REFERENCES

Aebersold, R. and Mann, M. 2003. Mass spectrometry-based proteomics. *Nature*, 422(6928):198–207.

Akoolo, L., Rocha, S.C. and Parveen, N. 2022. Protozoan co-infections and parasite influence on the efficacy of vaccines against bacterial and viral pathogens. *Frontiers in Microbiology*, 13:1020029.

Allen, J.E. and Maizels, R.M. 2011. Diversity and dialogue in immunity to helminths. *Nature Reviews Immunology*, 11(6):375–388.

Amato, R., Pearson, R.D., Almagro-Garcia, J., Amaratunga, C., Lim, P., Suon, S., Sreng, S., Drury, E., Stalker, J., Miotto, O. and Fairhurst, R.M. 2018. Origins of the current outbreak of multidrug-resistant malaria in southeast Asia: a retrospective genetic study. *The Lancet Infectious Diseases*, 18(3):337–345.

Angel, T.E., Aryal, U.K., Hengel, S.M., Baker, E.S., Kelly, R.T., Robinson, E.W. and Smith, R.D. 2012. Mass spectrometry-based proteomics: existing capabilities and future directions. *Chemical Society Reviews Journal*, 41(10):3912–3928.

Autino, B., Corbett, Y., Castelli, F. and Taramelli, D. 2012. Pathogenesis of malaria in tissues and blood. *Mediterranean Journal of Hematology and Infectious Diseases*, 4(1):e2012061.

Baker, M.J., Hussain, S.R., Lovergne, L., Untereiner, V., Hughes, C., Lukaszewski, R.A., Thiéfin, G. and Sockalingum, G.D. 2016. Developing and understanding biofluid vibrational spectroscopy: a critical review. *Chemical Society Reviews*, 45(7):1803–1818.

Balic, A., Bowles, V.M. and Meeusen, E.N. 2000. The immunobiology of gastrointestinal nematode infections in ruminants. *Advances in Parasitology*, 45:181–241.

Balog, C.I., Meissner, A., Göraler, S., Bladergroen, M.R., Vennervald, B.J., Mayboroda, O.A. and Deelder, A.M. 2011. Metabonomic investigation of human *Schistosoma mansoni* infection. *Molecular Biosystems*, 7(5):1473–1480.

Barker, I.K. 1975. Intestinal pathology associated with *Trichostrongylus colubriformis* infection in sheep: histology. *Parasitology*, 70(2):165–171.

Belhaj, M.R., Lawler, N.G. and Hoffman, N.J. 2021. Metabolomics and lipidomics: expanding the molecular landscape of exercise biology. *Metabolites*, 11(3):151.

Bhattacharya, S.B. 2018. *Further development and application of an LC/MS analysis of plasma oxysterol*. Doctoral dissertation, State University of New York.

Bisanz, C., Bastien, O., Grando, D., Jouhet, J., Maréchal, E. and Cesbron-Delauw, M.F. 2006. *Toxoplasma gondii* acyl-lipid metabolism: de novo synthesis from apicoplast-generated fatty acids versus scavenging of host cell precursors. *Biochemistry Journal*, 394:197–205.

Blaxter, M.L., De Ley, P., Garey, J.R., Liu, L.X., Scheldeman, P., Vierstraete, A., Vanfleteren, J.R., Mackey, L.Y., Dorris, M., Frisse, L.M. and Vida, J.T. 1998. A molecular evolutionary framework for the phylum Nematoda. *Nature*, 392(6671):71–75.

Boité, M.C., Mauricio, I.L., Miles, M.A. and Cupolillo, E. 2012. New insights on taxonomy, phylogeny and population genetics of *Leishmania* (Viannia) parasites based on multi-locus sequence analysis. *PLoS Neglected Tropical Diseases*, 6(11):1888.

Broder, S. and Venter, J.C. 2000. Sequencing the entire genomes of free-living organisms: the foundation of pharmacology in the new millennium. *Annual Review of Pharmacology and Toxicology*, 40(1):97–132.

Cable, J., Barber, I., Boag, B., Ellison, A.R., Morgan, E.R., Murray, K., Pascoe, E.L., Sait, S.M., Wilson, A.J. and Booth, M. 2017. Global change, parasite transmission and disease control: lessons from ecology. *Philosophical Transactions of the Royal Society B: Biological Sciences*, 372(1719):20160088.

Cantacessi, C., Campbell, B.E., Jex, A.R., Young, N.D., Hall, R.S., Ranganathan, S. and Gasser, R.B. 2012. Bioinformatics meets parasitology. *Parasite Immunology*, 34(5):265–275.

Carlos, N., Tang, Y.W. and Pei, Z. 2012. Pearls and pitfalls of genomics-based microbiome analysis. *Emerging Microbes and Infections*, 1(12):e45.

Cheeseman, I.H., Miller, B.A., Nair, S., Nkhoma, S., Tan, A., Tan, J.C., Al Saai, S., Phyo, A.P., Moo, C.L., Lwin, K.M. and McGready, R. 2012. A major genome region underlying artemisinin resistance in malaria. *Science*, 336(6077):79–82.

Ciocan-Cartita, C.A., Jurj, A., Buse, M., Gulei, D., Braicu, C., Raduly, L., Cojocneanu, R., Pruteanu, L.L., Iuga, C.A., Coza, O. and Berindan-Neagoe, I. 2019. The relevance of mass spectrometry analysis for personalized medicine through its successful application in cancer "omics". *International Journal of Molecular Science*, 20(10):2576.

Consden, R., Gordon, A.H., Martin, A.J.P. and Synge, R.L.M. 1947. 'Gramicidin S: the sequence of the amino-acid residues'. *Biochemistry Journal*, 41(4):596–602.

Conway, D.J. 2007. Molecular epidemiology of malaria. *Clinical Microbiology Reviews*, 20(1):188–204.

Cowell, A.N. and Winzeler, E.A. 2018. Exploration of the *Plasmodium falciparum* resistome and druggable genome reveals new mechanisms of drug resistance and antimalarial targets. *Microbiology Insights*, 11:1178636118808529.

Cowell, A.N. and Winzeler, E.A. 2019. Advances in omics-based methods to identify novel targets for malaria and other parasitic protozoan infections. *Genome Medicine*, 11:1–17.

Dapper, A.L. and Payseur, B.A. 2017. Connecting theory and data to understand recombination rate evolution. *Philosophical Transactions of the Royal Society B: Biological Sciences*, 372(1736):20160469.

Dawson, M.A. and Kouzarides, T. 2012. Cancer epigenetics: from mechanism to therapy. *Cell*, 150(1):12–27.

Dinger, M.E., Pang, K.C., Mercer, T.R. and Mattick, J.S. 2008. Differentiating protein-coding and noncoding RNA: challenges and ambiguities. *PLoS Computational Biology*, 4(11):1000176.

DiStefano, J.K. 2018. The emerging role of long noncoding RNAs in human disease. *Disease Gene Identification: Methods and Protocols*, 1706:91–110.

Downing, T., Imamura, H., Decuypere, S., Clark, T.G., Coombs, G.H., Cotton, J.A., Hilley, J.D., de Doncker, S., Maes, I., Mottram, J.C. and Quail, M.A. 2011. Whole genome sequencing of multiple *Leishmania donovani* clinical isolates provides insights into population structure and mechanisms of drug resistance. *Genome Research*, 21(12):2143–2156.

Dwivedi, S., Purohit, P., Misra, R., Pareek, P., Goel, A., Khattri, S., Pant, K.K., Misra, S. and Sharma, P. 2017. Diseases and molecular diagnostics: a step closer to precision medicine. *Indian Journal of Clinical Biochemistry*, 32(4):374–398.

Dziekan, J.M., Wirjanata, G., Dai, L., Go, K.D., Yu, H., Lim, Y.T., Chen, L., Wang, L.C., Puspita, B., Prabhu, N. and Sobota, R.M. 2020. Cellular thermal shift assay for the identification of drug–target interactions in the *Plasmodium falciparum* proteome. *Nature Protocols*, 15(6):1881–1921.

Ecker, J. and Liebisch, G. 2014. Application of stable isotopes to investigate the metabolism of fatty acids, glycerophospholipid and sphingolipid species. *Progress in Lipid Research*, 54:14–31.

Erkmen, C., Gebrehiwot, W.H. and Uslu, B. 2021. Hydrophilic interaction liquid chromatography (HILIC): latest applications in the pharmaceutical researches. *Current Pharmaceutical Analysis*, 17(3):316–345.

Escobar-Zepeda, A., Vera-Ponce de León, A. and Sanchez-Flores, A. 2015. The road to metagenomics: from microbiology to DNA sequencing technologies and bioinformatics. *Frontiers in Genetics*, 6:348.

Feinberg, A.P. and Vogelstein, B. 1983. Hypomethylation distinguishes genes of some human cancers from their normal counterparts. *Nature*, 301(5895):89–92.

Feinberg, A.P., Ohlsson, R. and Henikoff, S. 2006. The epigenetic progenitor origin of human cancer. *Nature Reviews Genetics*, 7(1):21–33.

Fernandez-Becerra, C., Xander, P., Alfandari, D., Dong, G., Aparici-Herraiz, I., Rosenhek-Goldian, I., Shokouhy, M., Gualdron-Lopez, M., Lozano, N., Cortes-Serra, N. and Karam, P.A. 2023. Guidelines for the purification and characterization of extracellular vesicles of parasites. *Journal of Extracellular Biology*, 2(10):117.

Fernández-García, M., Rojo, D., Rey-Stolle, F., García, A. and Barbas, C. 2018. Metabolic-based methods in diagnosis and monitoring infection progression. *Metabolic Interaction in Infection*, 109:283–315.

Fernie, A.R., Trethewey, R.N., Krotzky, A.J. and Willmitzer, L. 2004. Metabolite profiling: from diagnostics to systems biology. *Nature Reviews Molecular Cell Biology*, 5(9):763–769.

Fiehn, O. 2002. Metabolomics--the link between genotypes and phenotypes. *Plant Molecular Biology,* 48(1–2):155–171.

Galen, S.C., Borner, J., Williamson, J.L., Witt, C.C. and Perkins, S.L. 2020. Metatranscriptomics yields new genomic resources and sensitive detection of infections for diverse blood parasites. *Molecular Ecology Resources*, 20(1):14–28.

Garçon, N., Chomez, P. and Van Mechelen, M. 2007. GlaxoSmithKline Adjuvant Systems in vaccines: concepts, achievements and perspectives. *Expert Review of Vaccines*, 6(5):723–739.

Gause, W.C., Urban, J.F. and Stadecker, M.J. 2003. The immune response to parasitic helminths: insights from murine models. *Trends in Immunology*, 24(5):269–277.

Gilchrist, C.A., Ali, I.K.M., Kabir, M., Alam, F., Scherbakova, S., Ferlanti, E., Weedall, G.D., Hall, N., Haque, R., Petri, W.A. and Caler, E. 2012. A Multilocus Sequence Typing System (MLST) reveals a high level of diversity and a genetic component to Entamoeba histolytica virulence. *BMC Microbiology*, 12(1):1–14.

Gowda, G.N., Zhang, S., Gu, H., Asiago, V., Shanaiah, N. and Raftery, D. 2008. Metabolomics-based methods for early disease diagnostics. *Expert Review of Molecular Diagnostics*, 8(5):617–633.

Guijas, C., Montenegro-Burke, J.R., Warth, B., Spilker, M.E. and Siuzdak, G. 2018. Metabolomics activity screening for identifying metabolites that modulate phenotype. *Nature Biotechnology*, 36(4):316–320.

Gurunathan, S., Kang, M.H., Jeyaraj, M., Qasim, M. and Kim, J.H. 2019. Review of the isolation, characterization, biological function, and multifarious therapeutic approaches of exosomes. *Cells*, 8(4):307.

Haçarız, O. and Sayers, G.P. 2016. The omic approach to parasitic trematode research—a review of techniques and developments within the past 5 years. *Parasitology Research*, 115(7):2523–2543.

Han, X. and Gross, R.W. 2003. Global analyses of cellular lipidomes directly from crude extracts of biological samples by ESI mass spectrometry: a bridge to lipidomics. *Journal of Lipid Research*, 44(6):1071–1079.

Han, Y., Gao, S., Muegge, K., Zhang, W. and Zhou, B. 2015. Advanced applications of RNA sequencing and challenges. *Bioinformatics and Biology Insights*, 9:BBI–S28991.

Hänscheid, T. 2003. Current strategies to avoid misdiagnosis of malaria. *Clinical Microbiology and Infection*, 9(6):497–504.

Hartl, D.L. 2014. *Essential genetics: A genomics perspective*. Jones & Bartlett Publishers.

Harvey, D.J. 2012. Analysis of carbohydrates and glycoconjugates by matrix-assisted laser desorption/ionization mass spectrometry: an update for 2007-2008. *Mass Spectrometry Review*, 31(2):183–311.

Heather, J.M. and Chain, B. 2016. The sequence of sequencers: The history of sequencing DNA. *Genomics*, 107(1):1–8.

Heinson, A.I., Woelk, C.H. and Newell, M.L. 2015. The promise of reverse vaccinology. *International Health*, 7(2):85–89.

Hellani, F. 2022. *Induction of astrocytes senescence by Plasmodium infection: Role in cerebral malaria*. Doctoral dissertation, Université de Lille.

Holden-Dye, L. and Walker, R. 2014. Anthelmintic drugs and nematocides: studies in *Caenorhabditis elegans*. *WormBook*: the online review of *C. elegans* biology. 1–29.

Holmes, E., Wilson, I.D. and Nicholson, J.K. 2008. Metabolic phenotyping in health and disease. *Cell*, 134(5):714–717.

Hopkins, A.D. 2016. Neglected tropical diseases in Africa: a new paradigm. *International Health*, 8(suppl_1):i28–i33.

Horgan, R.P. and Kenny, L.C. 2011. 'Omic' technologies: genomics, transcriptomics, proteomics and metabolomics. *The Obstetrician & Gynaecologist*, 13(3):189–195.

Hu, L., Liu, J., Zhang, W., Wang, T., Zhang, N., Lee, Y.H. and Lu, H. 2020. Functional metabolomics decipher biochemical functions and associated mechanisms underlie small-molecule metabolism. *Mass Spectrometry Reviews*, 39(5–6):417–433.

Hupalo, D.N., Bradic, M. and Carlton, J.M. 2015. The impact of genomics on population genetics of parasitic diseases. *Current Opinion in Microbiology*, 23:49–54.

Jain, K.K. 2010. Role of biomarkers in health care. In: Jain, K.K. (ed.) *The handbook of biomarkers*, 1st edn. Humana Press, pp. 134–149.

Janda, J.M. and Abbott, S.L. 2007. 16S rRNA gene sequencing for bacterial identification in the diagnostic laboratory: pluses, perils, and pitfalls. *Journal of Clinical Microbiology*, 45(9):2761–2764.

Jin, P., Wang, K., Huang, C. and Nice, E.C. 2017. Mining the fecal proteome: from biomarkers to personalised medicine. *Expert Review of Proteomics*, 14(5):445–459.

Joachim, A., Ruttkowski, B., Christensen, C.M. and Daugschies, A. 1999. Identification, isolation, and characterization of a species-specific 30-kDa antigen of *Oesophagostomum dentatum*. *Parasitology Research*, 85:307–311.

Kanai, M., Yeo, T., Asua, V., Rosenthal, P.J., Fidock, D.A. and Mok, S. 2022. Comparative analysis of *Plasmodium falciparum* genotyping via SNP detection, microsatellite profiling, and whole-genome sequencing. *Antimicrobial Agents and Chemotherapy*, 66(1):e01163–21

Karczewski, K.J. and Snyder, M.P. 2018. Integrative omics for health and disease. *Nature Reviews Genetics,* 19(5):299–310.

Keiser, J. and Utzinger, J. 2008. Efficacy of current drugs against soil-transmitted helminth infections: systematic review and meta-analysis. *Jama*, 299(16):1937–1948.

Kim, D.H., Kim, Y.S., Son, N.I., Kang, C.K. and Kim, A.R. 2017. Recent omics technologies and their emerging applications for personalised medicine. *IET System Biology*, 11(3):87–98.

Klug, A. 2004. The discovery of the DNA double helix. *Journal of Molecular Biology*, 335:3–26.

Korhonen, P.K., Young, N.D. and Gasser, R.B. 2016. Making sense of genomes of parasitic worms: tackling bioinformatic challenges. *Biotechnology Advances*, 34(5):663–686.

Kosmides, A.K., Kamisoglu, K., Calvano, S.E., Corbett, S.A. and Androulakis, I. 2013. Metabolomic fingerprinting: challenges and opportunities. *Critical Review in Biomedical Engineering*, 41(3):205–221.

Kumar, A., Deepika, S.S. and Avasthi, A. 2023. Recent advances in the treatment of parasitic diseases: Current status and future. In: Singh, A., Rathi, B., Verma, A.K. and Singh, I.K. (eds.) *Natural product based drug discovery against human parasites: Opportunities and challenges*. Springer Singapore, pp. 249–286.

Lage, O.M., Ramos, M.C., Calisto, R., Almeida, E., Vasconcelos, V. and Vicente, F., 2018. Current screening methodologies in drug discovery for selected human diseases. *Marine Drugs*, 16(8):279.

Lakshmanan, V., Rhee, K.Y., Wang, W., Yu, Y., Khafizov, K., Fiser, A., Wu, P., Ndir, O., Mboup, S., Ndiaye, D. and Daily, J.P. 2012. Metabolomic analysis of patient plasma yields evidence of plant-like alpha-linolenic acid metabolism in *Plasmodium falciparum*. *Journal of Infectious Diseases*, 206(2):238–248.

Lander, E.S., Linton, L.M., Birren, B., Nusbaum, C., Zody, M.C., Baldwin, J., ... International Human Genome Sequencing Consortium. (2001). Initial sequencing and analysis of the human genome. *Nature*, 409(6822):860–921.

Lavelle, A. and Sokol, H. 2018. Beyond metagenomics, metatranscriptomics illuminates microbiome functionality in IBD. *Nature Reviews Gastroenterology & Hepatology,* 15(4):193–194.

Lee, C.H. 2017. A simple outline of methods for protein isolation and purification. *Endocrinology and Metabolism (Seoul)*. 32(1):18–22.

Letertre, M.P., Giraudeau, P. and De Tullio, P. 2021. Nuclear magnetic resonance spectroscopy in clinical metabolomics and personalized medicine: current challenges and perspectives. *Frontiers in Molecular Biosciences*, 8:698337.

Lin, C.Y., Viant, M.R. and Tjeerdema, R.S. 2006. Metabolomics: methodologies and applications in the environmental sciences. *Journal of Pesticide Science*, 31(3):245–251.

Liu, Q., Kreider, T., Bowdridge, S., Liu, Z., Song, Y., Gaydo, A.G., Urban, J.F. and Gause, W.C. 2010. B cells have distinct roles in host protection against different nematode parasites. *The Journal of Immunology*, 184(9):5213–5223.

Lohmann, K. and Klein, C. 2014. Next generation sequencing and the future of genetic diagnosis. *Neurotherapeutics*, 11:699–707.

Loker, E.S. and Hofkin, B.V. 2022. *Parasitology: A conceptual approach*. CRC Press.

Loukas, A. and Prociv, P., 2001. Immune responses in hookworm infections. *Clinical Microbiology Reviews*, 14(4):689–703.

Maizels, R.M., Balic, A., Gomez-Escobar, N., Nair, M., Taylor, M.D. and Allen, J.E. 2004. Helminth parasites–masters of regulation. *Immunological Reviews*, 201(1):89–116.

Manolio, T.A., Collins, F.S., Cox, N.J., Goldstein, D.B., Hindorff, L.A., Hunter, D.J., McCarthy, M.I., Ramos, E.M., Cardon, L.R., Chakravarti, A., Cho, J.H., Guttmacher, A.E., Kong, A., Kruglyak, L., Mardis, E., Rotimi, C.N., Slatkin, M., Valle, D., Whittemore, A.S., Boehnke, M., Clark, A.G., Eichler, E.E., Gibson, G., Haines, J.L., Mackay, T.F., McCarroll, S.A. and Visscher, P.M. 2009. Finding the missing heritability of complex diseases. *Nature*, 461(7265):747–53.

Martin, M.O. 2002. Predatory prokaryotes: an emerging research opportunity. *Journal of Molecular Microbiology and Biotechnology*, 4(5):467–478.

Matthews, H., Hanison, J. and Nirmalan, N. 2016. "Omics"-informed drug and biomarker discovery: opportunities, challenges and future perspectives. *Proteomes*, 4(3):28.

Maxwell, C., Hussain, R., Nutman, T.B., Poindexter, R.W., Little, M.D., Schad, G.A. and Ottesen, E.A. 1987. The clinical and immunologic responses of normal human volunteers to low dose hookworm (*Necator americanus*) infection. *The American Journal of Tropical Medicine and Hygiene*, 37(1):126–134.

Mayeux, R. 2004. Biomarkers: potential uses and limitations. *NeuroRx*, 1(2):182–188.

McCue, M.E. and McCoy, A.M. 2017. The scope of big data in one medicine: unprecedented opportunities and challenges. *Frontiers in Veterinary Science*, 4:194.

Mertins, P., Mani, D.R., Ruggles, K.V., Gillette, M.A., Clauser, K.R., Wang, P., Wang, X., Qiao, J.W., Cao, S., Petralia, F., et al.; NCI CPTAC. 2016. Proteogenomics connects somatic mutations to signalling in breast cancer. *Nature*, 534:55–62.

Metzker, M.L. 2010. Sequencing technologies—The next generation. *Nature Reviews Genetics*, 11(1):31–46.

Miller, J.E. and Horohov, D.W. 2006. Immunological aspects of nematode parasite control in sheep. *Journal of Animal Science*, 84(suppl_13):E124–E132.

Miotto, O., Almagro-Garcia, J., Manske, M., MacInnis, B., Campino, S., Rockett, K.A., Amaratunga, C., Lim, P., Suon, S., Sreng, S. and Anderson, J.M. 2013. Multiple populations of artemisinin-resistant *Plasmodium falciparum* in Cambodia. *Nature Genetics*, 45(6):648–655.

Miotto, O., Sekihara, M., Tachibana, S.I., Yamauchi, M., Pearson, R.D., Amato, R., Gonçalves, S., Mehra, S., Noviyanti, R., Marfurt, J. and Auburn, S. 2020. Emergence of artemisinin-resistant *Plasmodium falciparum* with kelch13 C580Y mutations on the island of New Guinea. *PLoS Pathogens*, 16(12):1009133.

Mirnaghi, F.S. and Caudy, A.A. 2014. Challenges of analyzing different classes of metabolites by a single analytical method. *Bioanalysis*, 6(24):3393–3416.

Mitchell, M.I., Ma, J., Carter, C.L. and Loudig, O. 2022. Circulating exosome cargoes contain functionally diverse cancer biomarkers: from biogenesis and function to purification and potential translational utility. *Cancers*, 14(14):3350.

Mitreva, M. 2022. Parasite OMICS, the grand challenges ahead. *Frontiers in Parasitology*, 1:995302.

Morales-Montor, J., Del Río-Araiza, V.H. and Hernandéz-Bello, R. 2022. *Parasitic helminths and zoonoses: From basic to applied research*. IntechOpen.

Müller, J.B., Geyer, P.E., Colaco, A.R., Treit, P.V., Strauss, M.T., Oroshi, M., Doll, S., Virreira Winter, S., Bader, J.M., Köhler, N. and Theis, F. 2020. The proteome landscape of the kingdoms of life. *Nature*, 582(7813):592–596.

Nakayasu, E.S., Gritsenko, M., Piehowski, P.D., Gao, Y., Orton, D.J., Schepmoes, A.A., Fillmore, T.L., Frohnert, B.I., Rewers, M., Krischer, J.P. and Ansong, C. 2021. Tutorial: best practices and considerations for mass-spectrometry-based protein biomarker discovery and validation. *Nature Protocols*, 16(8):3737–3760.

Navarro, M., Gabbiani, C., Messori, L. and Gambino, D. 2010. Metal-based drugs for malaria, trypanosomiasis and leishmaniasis: recent achievements and perspectives. *Drug Discovery Today*, 15(23–24):1070–1078.

Neafsey, D.E., Galinsky, K., Jiang, R.H., Young, L., Sykes, S.M., Saif, S., Gujja, S., Goldberg, J.M., Young, S., Zeng, Q. and Chapman, S.B. 2012. The malaria parasite *Plasmodium vivax* exhibits greater genetic diversity than *Plasmodium falciparum*. *Nature Genetics*, 44(9):1046–1050.

Njuguna, P.W. and Newton, C.R. 2004. Management of severe *falciparum malaria*. *Journal of Postgraduate Medicine*, 50(1):45–50.

Nyame, A.K., Kawar, Z.S. and Cummings, R.D. 2004. Antigenic glycans in parasitic infections: implications for vaccines and diagnostics. *Archives of Biochemistry and Biophysics*, 426(2):182–200.

O'Farrell, P.H. 1975. High resolution two-dimensional electrophoresis of proteins. *Journal of Biological Chemistry*, 250(10):4007–21.

Ohtsubo, K. and Marth, J.D. (2006). Glycosylation in cellular mechanisms of health and disease. *Cell*, 126(5):855–867.

Oliver, S.G., Winson, M.K., Kell, D.B. and Baganz, F. 1998. Systematic functional analysis of the yeast genome. *Trends in Biotechnology*, 16:373–378.

Olsen, O.W. 1986. *Animal parasites: Their life cycles and ecology.* Dover Publications.

Ozturk, E.A. and Caner, A. 2022. Liquid biopsy for promising non-invasive diagnostic biomarkers in parasitic infections. *Acta Parasitologica*, 67(1):1–17.

Pang, J.M.B., Byrne, D.J., Bergin, A.R., Caramia, F., Loi, S., Gorringe, K.L. and Fox, S.B. 2023. Spatial transcriptomics and the anatomical pathologist: molecular meets morphology. *Histopathology*, 84(4):577–586.

Pappa, V., Seydel, K., Gupta, S., Feintuch, C.M., Potchen, M.J., Kampondeni, S., Goldman-Yassen, A., Veenstra, M., Lopez, L., Kim, R.S., Berman, J.W., Taylor, T. and Daily, J.P. 2015. Lipid metabolites of the phospholipase A2 pathway and inflammatory cytokines are associated with brain volume in paediatric cerebral malaria. *Malar Journal*, 14:513.

Patel, N., Kreider, T., Urban Jr, J.F. and Gause, W.C. 2009. Characterisation of effector mechanisms at the host: parasite interface during the immune response to tissue-dwelling intestinal nematode parasites. *International Journal for Parasitology*, 39(1):13–21.

Patti, G.J., Yanes, O. and Siuzdak, G. 2012. Innovation: metabolomics: the apogee of the omics trilogy. *Nature Reviews Molecular Cell Biology*, 13(4):263–269.

Pearson, M.S., Tribolet, L., Cantacessi, C., Periago, M.V., Valerio, M.A., Jariwala, A.R., Hotez, P., Diemert, D., Loukas, A. and Bethony, J. 2012. Molecular mechanisms of hookworm disease: stealth, virulence, and vaccines. *Journal of Allergy and Clinical Immunology*, 130(1):13–21.

Quince, C., Walker, A.W., Simpson, J.T., Loman, N.J. and Segata, N. 2017. Shotgun metagenomics, from sampling to analysis. *Nature Biotechnology*, 35(9):833–844.

Ramakrishnan, S., Docampo, M.D., MacRae, J.I., Pujol, F.M., Brooks, C.F., van Dooren, G.G., Hiltunen, J.K., Kastaniotis, A.J., McConville, M.J. and Striepen, B. 2012. Apicoplast and endoplasmic reticulum cooperate in fatty acid biosynthesis in apicomplexan parasite *Toxoplasma gondii*. *Journal of Biological Chemistry*, 287(7):4957–4971.

Reck, M., Tomasch, J., Deng, Z., Jarek, M., Husemann, P., Wagner-Döbler, I. and COMBACTE Consortium. 2015. Stool metatranscriptomics: a technical guideline for mRNA stabilisation and isolation. *BMC Genomics*, 16:1–18.

Rivara-Espasandín, M., Palumbo, M.C., Sosa, E.J., Radío, S., Turjanski, A.G., Sotelo-Silveira, J., Fernandez Do Porto, D. and Smircich, P. 2023. Omics data integration facilitates target selection for new anti-parasitic drugs against *TriTryp infections*. *Frontiers in Pharmacology*, 14:1136321.

Robertson, A.P., Clark, C.L. and Martin, R.J. 2010. Levamisole and ryanodine receptors (I): a contraction study in *Ascaris suum*. *Molecular and Biochemical Parasitology*, 171(1):1–7.

Rogers, M.B., Hilley, J.D., Dickens, N.J., Wilkes, J., Bates, P.A., Depledge, D.P., Harris, D., Her, Y., Herzyk, P., Imamura, H. and Otto, T.D. 2011. Chromosome and gene copy number variation allow major structural change between species and strains of *Leishmania*. *Genome Research*, 21(12):2129–2142.

Rogers, W.P. and Sommerville, R.I. 1968. The infectious process, and its relation to the development of early parasitic stages of nematodes. *Advances in Parasitology*, 6:327–348.

Rojo, D. 2014. *Metabolómica e integración multiómica en organismos unicelulares. Hacia la comprensión de sistemas biológicos.* Dissertation, CEU San Pablo University.

Ronan, T., Qi, Z. and Naegle, K.M. 2016. Avoiding common pitfalls when clustering biological data. *Science Signaling*, 9(432):re6.

Ruiz-Romero, C. and Blanco, F.J. 2010. Proteomics role in the search for improved diagnosis, prognosis and treatment of osteoarthritis. *Osteoarthritis and Cartilage*, 18(4):500–509.

Sánchez-Ovejero, C., Benito-Lopez, F., Díez, P., Casulli, A., Siles-Lucas, M., Fuentes, M. and Manzano-Román, R. 2016. Sensing parasites: Proteomic and advanced bio-detection alternatives. *Journal of Proteomics*, 136:145–156.

Sanger, F., Coulson, A. 1975. A rapid method for determining sequences in DNA by primed synthesis with DNA polymerase. *Journal of Molecular Biology*, 94:441–448.

Scalese, G., Kostenkova, K., Crans, D.C. and Gambino, D. 2022. Metallomics and other omics approaches in anti-parasitic metal-based drug research. *Current Opinion in Chemical Biology*, 67:102127.

Schena, M., Shalon, D., Davis, R.W. and Brown, P.O. 1995. Quantitative monitoring of gene expression patterns with a complementary DNA microarray. *Science*, 270(5235):467–470.

Schmidt, H., Mauer, K., Glaser, M., Dezfuli, B.S., Hellmann, S.L., Silva Gomes, A.L., Butter, F., Wade, R.C., Hankeln, T. and Herlyn, H. 2022. Identification of antiparasitic drug targets using a multi-omics workflow in the acanthocephalan model. *BMC Genomics*, 23(1):1–16.

Schmidt, M. F. 2022. DNA: Blueprint of the proteins. In: Schmidt, M.F. (ed.) *Chemical biology: And drug discovery.* Springer Berlin Heidelberg, pp. 33–47.

Selbach, C., Jorge, F., Dowle, E., Bennett, J., Chai, X., Doherty, J.F., Eriksson, A., Filion, A., Hay, E., Herbison, R. and Lindner, J. 2019. Parasitological research in the molecular age. *Parasitology*, 146(11):1361–1370.

Sengupta, A., Ghosh, S., Das, B.K., Panda, A., Tripathy, R., Pied, S., Ravindran, B., Pathak, S., Sharma, S. and Sonawat, H.M. 2016. Host metabolic responses to *Plasmodium falciparum* infections evaluated by 1H NMR metabolomics. *Molecular BioSystems*, 12(11):3324–3332.

Sengupta, A., Ghosh, S., Pathak, S., Gogtay, N., Thatte, U., Doshi, M., Sharma, S. and Sonawat, H.M. 2015. Metabolomic analysis of urine samples of vivax malaria in-patients for biomarker identification. *Metabolomics*, 11(5):1351–1362.

Shalaby, H.A. 2013. Anthelmintics resistance; how to overcome it? *Iranian Journal of Parasitology*, 8(1):18.

Skrjabinet, K.I., Sobolev, A.A. and Ivashkin, V.M. 1967. *Principles of Nematology 19. Spirurata of animals and man and the diseases caused by them.* Part 5. Supplement (In Russian). Izdatel'stvo Nauka, p. 240.

Sommerville, R.I. 1957. The exsheathing mechanism of oematode infective larvae. *Experimental Parasitology*, 6(1):18–30.

Sonawat, H.M. and Sharma, S. 2012. Host responses in malaria disease evaluated through nuclear magnetic resonance-based metabonomics. *Clinics in Laboratory Medicine*, 32(2):129–142.

Stanley, S.L. 2005. The *Entamoeba histolytica* genome: something old, something new, something borrowed and sex too? *Trends in Parasitology,* 21(10):451–453.

Su, C., Howe, D.K., Dubey, J.P., Ajioka, J.W. and Sibley, L.D. 2002. Identification of quantitative trait loci controlling acute virulence in *Toxoplasma gondii*. *Proceedings of the National Academy of Sciences*, 99(16):10753–10758.

Subramanian A, Tamayo P, Mootha VK, Mukherjee S, Ebert BL, Gillette MA, Paulovich A, Pomeroy SL, Golub TR, Lander ES, et al. (2005). Gene set enrichment analysis: A knowledge-based approach for interpreting genome-wide expression profiles. *Proceedings of the National Academy of Sciences of the United States of America*, 102:15545–15550.

Sun, J. and Chang, E.B. 2014. Exploring gut microbes in human health and disease: pushing the envelope. *Genes & Diseases*, 1(2):132–139.

Surowiec, I., Orikiiriza, J., Karlsson, E., Nelson, M., Bonde, M., Kyamanwa, P., Karenzi, B., Bergström, S., Trygg, J. and Normark, J. 2015. Metabolic signature profiling as a diagnostic and prognostic tool in pediatric *Plasmodium falciparum* malaria. *Open Forum Infectious Diseases*, 2(2):ofv062.

Takala-Harrison, S., Clark, T.G., Jacob, C.G., Cummings, M.P., Miotto, O., Dondorp, A.M., Fukuda, M.M., Nosten, F., Noedl, H., Imwong, M. and Bethell, D. 2013. Genetic loci associated with delayed clearance of *Plasmodium falciparum* following artemisinin treatment in Southeast Asia. *Proceedings of the National Academy of Sciences*, 110(1):240–245.

Tenchov, R., Sasso, J.M., Wang, X., Liaw, W.S., Chen, C.A. and Zhou, Q.A. 2022. Exosomes—nature's lipid nanoparticles, a rising star in drug delivery and diagnostics. *ACS Nano*, 16(11):17802–17846.

Tomescu, O.A., Mattanovich, D. and Thallinger, G.G. 2014. Integrative omics analysis. A study based on *Plasmodium falciparum* mRNA and protein data. *BMC Systems Biology*, 8(2):1–16.

Tyagi, R., Rosa, B.A. and Mitreva, M. 2019. Omics-driven knowledge-based discovery of anthelmintic targets and drugs. In: Roy, K. (ed.) *In Silico Drug Design*. Academic Press, pp. 329–358.

Varki, A. 2017. Biological roles of glycans. *Glycobiology*, 27(1):3–49.

Varki, A., Cummings, R.D., Esko, J.D., Freeze, H.H., Stanley, P., Bertozzi, C.R., ... Hart, G.W. 2009. Symbol nomenclature for glycan representation. *Proteomics*, 9(24):5398–5399.

Vayssier-Taussat, M., Albina, E., Citti, C., Cosson, J.F., Jacques, M.A., Lebrun, M.H., Le Loir, Y., Ogliastro, M., Petit, M.A., Roumagnac, P. and Candresse, T. 2014. Shifting the paradigm from pathogens to pathobiome: new concepts in the light of meta-omics. *Frontiers in Cellular and Infection Microbiology*, 4:29.

Waller, P.J. 1997. Anthelmintic resistance. *Veterinary Parasitology*, 72(3–4):391–412.

Wang, R.S., Maron, B.A. and Loscalzo, J. 2015. Systems medicine: evolution of systems biology from bench to bedside. *Wiley Interdisciplinary Reviews: Systems Biology and Medicine*, 7(4):141–161.

Wang, Z., Gerstein, M. and Snyder, M. 2009. RNA-Seq: a revolutionary tool for transcriptomics. *Nature Reviews Genetics*, 10(1):57–63.

Weedall, G.D., Clark, C.G., Koldkjaer, P., Kay, S., Bruchhaus, I., Tannich, E., Paterson, S. and Hall, N. 2012. Genomic diversity of the human intestinal parasite Entamoeba histolytica. *Genome Biology*, 13(5):1–13.

Wishart, D.S. 2019. Metabolomics for investigating physiological and pathophysiological processes. *Physiological Reviews*, 99(4):1819–1875.

Wu, K., He, X., Wang, J., Pan, T., He, R., Kong, F., Cao, Z., Ju, F., Huang, Z. and Nie, L. 2022. Recent progress of microfluidic chips in immunoassay. *Frontiers in Bioengineering and Biotechnology*, 10:1112327.

Xia, J., Broadhurst, D.I., Wilson, M. and Wishart, D.S. 2013. Translational biomarker discovery in clinical metabolomics: an introductory tutorial. *Metabolomics*, 9(2):280–299.

Yadav, S.P. and Shukla, G.C. 2007. P94-S fishing for RNA-binding proteins from the HeLa cell nuclear extract using biacore 3000. *Journal of Biomolecular Techniques*, 18(1):32.

Yan, S., Nagle, D.G., Zhou, Y. and Zhang, W. 2018. Application of systems biology in the research of TCM formulae. In: Zhang, W. (ed.), *Systems biology and its application in TCM formulas research*. Academic Press, pp. 31–67.

Zhang, W., Hankemeier, T. and Ramautar, R. 2017. Next-generation capillary electrophoresis–mass spectrometry approaches in metabolomics. *Current Opinion in Biotechnology*, 43:1–7.

Zhang, W., Ou, X. and Wu, X. 2019. Proteomics profiling of plasma exosomes in epithelial ovarian cancer: A potential role in the coagulation cascade, diagnosis and prognosis. *International Journal of Oncology*, 54(5):1719–1733.

Zhang, X. and Figeys, D. 2019. Perspective and guidelines for metaproteomics in microbiome studies. *Journal of Proteome Research*, 18(6):2370–2380.

Zhernakova, A., Kurilshikov, A., Bonder, M.J., Tigchelaar, E.F., Schirmer, M., Vatanen, T., Mujagic, Z., Vila, A.V., Falony, G., Vieira-Silva, S. and Wang, J. 2016. Population-based metagenomics analysis reveals markers for gut microbiome composition and diversity. *Science*, 352(6285):565–569.

3 Genomic Approaches in Parasitic Diagnosis

Shameeran Salman Ismael Bamarni[1]
and Mourad Ben Said[2,3]

[1]Head of Medical Laboratory Sciences
Department, University Of Duhok, College
Of Health Science, Duhok, Iraq

[2]Laboratory of Microbiology, National School of Veterinary
Medicine of Sidi Thabet, University of Manouba,
Manouba, Tunisia

[3]Department of Basic Sciences, Higher Institute
of Biotechnology of Sidi Thabet, University
of Manouba, Manouba, Tunisia

3.1 INTRODUCTION

In the eukaryotic tree of life, parasites constitute a diverse group of eukaryotic microorganisms that impact both human and animal health (Parfrey et al., 2010). The inherent diversity of these organisms, historically challenging to study due to their complex life cycles and associations with underdeveloped environments, is now being unveiled through genome sequencing (Auld & Tinsley, 2015). Over the past decade, numerous parasitic reference genomes and field isolates from patient populations have been sequenced, stemming from initiatives in large-scale sequencing facilities and, increasingly, in individual research labs. This "tsunami" of genomic data is addressing questions regarding the genetic variety of parasites, evolutionary patterns influenced by host immune pressure and anti-parasitic medication pressure, and population characteristics (Hupalo et al., 2015).

About 65 reference genomes of parasitic organisms belonging to the kingdom Protista were submitted to GenBank in 2014 (Hupalo et al., 2015). The majority of these genomes are attributed to two phyla: Kinetoplastidae and Apicomplexa. Kinetoplastidae encompasses parasites causing diseases such as African sleeping sickness (*Trypanosoma brucei*), Chagas disease (*Trypanosoma cruzi*), and visceral leishmaniasis (*Leishmania* spp.). The second phylum, Apicomplexa, includes the genus *Plasmodium*, responsible for malaria in over 100 countries (Carlton et al., 2002).

The clades containing *Plasmodium* (Carlton et al., 2002), *Leishmania* (Peacock et al., 2007), and *Trypanosoma* (El-Sayed et al., 2005) have been the primary focus of "comparative genomics" studies on parasite genomes. Initially, most of these

DOI: 10.1201/9781032651071-3

genomes were sequenced using first-generation Sanger technology, requiring significant time for gene discovery, assembly, and annotation processes (Forrester & Hall, 2014).

Advancements in sequencing technologies, such as next-generation platforms from Life Technologies (Ion Torrent Personal Genome Machine), Roche 454 (GS Junior), and Illumina (HiSeq series), have facilitated more cost-effective, rapid, and accurate whole-genome sequencing of numerous field isolates from patients. These incomplete genomes are archived in either the European Bioinformatics Institute's European Nucleotide Archive or GenBank's Sequence Read Archive (Aurrecoechea et al., 2013).

In the past two decades, omics investigations, encompassing genomes, transcriptomes, proteomics, and metabolomics, have marked a revolutionary leap in datasets for studying parasite system biology, host–parasite interactions, and phylogenetic analysis in the field of medical parasitology (Zhang & Wang, 2015). Genome-wide association studies (GWASs), coupled with bioinformatics, have empowered researchers to unearth diagnostic biomarkers, potential therapeutic targets, and viable vaccine candidates for the diagnosis, treatment, and prevention of various neglected tropical diseases. Omics approaches can be broadly categorised into two types: genomics and post-genomics (Diab & Younis, 2022).

Parasite omics' extensive databases hold immense promise for numerous domains, including molecular epidemiology, diagnostic biomarkers, medication resistance, and the identification of potential therapeutic targets or vaccine candidates (Qiu et al., 2023). This comprehensive field incorporates knowledge from genomics and other biological subfields, covering aspects such as sequencing, function, evolution, and editing (Satam et al., 2023). The GWASs, also referred to as genetic mapping by linkage, involve selecting genomic regions recently subject to strong selection, like candidate resistance loci. Subsequent genetic manipulations demonstrate causality or broad expression analyses to identify genetic variation mapping (Gunawardena & Karunaweera, 2015).

Functional omics studies, including transcriptomics and proteomics, explore protein expression and RNA transcription, respectively. These studies aim to determine the critical impact of protein expression and gene transcription on the parasite's survival, development, and/or virulence (Lee et al., 2018). To comprehensively analyse the full spectrum of epigenetic alterations or stable changes influencing gene expression, epigenomics, also known as GWAS, is conducted (Li, 2021). A deep understanding of biological processes requiring DNA alteration and expression heavily relies on the epigenetic environment (Arama et al., 2018).

In the last two decades, the field of bioinformatics has seen remarkable advancements through novel methodological approaches, such as aptamers and cell-free expression systems. Aptamers, comprising DNA or RNA oligonucleotides or peptides, possess high-affinity protein-binding properties and are instrumental in interacting with specific targets like diagnostic biomarkers, therapeutic targets, or vaccine candidates (Ospina-Villa et al., 2016).

Bioinformatics, a vital component of the broader omics field, is an interdisciplinary digital approach that employs physical, mathematical, computational, and statistical analyses to dissect sequencing and functional data from genomic and post-genomic research studies (Orlov et al., 2020). This analytical process transforms complex data into actionable information, offering various practical applications (Cai et al., 2013). Within the field of medical parasitology, bioinformatics plays a crucial role in addressing several key aspects: first, it aids in uncovering the molecular basis and mechanisms underlying host–parasite interactions and integrated parasite systems biology. This knowledge is pivotal for the development of more effective diagnostic tools, drugs, and vaccines (Mahanta et al., 2018). Second, the study of specific amino acid modifications resulting from host-parasite interactions, including post-translational modifications (PTMs) like methylation, glycosylation, phosphorylation, deacetylation, and acetylation, has emerged as a valuable tool. The PTMs act as biosensors or metabolic fingerprints, contributing to diagnosis and the creation of portable ultrasensitive protein detection devices (Sin et al., 2014). Thirdly, bioinformatics facilitates phylogenetic analysis by leveraging sequencing techniques across various genomic sources. This approach eliminates spurious homology caused by natural selection, enhancing the accuracy of evolutionary studies (Abaza, 2020). In the context of molecular epidemiology investigations, bioinformatics tools prove invaluable in determining the causative pathogen, species, and origin of infection during aquatic outbreaks (Feng et al., 2018; Thompson & Ash, 2019).

The application of metabarcoding is another significant contribution, allowing high-throughput screening through parallel DNA sequencing of multiple parasites in diverse samples, whether biological or environmental. This innovative approach enables the identification of short DNA sequences or barcodes of specific genes (Burki et al., 2021). Furthermore, the interdisciplinary field of landscape genetics explores the intricate relationship between population genetics and landscape ecology. Leveraging data from landscape population genetics, researchers can unveil how ecological changes impact genetic structures, shedding light on the origins of disease resistance and vulnerability (Schwabl et al., 2017).

In the realm of omics investigations, additional technologies such as RNA sequencing-based research have been applied. This has revealed the significance of non-coding protein RNA (ncRNA) transcriptomes in understanding parasite virulence (Raabe et al., 2010). Notably, ncRNAs, encompassing diverse types such as ribosomal RNA, transfer RNA, short nucleolar RNA, and long non-coding RNA, play essential biological roles in eukaryotes without encoding proteins (Diamantopoulos et al., 2018). The integration of these diverse technologies and methodologies into the study of parasites showcases the dynamic and interdisciplinary nature of contemporary research in the field of medical and veterinary parasitology.

3.2   WHOLE-GENOME SEQUENCING (WGS)

Genomic sequencing, the process of determining the precise nucleotide sequence within a DNA molecule, spans techniques that establish the order of bases in a DNA strand, including the sequence of operons, single genes, entire genomes, or whole chromosomes (Church & Gilbert, 1984). Whole-genome sequencing (WGS) stands out as a powerful tool in this domain, playing a pivotal role in various aspects of research and public health (Satam et al., 2023). When integrated into surveillance and response systems, WGS accelerates threat detection and response times, enabling quicker and more precise interventions. This approach enhances our understanding of hazards and facilitates targeted responses, particularly in the context of monitoring and responding to foodborne diseases, offering the highest microbial sub-typing resolution for public health authorities (Francis et al., 2022).

Various methods are employed for genome sequencing, with some of the most frequently used ones being polymerase chain reaction (PCR) sequencing, 454 sequencing, Sanger sequencing, shotgun sequencing, and Illumina sequencing (Hall, 2001). Genomic sequencing serves as a valuable tool for identifying therapeutic targets and understanding gene mutations or deletions that contribute to the emergence of antiparasitic drug resistance (Ekblom & Wolf, 2014). Researchers leverage genome-wide approaches to investigate the genetics of anthelmintic resistance, comparing phenotypically distinct strains throughout the entire genome to pinpoint regions associated with resistance (McVeigh, 2020). Moreover, genomic sequencing has played a critical role in identifying vaccine targets for parasitic diseases like malaria (Su, 2015).

The advent of Next-Generation Sequencing has significantly improved public health and clinical microbiology. High-throughput technologies and bioinformatics not only expedite the identification of pathogens compared to conventional techniques but also offer new insights into disease transmission, virulence, and antiparasitic resistance (Gwinn et al., 2017). The integration of WGS into these research and public health practices represents a powerful approach that continues to advance our understanding of genomics and contribute to various aspects of disease detection, intervention, and vaccine development (Cowell & Winzeler, 2019).

3.3   NEXT-GENERATION SEQUENCING (NGS)

NGS, also known as high-throughput or deep sequencing, has emerged as a revolutionary DNA sequencing technology that has transformed genetic research. NGS has the capability to sequence the entire human or parasite genome in just one day (Behjati & Tarpey, 2013). This technology not only provides precise data but is also more cost-effective than microarrays, making it a viable choice for genome, transcriptome, or proteome sequencing. In comparison to previous technologies, NGS simplifies the synthesis and sequencing of a large number of DNA fragments simultaneously, eliminating the need for bacterial cloning (Le Roch et al., 2012).

One significant application of NGS is transcriptome sequencing, known as RNA-seq. This technique enables the reconstruction of the entire transcriptome in a chosen species, providing quantitative expression scores for each transcript. RNA-seq data analysis allows for a quantitative examination of RNA expression patterns at comparative genome levels and the identification of additional molecular markers (Gunawardena & Karunaweera, 2015). Recent technological advancements have further allowed the development of in situ single-cell RNA sequencing, referred to as spatial transcriptomics. This involves sequencing RNA within a tissue or organ using either sequential-fluorescent *in situ* hybridisation or fluorescent-labelled cDNA. These applications have been instrumental in identifying new anti-parasitic drugs that specifically target essential parasites for their survival and virulence (Goh et al., 2020; Liao et al., 2021).

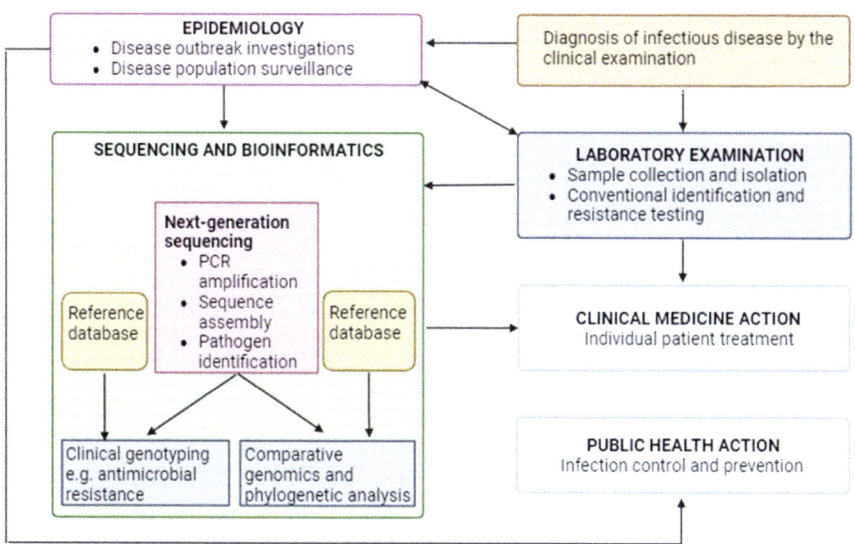

FIGURE 3.1   How Next-Generation Sequencing works against microorganisms.

Converting raw sequence data into usable information poses challenges. The assembly of shorter pieces into whole sequences is typically the first step, achieved either by mapping against a known reference genome or by creating the sequence from scratch using overlapping reads (Ekblom & Wolf, 2014). Comparing the assembled genome with reference strains enables various conclusions, including pathogen identification, prediction of significant phenotypic traits, and high-resolution strain typing. Given the rapid evolution of microbial pathogens and the exchange of plasmids among bacteria, often encoding virulence and anti-parasitic resistance traits, well-curated and current reference databases are crucial (Morschhäuser et al., 2000). Phylogenetic clustering, indicative of transmission, can be identified by comparing assembled genomes with those of other organisms. This complex process requires the synchronisation of multiple bioinformatics tools for each step (assembly, strain typing, phenotyping, and clustering) into a unified workflow, as illustrated in Figure 3.1 (Besser et al., 2018; Quainoo et al., 2017). The integration of NGS into parasitology research has significantly enhanced our understanding of genomic and functional aspects, paving the way for innovative discoveries and applications in the field.

3.4   METAGENOMICS

The application of Metagenomic Next-Generation Sequencing (MNGS) has become increasingly prevalent in the etiological diagnosis of infectious disorders, including parasitic infections, with advancements in NGS technology (Thoendel et al., 2018; Blauwkamp et al., 2019; Kounosu et al., 2019). Leveraging high-throughput sequencing and database comparison, MNGS has the capacity to directly identify potential pathogens, encompassing bacteria, fungi, viruses, and parasites, in DNA samples without the need for prior pathogen isolation. This proves particularly advantageous for identifying pathogens that are challenging to cultivate or cannot be cultured at all (Li et al., 2021). The MNGS has demonstrated clear advantages over conventional pathogen detection techniques, especially in cases where pathogens are difficult to culture (Liu et al., 2022). A notable example is the critical role of MNGS in the clinical diagnosis and management of visceral leishmaniasis, where *Leishmania* was identified in the bone marrow of three patients, marking the first report of leishmaniasis diagnosis by MNGS in China (Chen et al., 2020).

The versatility of MNGS in identifying a broad spectrum of probable causes, spanning parasitic, bacterial, fungal, and viral origins, positions it as a promising method for diagnosing infectious diseases (Goldberg et al., 2015; Forbes et al., 2017). However, studies detailing the use of MNGS in patients with meningitis or encephalitis are currently limited to case reports involving either a single patient or a small number of retrospective cases (Simner et al., 2018). The expanding applications of MNGS offer significant potential for enhancing diagnostic capabilities, especially in scenarios where traditional methods face limitations or challenges in pathogen identification (Batool & Galloway-Peña, 2023).

3.5 CHALLENGES AND LIMITATIONS OF GENOMIC DIAGNOSTICS IN PARASITIC INFECTIONS

The genomes of parasites exhibit remarkable diversity in their architectures, presenting unique challenges for genomic diagnostics. Varied characteristics, such as nucleotide bias and isochore structure, contribute to this diversity (Gardner et al., 2002). Additionally, many parasite genomes contain a significant number of transposable elements or exhibit high repetitiveness, as seen in *Entamoeba (E.) histolytica* (Loftus et al., 2005). Parasite genome sizes also vary widely, ranging from the relatively small genome of the microsporidian *Encephalitozoon cuniculi* (2.3 Mb) to the considerably larger genome of *Trichomonas (T.) vaginalis* (over 160 Mb) (Katinka et al., 2001; Carlton et al., 2007).

The immense variation in parasite genomes poses specific challenges for WGS, particularly in terms of achieving sufficient genome coverage, detecting polymorphisms, and obtaining accurate readings of population genetic factors (Hupalo et al., 2015). To address these challenges, new sequencing techniques have been developed for patient isolate samples, including "reduced representation" methods utilised to create genetic markers for population genomic studies (Davey et al., 2011). One such technique, restriction-site-associated DNA (RAD) sequencing, has been applied to re-sequence approximately 180 *T. vaginalis* genomes, using either one (RAD) or a pair (ddRAD) of restriction enzymes (Baird et al., 2008; Peterson et al., 2012; Conrad et al., 2013).

Despite the widespread use of various metagenomic methods, the application of metagenomics on protozoan parasites remains limited (Maritz et al., 2019). The complexities of eukaryotic genomes, their substantial sizes, increased variability in certain genes, and the presence of multiple copies of some genes pose significant challenges for metagenomic investigations on protozoan parasites. Examples like *Toxoplasma gondii* (110 copies) and *Cryptosporidium (C.) parvum* (five copies) illustrate the numerous gene copy counts in the 18S small subunit ribosomal DNA gene (Huang et al., 2016). Additionally, the presence of repeated non-coding DNA sequences in eukaryotic genomes further complicates the creation of reliable standard techniques for metagenomic profiling of protozoans. These challenges contribute to fewer research initiatives and a limited number of fully sequenced genomes in reference databases for protozoan parasites. The ongoing exploration of advanced sequencing methods and innovative approaches is crucial to overcoming these obstacles and advancing genomic diagnostics in the study of parasitic infections (Handelsman, 2004).

3.6 INTEGRATION OF GENOMIC DIAGNOSTICS IN CLINICAL PRACTICE

Genomic diagnostics, including WGS, exome genome sequencing, and array comparative genomic hybridisation, have become pivotal tools in various academic, medical, and genetic laboratories within the field of human and veterinary genetics. NGS, although reliant on the human and veterinary genome sequence for fundamental analyses, presents challenges such as high costs, time-consuming procedures, and reduced specificity when used in isolation (Miller, 2013; Adeyemo et al., 2018). Sanger sequencing, another traditional method, is limited in its ability to study single fragments and estimate small sequence lengths (300–1000 bases) without prior knowledge of the target sequence (Dulanto & Dekker, 2020). The difficulty in distinguishing host-specific protozoan species, which often share high genetic similarity, using conventional techniques further emphasises the need for novel identification and analysis methods (Ricciardi & Ndao, 2015).

Protozoan parasites, like *C. parvum* and *C. hominis*, exhibit DNA sequence similarities of 95–97%, making it challenging to differentiate them using traditional methods (Widmer & Sullivan, 2012). Additionally, morphological similarities between species, as seen in *E. histolytica* and *E. dispar*, can lead to misdiagnoses (Ricciardi & Ndao, 2015). Even oocysts of the same species, such as those from the *Eimeria* species, may vary in form, highlighting the limitations of conventional techniques and the necessity for advanced genetic diversity analysis methods (Vermeulen et al., 2016).

Metagenomics, heavily utilised in microbiome studies with the aid of NGS technologies, offers valuable insights without prior knowledge of microbial communities in a sample. It is not culture-dependent, enables identification in populations with low abundance, provides rapid microbial assessment, and aids in the recovery of novel species (Alves et al., 2018). Two primary methods for metagenomic profiling include deep amplicon metagenomics, involving PCR amplification before NGS sequencing, and the shotgun metagenomic method, which shears DNA sequences into fragments before sequencing all nucleic acids in a sample (Miller, 2013; Quince et al., 2017). The integration of these genomic diagnostic techniques into clinical practice holds immense promise for enhancing accuracy, speed, and the scope of infectious disease diagnosis and management (Sperber et al., 2021).

3.7   CASE STUDIES AND SUCCESS STORIES IN GENOMIC PARASITIC DIAGNOSIS

Numerous studies have utilised genomic approaches for the diagnosis of various parasites, including helminths, protozoa, and arthropods, showcasing the potential and success of these techniques in advancing our understanding of parasitic infections. One significant case involves the first reference genome analysis of *E. histolytica*, which uncovered a complement of genes associated with meiosis, suggesting the potential for sexual reproduction in wild populations (Stanley, 2005). Building on this, Weedall et al. (2012) developed a substantial NGS dataset from ten lab-cultured *E. histolytica* lines worldwide, offering more reliable data. Gilchrist et al. (2012) genotyped 84 samples using 16 marker loci discovered from NGS datasets, revealing significant diversity and connecting specific loci to clinical symptoms, supporting the link between *E. histolytica* genotype and virulence. In the realm of malaria research, Tachibana et al. (2012) demonstrated the impact of NGS data on population genetic analyses within the monkey malaria clade. Sequencing *Trypanosoma brucei* subspecies has allowed more recent genomic research in Kinetoplastidae to explore recombination within the *Trypanosoma* genus (Goodhead et al., 2013).

In the context of arthropods, Ismael and Omer (2020) used conventional PCR and DNA sequencing to identify three species of hard ticks in goats and sheep in Duhok City, Iraq. In another study, Ismael and Omer (2021) employed 16S rRNA and DNA sequencing for the identification of *Hyalomma asiaticum asiaticum* (hard tick) from small ruminants in the same area, marking the first such study in Iraq and Duhok City. He et al. (2022) utilised real-time sequencing and Illumina sequencing for transcriptome analysis of mites, revealing over 2000 differentially expressed genes between adult mites and nymphs/larvae. This research provides valuable insights into the biology of the parasite and the diseases it causes. Additionally, Kemp and Maiers (2022) highlighted the utility of NGS in fundamental microbiology research, infectious disease diagnosis, and surveillance. As NGS becomes more accessible, cost-effective, rapid, and scalable, it is expected to play an increasing role in preventing and managing infections in the future. These case studies collectively illustrate the transformative impact of genomic approaches in advancing our knowledge of parasitic infections and improving diagnostic capabilities.

3.8   CONCLUSION

In conclusion, the integration of genomic diagnostics has significantly advanced the understanding and diagnosis of parasitic infections. The vast diversity in parasite genomes, spanning helminths, protozoa, and arthropods, poses unique challenges that have been effectively addressed through innovative genomic techniques. Case studies, such as the comprehensive analysis of *E. histolytica*, highlight the power of genomics in uncovering genetic features related to meiosis and clinical symptoms. The utilisation of NGS technologies, as demonstrated in various studies, has facilitated population genetic analyses, uncovering diversity and recombination within parasite species like *Plasmodium* and *Trypanosoma*. Notably, the application of NGS in arthropod studies, exemplified by the identification of hard ticks, showcases the versatility of genomic approaches in understanding diverse host-parasite interactions. Furthermore, the success stories extend to mite transcriptome analysis, revealing thousands of differentially expressed genes and providing valuable insights into the biology of parasitic illnesses. The continued evolution and accessibility of NGS are poised to play a pivotal role in fundamental microbiology research, infectious disease diagnosis, and surveillance, thereby contributing to the prevention and management of infections. In essence, the integration of genomic diagnostics into clinical practice holds tremendous promise for enhancing accuracy, speed, and the depth of infectious disease diagnosis. The presented case studies and success stories underscore the transformative impact of genomics in unravelling the intricacies of parasitic infections, paving the way for more effective strategies in their detection, treatment, and prevention. As technology progresses, genomics is poised to play an increasingly vital role in the ongoing battle against parasitic diseases.

REFERENCES

Abaza, S. M. 2020. What is and why do we have to know phylogenetic tree? *Parasitologists United Journal,* 13(2), 68–71.

Adeyemo, F. E., Singh, G., Reddy, P., & Stenström, T. A. 2018. Methods for the detection of Cryptosporidium and Giardia: From microscopy to nucleic acid based tools in clinical and environmental regimes. *Acta Tropica*, 184, 15–28. https://doi.org/10.1016/j.actatropica.2018.01.011

Alves, L. F., Westmann, C. A., Lovate, G. L., de Siqueira, G. M. V., Borelli, T. C., & Guazzaroni, M. E. 2018. Metagenomic approaches for understanding new concepts in microbial science. *International Journal of Genomics*, 2018, 2312987. https://doi.org/10.1155/2018/2312987

Arama, C., Quin, J. E., Kouriba, B., Östlund Farrants, A. K., Troye-Blomberg, M., & Doumbo, O. K. 2018. Epigenetics and Malaria susceptibility/protection: A missing piece of the puzzle. *Frontiers in Immunology*, 9, 1733. https://doi.org/10.3389/fimmu.2018.01733

Auld, S. K., & Tinsley, M. C. 2015. The evolutionary ecology of complex lifecycle parasites: linking phenomena with mechanisms. *Heredity*, 114(2), 125–132. https://doi.org/10.1038/hdy.2014.84

Aurrecoechea, C., Barreto, A., Brestelli, J., Brunk, B. P., Cade, S., Doherty, R., Fischer, S., Gajria, B., Gao, X., Gingle, A., Grant, G., Harb, O. S., Heiges, M., Hu, S., Iodice, J., Kissinger, J. C., Kraemer, E. T., Li, W., Pinney, D. F., Pitts, B., … Warrenfeltz, S. 2013. EuPathDB: the eukaryotic pathogen database. *Nucleic Acids Research*, 41(Database issue), D684–D691. https://doi.org/10.1093/nar/gks1113

Baird, N. A., Etter, P. D., Atwood, T. S., Currey, M. C., Shiver, A. L., Lewis, Z. A., Selker, E. U., Cresko, W. A., & Johnson, E. A. 2008. Rapid SNP discovery and genetic mapping using sequenced RAD markers. *PLoS One*, 3(10), e3376. https://doi.org/10.1371/journal.pone.0003376

Batool, M., & Galloway-Peña, J. 2023. Clinical metagenomics-challenges and future prospects. *Frontiers in Microbiology*, 14, 1186424. https://doi.org/10.3389/fmicb.2023 .1186424

Behjati, S., & Tarpey, P. S. 2013. What is next generation sequencing? Archives of disease in childhood. *Education and Practice Edition*, 98(6), 236–238. https://doi.org/10.1136 /archdischild-2013-304340

Besser, J., Carleton, H. A., Gerner-Smidt, P., Lindsey, R. L., & Trees, E. 2018. Next-generation sequencing technologies and their application to the study and control of bacterial infections. *Clinical Microbiology and Infection: the Official Publication of the European Society of Clinical Microbiology and Infectious Diseases*, 24(4), 335–341. https://doi .org/10.1016/j.cmi.2017.10.013

Blauwkamp, T. A., Thair, S., Rosen, M. J., Blair, L., Lindner, M. S., Vilfan, I. D., Kawli, T., Christians, F. C., Venkatasubrahmanyam, S., Wall, G. D., Cheung, A., Rogers, Z. N., Meshulam-Simon, G., Huijse, L., Balakrishnan, S., Quinn, J. V., Hollemon, D., Hong, D. K., Vaughn, M. L., Kertesz, M., & Yang, S. 2019. Analytical and clinical validation of a microbial cell-free DNA sequencing test for infectious disease. *Nature Microbiology*, 4(4), 663–674. https://doi.org/10.1038/s41564-018-0349-6

Burki, F., Sandin, M. M., & Jamy, M. 2021. Diversity and ecology of protists revealed by metabarcoding. *Current Biology: CB*, 31(19), R1267–R1280. https://doi.org/10.1016/j .cub.2021.07.066

Cai, Y., Huang, T., Chen, L., & Niu, B. 2013. Application of systems biology and bioinformatics methods in biochemistry and biomedicine. *BioMed Research International*, 2013, 651968. https://doi.org/10.1155/2013/651968

Carlton, J. M., Angiuoli, S. V., Suh, B. B., Kooij, T. W., Pertea, M., Silva, J. C., Ermolaeva, M. D., Allen, J. E., Selengut, J. D., Koo, H. L., Peterson, J. D., Pop, M., Kosack, D. S., Shumway, M. F., Bidwell, S. L., Shallom, S. J., van Aken, S. E., Riedmuller, S. B., Feldblyum, T. V., Cho, J. K., … Carucci, D. J. 2002. Genome sequence and comparative analysis of the model rodent malaria parasite Plasmodium yoelii yoelii. *Nature*, 419(6906), 512–519. https://doi.org/10.1038/nature01099

Carlton, J. M., Hirt, R. P., Silva, J. C., Delcher, A. L., Schatz, M., Zhao, Q., Wortman, J. R., Bidwell, S. L., Alsmark, U. C., Besteiro, S., Sicheritz-Ponten, T., Noel, C. J., Dacks, J. B., Foster, P. G., Simillion, C., Van de Peer, Y., Miranda-Saavedra, D., Barton, G. J., Westrop, G. D., Müller, S., … Johnson, P. J. 2007. Draft genome sequence of the sexually transmitted pathogen Trichomonas vaginalis. *Science* (New York, N.Y.), 315(5809), 207–212. https://doi.org/10.1126/science.1132894

Chen, H., Fan, C., Gao, H., Yin, Y., Wang, X., Zhang, Y., & Wang, H. 2020. Leishmaniasis Diagnosis via Metagenomic Next-Generation Sequencing. *Frontiers in Cellular and Infection Microbiology*, 10, 528884. https://doi.org/10.3389/fcimb.2020.528884

Church, G. M., & Gilbert, W. 1984. Genomic sequencing. *Proceedings of the National Academy of Sciences of the United States of America*, 81(7), 1991–1995. https://doi.org /10.1073/pnas.81.7.1991

Conrad, M. D., Bradic, M., Warring, S. D., Gorman, A. W., & Carlton, J. M. 2013. Getting trichy: Tools and approaches to interrogating *Trichomonas vaginalis* in a post-genome world. *Trends in Parasitology*, 29(1), 17–25. https://doi.org/10.1016/j.pt.2012.10.004

Cowell, A. N., & Winzeler, E. A. 2019. The genomic architecture of antimalarial drug resistance. *Briefings in Functional Genomics*, 18(5), 314–328. https://doi.org/10.1093/bfgp /elz008

Davey, J. W., Hohenlohe, P. A., Etter, P. D., Boone, J. Q., Catchen, J. M., & Blaxter, M. L. 2011. Genome-wide genetic marker discovery and genotyping using next-generation sequencing. *Nature Reviews. Genetics*, 12(7), 499–510. https://doi.org/10.1038/nrg3012

Diab, R.G., & Younis, S.S. 2022. Omics: Approaches and applications related to diagnosis, treatment, and control of parasitic diseases. Part I: Plasmodium spp. *Parasitologists United Journal,* 15(2), 144–153.

Diamantopoulos, M. A., Tsiakanikas, P., & Scorilas, A. 2018. Non-coding RNAs: the riddle of the transcriptome and their perspectives in cancer. *Annals of Translational Medicine,* 6(12), 241. https://doi.org/10.21037/atm.2018.06.10

Dulanto Chiang, A., & Dekker, J. P. 2020. From the Pipeline to the Bedside: Advances and Challenges in Clinical Metagenomics. *The Journal of Infectious Diseases,* 221(Suppl 3), S331–S340. https://doi.org/10.1093/infdis/jiz151

Ekblom, R., & Wolf, J. B. 2014. A field guide to whole-genome sequencing, assembly and annotation. *Evolutionary Applications,* 7(9), 1026–1042. https://doi.org/10.1111/eva.12178

El-Sayed, N. M., Myler, P. J., Blandin, G., Berriman, M., Crabtree, J., Aggarwal, G., Caler, E., Renauld, H., Worthey, E. A., Hertz-Fowler, C., Ghedin, E., Peacock, C., Bartholomeu, D. C., Haas, B. J., Tran, A. N., Wortman, J. R., Alsmark, U. C., Angiuoli, S., Anupama, A., Badger, J., ... Hall, N. 2005). Comparative genomics of trypanosomatid parasitic protozoa. *Science* (New York, N.Y.), 309(5733), 404–409. https://doi.org/10.1126/science.1112181

Feng, Y., Ryan, U. M., & Xiao, L. 2018. Genetic diversity and population structure of cryptosporidium. *Trends in Parasitology,* 34(11), 997–1011. https://doi.org/10.1016/j.pt.2018.07.009

Forbes, J. D., Knox, N. C., Ronholm, J., Pagotto, F., & Reimer, A. 2017. Metagenomics: The next culture-independent game changer. *Frontiers in Microbiology,* 8, 1069. https://doi.org/10.3389/fmicb.2017.01069

Forrester, S. J., & Hall, N. 2014. The revolution of whole genome sequencing to study parasites. *Molecular and Biochemical Parasitology,* 195(2), 77–81. https://doi.org/10.1016/j.molbiopara.2014.07.008

Francis, R. V., Billam, H., Clarke, M., Yates, C., Tsoleridis, T., Berry, L., Mahida, N., Irving, W. L., Moore, C., Holmes, N., Ball, J. K., Loose, M., McClure, C. P., & COVID-19 Genomics UK (COG-UK) consortium. 2022. The impact of real-time whole-genome sequencing in controlling healthcare-associated SARS-CoV-2 outbreaks. *The Journal of Infectious Diseases,* 225(1), 10–18. https://doi.org/10.1093/infdis/jiab483

Gardner, M. J., Hall, N., Fung, E., White, O., Berriman, M., Hyman, R. W., Carlton, J. M., Pain, A., Nelson, K. E., Bowman, S., Paulsen, I. T., James, K., Eisen, J. A., Rutherford, K., Salzberg, S. L., Craig, A., Kyes, S., Chan, M. S., Nene, V., Shallom, S. J., ... Barrell, B. (2002. Genome sequence of the human malaria parasite Plasmodium falciparum. *Nature,* 419(6906), 498–511. https://doi.org/10.1038/nature01097

Gilchrist, C. A., Ali, I. K., Kabir, M., Alam, F., Scherbakova, S., Ferlanti, E., Weedall, G. D., Hall, N., Haque, R., Petri, W. A., Jr, & Caler, E. 2012. A Multilocus Sequence Typing System (MLST) reveals a high level of diversity and a genetic component to Entamoeba histolytica virulence. *BMC Microbiology,* 12, 151. https://doi.org/10.1186/1471-2180-12-151

Goh, J. J. L., Chou, N., Seow, W. Y., Ha, N., Cheng, C. P. P., Chang, Y. C., Zhao, Z. W., & Chen, K. H. 2020. Highly specific multiplexed RNA imaging in tissues with split-FISH. *Nature Methods,* 17(7), 689–693. https://doi.org/10.1038/s41592-020-0858-0

Goldberg, B., Sichtig, H., Geyer, C., Ledeboer, N., & Weinstock, G. M. 2015. Making the leap from research laboratory to clinic: Challenges and opportunities for next-generation sequencing in infectious disease diagnostics. *mBio,* 6(6), e01888-15. https://doi.org/10.1128/mBio.01888-15

Goodhead, I., Capewell, P., Bailey, J. W., Beament, T., Chance, M., Kay, S., Forrester, S., MacLeod, A., Taylor, M., Noyes, H., & Hall, N. 2013. Whole-genome sequencing of Trypanosoma brucei reveals introgression between subspecies that is associated with virulence. *mBio*, 4(4), e00197-13. https://doi.org/10.1128/mBio.00197-13

Gunawardena, S., & Karunaweera, N. D. 2015. Advances in genetics and genomics: use and limitations in achieving malaria elimination goals. *Pathogens and Global Health*, 109(3), 123–141. https://doi.org/10.1179/2047773215Y.0000000015

Gwinn, M., MacCannell, D. R., & Khabbaz, R. F. 2017. Integrating advanced molecular technologies into public health. *Journal of Clinical Microbiology*, 55(3), 703–714. https://doi.org/10.1128/JCM.01967-16

Hall, N. 2001. Royal Society discussion meeting: utilising the genome sequence of parasitic protozoa. *Comparative and Functional Genomics*, 2(4), 257–262. https://doi.org/10.1002/cfg.88

Handelsman, J. 2004. Metagenomics: application of genomics to uncultured microorganisms. *Microbiology and Molecular Biology Reviews*, 68(4), 669–685.

He, R., Zhang, Q., Gu, X., Xie, Y., Xu, J., Peng, X., & Yang, G. 2022. Transcriptome analysis of otodectes cynotis in different developmental stages. *Frontiers in Microbiology*, 13, 687387. https://doi.org/10.3389/fmicb.2022.687387

Huang, Y., Chen, S. Y., & Deng, F. 2016. Well-characterized sequence features of eukaryote genomes and implications for ab initio gene prediction. *Computational and Structural Biotechnology* Journal, 14, 298–303. https://doi.org/10.1016/j.csbj.2016.07.002

Hupalo, D. N., Bradic, M., & Carlton, J. M. 2015. The impact of genomics on population genetics of parasitic diseases. *Current Opinion in Microbiology*, 23, 49–54. https://doi.org/10.1016/j.mib.2014.11.001

Ismael, S. S., & Omer, L. T. 2020. Morphologcal and molecular study of hard ticks species that infested small ruminants in Duhok Governorate, Kurdistan region, IRAQ. *Basrah Journal of Veterinary Research,* 19(1), 88–108.

Ismael, S. S., & Omer, L. T. 2021. Molecular identification of new circulating *Hyalomma asiaticum asiaticum* from sheep and goats in Duhok governorate, Iraq. *Iraqi Journal of Veterinary Sciences*, 35(1), 79–83.

Katinka, M. D., Duprat, S., Cornillot, E., Méténier, G., Thomarat, F., Prensier, G., Barbe, V., Peyretaillade, E., Brottier, P., Wincker, P., Delbac, F., El Alaoui, H., Peyret, P., Saurin, W., Gouy, M., Weissenbach, J., & Vivarès, C. P. 2001. Genome sequence and gene compaction of the eukaryote parasite Encephalitozoon cuniculi. *Nature*, 414(6862), 450–453. https://doi.org/10.1038/35106579

Kemp, M., & Maiers, M. 2022. Editorial: Application of Next Generation Sequencing (NGS) in infection prevention. *Frontiers in Public Health*, 10, 945595. https://doi.org/10.3389/fpubh.2022.945595

Kounosu, A., Murase, K., Yoshida, A., Maruyama, H., & Kikuchi, T. 2019. Improved 18S and 28S rDNA primer sets for NGS-based parasite detection. *Scientific Reports*, 9(1), 15789. https://doi.org/10.1038/s41598-019-52422-z

Le Roch, K. G., Chung, D. W., & Ponts, N. 2012. Genomics and integrated systems biology in Plasmodium falciparum: a path to malaria control and eradication. *Parasite Immunology*, 34(2–3), 50–60. https://doi.org/10.1111/j.1365-3024.2011.01340.x

Lee, H. J., Georgiadou, A., Otto, T. D., Levin, M., Coin, L. J., Conway, D. J., & Cunnington, A. J. 2018. Transcriptomic studies of Malaria: a paradigm for investigation of systemic host-pathogen interactions. *Microbiology and Molecular Biology Reviews: MMBR*, 82(2), e00071-17. https://doi.org/10.1128/MMBR.00071-17

Li, Y. 2021. Modern epigenetics methods in biological research. *Methods* (San Diego, Calif.), 187, 104–113. https://doi.org/10.1016/j.ymeth.2020.06.022

Liao, J., Lu, X., Shao, X., Zhu, L., & Fan, X. 2021. Uncovering an organ's molecular architecture at single-cell resolution by spatially resolved transcriptomics. *Trends in Biotechnology*, 39(1), 43–58. https://doi.org/10.1016/j.tibtech.2020.05.006

Liu, J., Zhang, Q., Dong, Y. Q., Yin, J., & Qiu, Y. Q. 2022. Diagnostic accuracy of metagenomic next-generation sequencing in diagnosing infectious diseases: a meta-analysis. *Scientific Reports*, 12(1), 21032. https://doi.org/10.1038/s41598-022-25314-y

Loftus, B., Anderson, I., Davies, R., Alsmark, U. C., Samuelson, J., Amedeo, P., Roncaglia, P., Berriman, M., Hirt, R. P., Mann, B. J., Nozaki, T., Suh, B., Pop, M., Duchene, M., Ackers, J., Tannich, E., Leippe, M., Hofer, M., Bruchhaus, I., Willhoeft, U., … Hall, N. 2005. The genome of the protist parasite Entamoeba histolytica. *Nature*, 433(7028), 865–868. https://doi.org/10.1038/nature03291

Mahanta, A., Ganguli, P., Barah, P., Sarkar, R. R., Sarmah, N., Phukan, S., Bora, M., & Baruah, S. 2018. Integrative approaches to understand the mastery in manipulation of host Cytokine networks by protozoan parasites with emphasis on plasmodium and leishmania species. *Frontiers in Immunology*, 9, 296. https://doi.org/10.3389/fimmu.2018.00296

Maritz, J. M., Ten Eyck, T. A., Elizabeth Alter, S., & Carlton, J. M. 2019. Patterns of protist diversity associated with raw sewage in New York City. *The ISME Journal*, 13(11), 2750–2763. https://doi.org/10.1038/s41396-019-0467-z

McVeigh P. 2020. Post-genomic progress in helminth parasitology. *Parasitology*, 147(8), 835–840. https://doi.org/10.1017/S0031182020000591

Miller, R. K. 2013. Helping new librarians find success and satisfaction in the academic library. In *Book: Workplace culture in academic libraries,* pp. 81–96. https://doi.org/10.1016/B978-1-84334-702-6.50005-8

Morschhäuser, J., Köhler, G., Ziebuhr, W., Blum-Oehler, G., Dobrindt, U., & Hacker, J. 2000. Evolution of microbial pathogens. *Philosophical Transactions of the Royal Society of London. Series B, Biological Sciences*, 355(1397), 695–704. https://doi.org/10.1098/rstb.2000.0609

Orlov, Y. L., Baranova, A. V., & Tatarinova, T. V. 2020. Bioinformatics methods in medical genetics and genomics. *International Journal of Molecular Sciences*, 21(17), 6224. https://doi.org/10.3390/ijms21176224

Ospina-Villa, J. D., Zamorano-Carrillo, A., Castañón-Sánchez, C. A., Ramírez-Moreno, E., & Marchat, L. A. 2016. Aptamers as a promising approach for the control of parasitic diseases. *The Brazilian Journal of Infectious Diseases: An Official Publication of the Brazilian Society of Infectious Diseases*, 20(6), 610–618. https://doi.org/10.1016/j.bjid.2016.08.011

Parfrey, L. W., Grant, J., Tekle, Y. I., Lasek-Nesselquist, E., Morrison, H. G., Sogin, M. L., Patterson, D. J., & Katz, L. A. 2010. Broadly sampled multigene analyses yield a well-resolved eukaryotic tree of life. *Systematic Biology*, 59(5), 518–533. https://doi.org/10.1093/sysbio/syq037

Peacock, C. S., Seeger, K., Harris, D., Murphy, L., Ruiz, J. C., Quail, M. A., Peters, N., Adlem, E., Tivey, A., Aslett, M., Kerhornou, A., Ivens, A., Fraser, A., Rajandream, M. A., Carver, T., Norbertczak, H., Chillingworth, T., Hance, Z., Jagels, K., Moule, S., … Berriman, M. 2007. Comparative genomic analysis of three Leishmania species that cause diverse human disease. *Nature Genetics*, 39(7), 839–847. https://doi.org/10.1038/ng2053

Peterson, B. K., Weber, J. N., Kay, E. H., Fisher, H. S., & Hoekstra, H. E. 2012. Double digest RADseq: an inexpensive method for de novo SNP discovery and genotyping in model and non-model species. *PLoS One*, 7(5), e37135. https://doi.org/10.1371/journal.pone.0037135

Qiu, S., Cai, Y., Yao, H., Lin, C., Xie, Y., Tang, S., & Zhang, A. 2023. Small molecule metabolites: discovery of biomarkers and therapeutic targets. *Signal Transduction and Targeted Therapy*, 8(1), 132. https://doi.org/10.1038/s41392-023-01399-3

Quainoo, S., Coolen, J. P. M., van Hijum, S. A. F. T., Huynen, M. A., Melchers, W. J. G., van Schaik, W., & Wertheim, H. F. L. 2017. Whole-genome sequencing of bacterial pathogens: the future of nosocomial outbreak analysis. *Clinical Microbiology Reviews*, 30(4), 1015–1063. https://doi.org/10.1128/CMR.00016-17

Quince, C., Walker, A. W., Simpson, J. T., Loman, N. J., & Segata, N. (2017). Shotgun metagenomics, from sampling to analysis. *Nature Biotechnology*, 35(9), 833–844. https://doi.org/10.1038/nbt.3935

Raabe, C. A., Sanchez, C. P., Randau, G., Robeck, T., Skryabin, B. V., Chinni, S. V., Kube, M., Reinhardt, R., Ng, G. H., Manickam, R., Kuryshev, V. Y., Lanzer, M., Brosius, J., Tang, T. H., & Rozhdestvensky, T. S. 2010. A global view of the nonprotein-coding transcriptome in Plasmodium falciparum. *Nucleic Acids Research*, 38(2), 608–617. https://doi.org/10.1093/nar/gkp895

Ricciardi, A., & Ndao, M. 2015. Diagnosis of parasitic infections: what's going on? *Journal of Biomolecular Screening*, 20(1), 6–21. https://doi.org/10.1177/1087057114548065

Satam, H., Joshi, K., Mangrolia, U., Waghoo, S., Zaidi, G., Rawool, S., Thakare, R. P., Banday, S., Mishra, A. K., Das, G., & Malonia, S. K. 2023. Next-generation sequencing technology: Current trends and advancements. *Biology*, 12(7), 997. https://doi.org/10.3390/biology12070997

Schwabl, P., Llewellyn, M. S., Landguth, E. L., Andersson, B., Kitron, U., Costales, J. A., Ocaña, S., & Grijalva, M. J. 2017. Prediction and prevention of parasitic diseases using a landscape genomics framework. *Trends in Parasitology*, 33(4), 264–275. https://doi.org/10.1016/j.pt.2016.10.008

Simner, P. J., Miller, S., & Carroll, K. C. 2018. Understanding the promises and hurdles of metagenomic next-generation sequencing as a diagnostic tool for infectious diseases. *Clinical Infectious Diseases: An Official Publication of the Infectious Diseases Society of America*, 66(5), 778–788. https://doi.org/10.1093/cid/cix881

Sin, M. L., Mach, K. E., Wong, P. K., & Liao, J. C. 2014. Advances and challenges in biosensor-based diagnosis of infectious diseases. *Expert Review of Molecular Diagnostics*, 14(2), 225–244. https://doi.org/10.1586/14737159.2014.888313

Sperber, N. R., Dong, O. M., Roberts, M. C., Dexter, P., Elsey, A. R., Ginsburg, G. S., Horowitz, C. R., Johnson, J. A., Levy, K. D., Ong, H., Peterson, J. F., Pollin, T. I., Rakhra-Burris, T., Ramos, M. A., Skaar, T., & Orlando, L. A. 2021. Strategies to integrate genomic medicine into clinical care: Evidence from the IGNITE network. *Journal of Personalized Medicine*, 11(7), 647. https://doi.org/10.3390/jpm11070647

Stanley S. L., Jr. 2005. The *Entamoeba histolytica* genome: something old, something new, something borrowed and sex too?. *Trends in Parasitology*, 21(10), 451–453. https://doi.org/10.1016/j.pt.2005.08.006

Su, K. 2015. Genome sequencing. *Journal of Current Research*, 7, 11260-3.

Tachibana, S., Sullivan, S. A., Kawai, S., Nakamura, S., Kim, H. R., Goto, N., Arisue, N., Palacpac, N. M., Honma, H., Yagi, M., Tougan, T., Katakai, Y., Kaneko, O., Mita, T., Kita, K., Yasutomi, Y., Sutton, P. L., Shakhbatyan, R., Horii, T., Yasunaga, T., … Tanabe, K. 2012. Plasmodium cynomolgi genome sequences provide insight into Plasmodium vivax and the monkey malaria clade. *Nature Genetics*, 44(9), 1051–1055. https://doi.org/10.1038/ng.2375

Thoendel, M. J., Jeraldo, P. R., Greenwood-Quaintance, K. E., Yao, J. Z., Chia, N., Hanssen, A. D., Abdel, M. P., & Patel, R. 2018. Identification of prosthetic joint infection pathogens using a shotgun metagenomics approach. *Clinical Infectious Diseases: An Official Publication of the Infectious Diseases Society of America*, 67(9), 1333–1338. https://doi .org/10.1093/cid/ciy303

Thompson, R. C. A., & Ash, A. 2019. Molecular epidemiology of Giardia and Cryptosporidium infections - What's new?. *Infection, Genetics and Evolution: Journal of Molecular Epidemiology and Evolutionary Genetics in Infectious Diseases*, 75, 103951. https:// doi.org/10.1016/j.meegid.2019.103951

Vermeulen, E. T., Lott, M. J., Eldridge, M. D., & Power, M. L. 2016. Evaluation of next generation sequencing for the analysis of Eimeria communities in wildlife. *Journal of Microbiological Methods*, 124, 1–9. https://doi.org/10.1016/j.mimet.2016.02.018

Weedall, G. D., Clark, C. G., Koldkjaer, P., Kay, S., Bruchhaus, I., Tannich, E., Paterson, S., & Hall, N. 2012. Genomic diversity of the human intestinal parasite Entamoeba histolytica. *Genome Biology*, 13(5), R38. https://doi.org/10.1186/gb-2012-13-5-r38

Widmer, G., & Sullivan, S. 2012. Genomics and population biology of Cryptosporidium species. *Parasite Immunology*, 34(2–3), 61–71. https://doi.org/10.1111/j.1365-3024.2011 .01301.x

Zhang, N., & Wang, Z. 2015. 3 pezizomycotina: sordariomycetes and leotiomycetes. In: McLaughlin, D., & Spatafora, J. (eds.) *Systematics and evolution. The Mycota (A comprehensive treatise on fungi as experimental systems for basic and applied research)*. Berlin, Heidelberg: Springer, pp. 57–88.

4 Transcriptomic Profiling of Parasites

Haider Abbas[1], Hafiz Muhammad Rizwan[1], HazratUllah Raheemi[2], and Usman Elahi[3]

[1]Section of Parasitology, Department of Pathobiology, KBCMA College of Veterinary and Animal Sciences, Narowal, Sub-campus University of Veterinary and Animal Sciences, Lahore, Pakistan

[2]Department of Health and Biological Sciences, Faculty of Life Sciences, Abasyn University, Peshawar, Pakistan

[3]Faculty of Agriculture and Veterinary Sciences, Superior University, Lahore, Pakistan

4.1 BACKGROUND

Major groups of parasites of veterinary and public health significance include protozoa, helminths, and arthropods. Chemotherapy is mainly used to control livestock parasites (McKellar and Jackson, 2004). However, the emergence of drug-resistant parasites, especially multidrug resistance, has had markedly negative impacts on the growth and production of livestock globally (Kaplan and Vidyashankar, 2012). Moreover, poor anti-parasitic treatment responses have been observed in parasites (Krücken et al., 2017). To cope with the development of anti-parasitic resistance, new drugs against parasites must be developed (Gearyet al., 2004). Studies are also being focused on the development of vaccines for the persistent mitigation of parasitic infections in humans and livestock (Hotez et al., 2016). Immunization through vaccines or in combination with anti-parasitic drug administration may help minimise the development of drug resistance (Lee et al., 2011). However, there are challenges faced in developing vaccines against parasites, including their immunoregulatory capability and complex antigenic variations of these parasites (Hewitson and Maizels, 2014).

For transcriptomic profiling, Next-Generation Sequencing (NGS) is considered a significant source. NGS has advantages over primitive DNA sequencing as it is comparatively less time-consuming and more efficient. It involves multiple sequencing reactions to mark millions or billions of base pair positions in genes, ultimately resulting in finding the desired genes expressed differentially in various genders, cells, tissues, and stages during initiation or development of immune reactions. Furthermore, this tool enables the sequencing of the whole genome both at the nuclear and organelle levels at the same time (Shendure and Ji, 2008). Helicos,

DOI: 10.1201/9781032651071-4

SOLiD, Roche 454, and Solexa/Illumina are among the NGS tools that modify the transcriptomes and genomes of parasites the way they are studied and described (Kulski, 2016; Gupta and Verma, 2019; Akoniyon et al., 2022). In addition, these sequencing tools have been considered to be linked with the evolution of computational methods related to the interpretation, assemblage, and pre-processing of the sequence datasets (Nagaraj et al., 2007).

Parasites have been extensively characterised through genomic and transcriptome investigations. These studies have identified numerous genes that exhibit differential expression throughout various phases of the parasite's life cycle. A large number of gene families have been recognised among differentially regulated genes (Basikaet al., 2019). Paraloges of genes that arise via replication make up gene families (Lallemand et al., 2020). Numerous functional classes, including ion channels, detoxifying proteins, proteases, and kinases, are transcribed by gene families that proliferate not only in other parasite species but also in numerous ancestral lines of parasites (Coghlan et al., 2019). Several kinds of parasites exhibit differential expression of duplicate genes in these categories over their life cycles. Recently, various parasite model systems are being utilised to establish genomic resources and techniques for examining gene expression (Lin et al., 2011; Olson et al., 2018). Analyses of transcriptomic profiling of parasites, including nematodes (*Haemonchus contortus*, *Ascaris suum*), trematodes (*Clonorchis sinensis*, *Schistosoma (S.) mansoni* and *S. japonicum*), and protozoa (*Eimeria brunette* and *Leishmania donovani*) by various technologies have generated knowledge of molecular and biochemical pathways associated with replication, growth, and parasite–host relationships (Jacob et al., 2008; Aarthi et al., 2011; Chelomina, 2017; Wang, 2021; Reyes-Guerrero et al., 2023). Transcriptomic profiling in parasitology provides the opportunity to add knowledge and new viewpoints on the biology and pathogenesis of parasites.

4.2   TRANSCRIPTOMIC PROFILING OF PROTOZOA

The quick development of single-cell RNA sequencing (scRNA-seq) techniques is causing a change in outlook in the assessment of cell populations, prompting significant advancements in fields like malignant growth research, immunology, and developmental science (Svensson et al., 2018). Single-cell transcriptomics offers a significant advantage: it allows for unbiased identification of cell populations based on global gene expression analysis. This means cells are grouped after analysis based on gene expression patterns, rather than being pre-sorted based on a biased set of markers. This approach ensures a fair and comprehensive representation of cell populations, improving the accuracy of the analysis. This enables measurement of the fluctuation in gene expression across diversified populations, providing the recognition of particular cell types or states, cellular reactions in response to stimuli, and insights into the differentiation process. While scRNA-seq can be a valuable technique, it may not always be the optimal choice for transcriptional profiling due to its higher cost and technological challenges associated with transcript capture, signal amplification, and analysis (Ziegenhain et al., 2017).

The ability of scRNA-seq in distinguishing differential quality articulation between subpopulations depends on both the transcript capture productivity per cell and the quantity of cells examined inside minor subpopulations for correlation (Svensson et al., 2017). Given the compromise between catch efficiency and per-cell sequencing cost, innovations with high capture efficiencies are well-suited for correlations involving multiple subpopulations, as underscored by Reid et al. (2018). Nonetheless, they may be restrictively costly for dissecting intriguing cell types because of the significant number of transcriptomes needed to capture an adequate portrayal of interesting cells. Additionally, it's important to consider organic diversity that doesn't relate to the research question. For example, a recent study on differentially expressed genes in physically distinct schizonts of *Plasmodium* (*P.*) *falciparum* required the ability to profile numerous transcriptomes, even though they represented a significant subpopulation (Poran et al., 2017).

The latest exploration into *Plasmodium* parasites has shown the possibility and the utilisation of single-cell expression profiling in portraying transcriptional variation in the protozoan parasite population (Reid et al., 2018). Exploring the transcriptional series involving bet-hedging strategies holds specific potential for utilisation of scRNAseq. Aside from sexual differentiation in *Plasmodium*, studies reported the development and reemergence of non-active hepatic stages in specific *Plasmodium* species (Witmer et al., 2021), development of a metabolically dormant form of *Giardia* (*G.*) *lamblia* (Kim and Park, 2019) or cyst development of *Toxoplasma* (*T.*) *gondii* in host tissues (Christiansen, 2022). Also, scRNA-seq might reveal new insights into transcriptional events related to exchanging gene expression between individuals from gene families that display totally unrelated gene expression, like vsp genes in *G. lamblia*, var genes in *P. falciparum,* and ves genes in *Babesia bovis* (Deitsch et al., 2009). Transcriptomic examination is an integral asset for disclosing metabolic pathways, clarifying connections among practical qualities in cells or parasites, and recognising key useful qualities under unambiguous circumstances (Chung et al., 2021). In the case of *T. gondii*, transcriptomic analysis revealed the potential role of small RNAs communicated by the parasite in influencing the response of host safe cells and the adaptation of *T. gondii* to its host environment. Additionally, some transcriptomic studies have been conducted on *Cryptosporidium* (Menard et al., 2019).

4.2.1 GIARDIA

Giardiasis can manifest as acute or chronic conditions, often accompanied by symptoms such as stomach cramps, gas, nausea, and weight loss. In severe cases, it can lead to malabsorptive diarrhoea characterised by fatty and watery stools (Nosala and Dawson, 2015). Throughout its life cycle, *Giardia* undergoes two distinct morphological stages: a motile trophozoite residing in the host's gastrointestinal (GI) tract and a cyst passed into the environment (Fink et al., 2020). The *Giardia* cyst features nuclei (typically four) and a dense outer cell wall containing cyst wall proteins (CWP 1, CWP 2, and CWP 3) alongside a unique β-1,3-linked N-acetylgalactosamine homopolymer. Other components include EGFP family proteins, disulphide isomerases, and high cysteine membrane protein (Ankarklev et al., 2015; Ebneter et al., 2016).

Easy imaging techniques for bioluminescent *Giardia* parasites provide valuable insights into host-parasite interactions (Barash et al., 2017). Bioluminescence imaging (BLI) allows sensitive assessment of transcriptional activity and protein expression (Stacer et al., 2013). Compared to axenic culture, high-density foci within the host exhibit significant up-regulation of specific genes, particularly those associated with oxidative stress, membrane transport, and metabolic and structural functions related to encystation (Pham et al., 2017). This suggests physiological adaptations due to high-density growth within intestinal segments. Additionally, novel *Giardia* cyst-specific proteins, including components of the cyst wall, show high expression in these foci.

4.2.2 *TOXOPLASMA GONDII*

Toxoplasma(T.) gondii, a GI parasite belonging to the coccidian group, primarily infects cats, serving as its definitive host (Tong et al., 2021). Upon infection, *Toxoplasma* triggers a robust Th1 immune response characterised by dendritic cell-mediated IL-12 production and the simultaneous promotion of counter-regulatory cytokines like IL-10 (Sasai et al., 2018). In murine models, a parasite protein called profilin acts as a microbial-associated molecular pattern molecule, stimulating IL-12 production through host Toll-like receptors 11 and 12 (Raetz et al., 2013; Yarovinsky, 2014). *Toxoplasma* also injects effector proteins into host cells, such as ROP16, TgIST, GRA18, and GRA24, which manipulate host signalling pathways by activating STAT3/6, NFκB, and p38 MAPK pathways (Rosowski et al., 2011; He et al., 2018). The parasite's success is attributed to its ability to deliver host-modulating effectors that maintain a balance between pro-inflammatory and anti-inflammatory responses. Additionally, the host's non-coding RNA responses, including various microRNAs and long non-coding RNAs activated by *Toxoplasma* infection, play crucial roles in cellular function regulation (Menard et al., 2019).

Hu et al. (2020) conducted a transcriptome study on mouse brains infected with *T. gondii* Pru strain oocysts at 11- and 33-days post-infection (dpi) using RNA sequencing (RNA-seq), comparing them to uninfected control mice. The study revealed that *T. gondii* altered the expression of 936 and 2081 transcripts at 11 and 33 dpi, respectively, with most showing elevated levels in the affected brains. At 11 dpi, there was a significant impact on genes involved in the immune response, particularly those responsive to interferon-gamma (IFN-γ). Similarly, at 33 dpi, changes were observed in transcripts associated with T cell activation, cytokine production, and immune cell proliferation. Some differentially expressed transcripts were linked to metabolic processes, immunological signalling, biosynthesis-related activities, and interactions between host and parasite (Table 4.1). These findings provide insights into the transcriptional regulation and signalling cascades during acute and chronic *T. gondii* infections.

The transcriptomes specific to merozoites and sporulated oocysts/sporozoites exhibit expression patterns that are intermediate between tachyzoites/bradyzoites and unsporulated oocysts (Hehl et al., 2015). Despite this, these transcriptomes display opposing expression patterns due to the diverse biological functions of these

TABLE 4.1
Transcriptomic Profiling of *Toxoplasma gondii* in Mouse

Gene Encoding Protein/Gene ID	Gene Up-Regulated (Yes or No)	Gene Down-Regulated (Yes or No)
Transcriptional repressor GATA binding 1/Trps1#	No	Yes
Activating transcription factor 3/Batf2*	Yes	No
Transcription factor AP-2, alpha/Tfap2a#	No	Yes
Basic leucine zipper transcription factor, ATF-like 2/Atf3*	Yes	No
Protein inhibitor of activated STAT 3/Pias3#	No	Yes
B cell leukaemia/lymphoma 3/Bcl3*	Yes	No
General transcription factor II I/Gtf2i#	No	Yes
Eukaryotic translation initiation factor 2-alpha kinase 2/Eif2ak2*	Yes	No
FBJ osteosarcoma oncogene/Fos#	No	Yes
IKAROS family zinc finger 1/Ikzf1*	Yes	No
Ets variant 1/Etv1#	No	Yes
Interferon regulatory factor 1/Irf1*	Yes	No
Transcription factor 3/Tcf3#	Yes	No
Interferon regulatory factor 8/Irf8*	Yes	No
Signal transducer and activator of transcription 3/Stat3#	Yes	No
Interferon regulatory factor 9/Irf9*	Yes	No
Spi-B transcription factor (Spi-1/PU.1 related)/Spib#	Yes	No
Spleen focus forming virus (SFFV) proviral integration oncogene/Spi1*	Yes	No
Runt related transcription factor 3/Runx3#	Yes	No
Signal transducer and activator of transcription 1/Stat1*	Yes	No
Runt related transcription factor 1/Runx1#	Yes	No
Signal transducer and activator of transcription 2/Stat2*	Yes	No
PR domain-containing 1, with ZNF domain/Prdm1#	Yes	No
Basic leucine zipper transcription factor, ATF-like 3/Batf3#	Yes	No
POU domain, class 2, associating factor 1/Pou2af1#	Yes	No
CD7 antigen/ Cd7#	Yes	No
Paired box 6/ Pax6#	Yes	No
Colony stimulating factor 1 (macrophage)/Csf1#	Yes	No
Nuclear factor of kappa light polypeptide gene enhancer in B cells 1, p105/Nfkb1#	Yes	No
E74-like factor 1/Elf1#	Yes	No
Minichromosome maintenance complex component 6/Mcm6#	Yes	No
ELK3, member of ETS oncogene family/Elk3#	Yes	No
Interferon regulatory factor 5/Irf5#	Yes	No
E26 avian leukaemia oncogene 1, 5′ domain/Ets1#	Yes	No
Interferon regulatory factor 4/Irf4#	Yes	No
Friend leukaemia integration 1/Fli1#	Yes	No
H2.0-like homeobox/Hlx#	Yes	No
Growth factor independent 1 transcription repressor/Gfi1#	Yes	No

developmental stages. While sporozoites prepare for host-related activities, merozoites and gametes produce genetically diverse offspring for a life cycle outside the host (Dubey, 2020). Expression patterns of known tachyzoite virulence factors, which influence host activities during infection and are involved in invasion and replication, are up-regulated in sporozoites but largely down-regulated in merozoites (Hehl et al., 2015).

4.2.3 *CRYPTOSPORIDIUM PARVUM*

Belonging to the phylum Apicomplexa, several parasitic protozoans include *Cryptosporidium (C.) parvum*, a globally distributed zoonotic pathogen known for causing severe watery diarrhoea in both animals and humans, particularly in immunocompromised individuals like those with HIV (Davies and Chalmers, 2009). Classified as a Category B agent in the National Institutes of Health's biodefence programme, *Cryptosporidium* poses significant health risks but has been relatively understudied due to limited tools for genetic analysis, such as reliable culture systems, transfection techniques, and parasite-specific microarrays (O'Connor et al., 2011).

The spread of *Cryptosporidium* occurs through oocysts, highly resilient structures capable of persisting in ecosystems for extended periods, even after exposure to disinfectants like chlorine (Robertson and Gjerde, 2007). Research on the oocyst stage has primarily focused on characterising the composition of the oocyst wall, including the family of oocyst wall proteins (Jenkins et al., 2010). However, the biochemical processes involved in this stage remain poorly understood. Understanding the global gene expression patterns in oocysts could provide insights into the biology and metabolic characteristics of this pathogen, shedding light on how oocysts withstand various stressors and nutrient deprivation in their natural habitats. For instance, *C. parvum* relies solely on glycolysis and fermentation for energy and carbon due to the lack of a citrate cycle and a respiratory chain based on cytochromes (Thompson et al., 2005; Rider and Zhu, 2010). Given their adaptation to anaerobic conditions within the host intestine, understanding how oocysts respond to oxygen-rich environments is crucial, especially considering their exposure to harsh environmental conditions for months or years.

Zhang et al. (2012) developed the first *C. parvum* Agilent microarray (CpArray15K), covering all expected open reading frames (ORFs) in the parasite genome. Using real-time qRT-PCR alongside global transcriptome analysis with CpArray15K, distinct metabolic characteristics in oocysts were identified. High transcript levels of genes associated with ribosome biogenesis, transcription, and translation indicate significant protein synthesis activity in oocysts. The presence of proteasome and ubiquitin-associated components suggests oocysts may utilise protein breakdown pathways to recycle amino acids due to their inability to synthesise them de novo. Notably, lactate dehydrogenase (LDH) emerged as the most highly expressed gene in oocyst energy metabolism (Table 4.2). Additionally, the response of parasites to UV light revealed intricate and dynamic gene expression regulation, with elevated transcript levels of genes involved in intracellular trafficking and DNA

TABLE 4.2

Transcriptome Analysis of *Cryptosporidium parvum* Oocysts

Highly Expressed Genes and Gene ID	Feature Description
Lactate dehydrogenase (LDH)—cgd7_480	Glycolytic enzymes
Predicted extracellular protein—cgd6_780	Predicted membrane proteins
Choline-phosphate cytidylyltransferase—cgd8_1150	Membrane remodelling
Possible apicomplexan-specific protein—cgd2_200	Conserved domain-containing
Nucleoside-diphosphate kinase domain—cgd5_1470	Nucleotide metabolic enzymes
HMG-box protein—cgd2_3070	Methytranferase, DNA-binding
Cyclin—cgd7_3780	Cyclin family protein
Ptc7p phosphatase (PP2C family)—cgd7_4790	Peptidase, kinase, phosphatase
T22E16.120 SC35-like splicing factor—cgd7_940	Methylase, Helicase, RNA-splicing, RNA-binding
Mitochondrial ATP synthase β-chain—cgd2_1360	IscU-like, F-ATPase headpiece
GNog1p. GTPase—cgd4_1700	GTPase, ribonucleoprotein
Putative fucose translocator—cgd3_510	ABC, ion, nutrients, V-type
60S ribosomal protein L37A—cgd3_2250	RPL, RPS, or associated proteins
Glutaredoxin related protein—cgd2_2540	Glutaredoxin/thioredoxin related
20S proteasome beta subunit D2—cgd1_420	Proteosome/ubiquitin subunits
HSP90—cgd3_3770	DnaJ, HSP20, HSP90
Eukaryotic initiation factor 4A—cgd1_880	Translation factors, RNA helicases
Actin—cgd5_3160	Microfilament elements
Cutinase negative acting protein—cgd3_4150	RNA Pol, transcription factors
Mucin-like glycoprotein—cgd2_430	All mucin-like proteins

repair, highlighting the importance of TCP-1 family members and thioredoxin-associated genes in UV-induced damage repair for oocysts (Zhang et al., 2012).

4.2.4 *Trypanosoma Congolense*

African trypanosomes, particularly *Trypanosoma (Tr.) congolense, Tr. brucei*, and *Tr. vivax*, are responsible for causing animal African trypanosomiasis (AAT), commonly known as nagana, which is transmitted by tsetse flies. Among these parasites, *Tr. congolense*, especially of the savannah subtype, is considered one of the most pathogenic species in Africa. The life cycle of *Tr. congolense* alternates between the circulatory system of mammalian hosts, typically cattle, and the tsetse fly vector (Bengaly et al., 2002).

Recent research on variant antigen profiling has enabled the characterisation and quantification of the variable surface glycoproteins (VSG) diversity of each isolate using sequencing data (Pereira et al., 2019). In a study aimed at determining whether the VSG genes of interest exhibit constitutive expression in natural populations of tsetse flies with varying strains and genetic backgrounds, Pereira et al. (2022)

TABLE 4.3

Transcriptomic Profiling of *Trypanosoma congolense* in Tsetse Flies

Genes Encoding Proteins	Up-Regulated Gene (Yes or No)	Down-Regulated Gene (Yes or No)
Hypothetical proteins	Yes	No
Zinc-finger proteins	Yes	No
GTPase-related genes	Yes	No
Histones	Yes	No
Fam50 (brucei alanine-rich proteins)	Yes	No
ESAG2-like (most likely transferrin receptors)	No	Yes
ISG and RHS genes	No	Yes
Adenylate cyclases	No	Yes
Trans-sialidases	No	Yes

investigated the metacyclic VSG expression. They analysed the expressed VSG repertoires by sequencing the transcriptomes of wild tsetse flies from the Shimba Hills National Reserve in Kenya, identifying infections in their mouthparts, and diagnosing *Tr. congolense* infections. Their findings revealed diverse gene expression profiles in trypanosomes from both experimental and natural fly infections, with several genes being expressed differently in bloodstream- and metacyclic-form parasites. Notably, a specific VSG gene from *Tr. congolense* phylotype 8 was found to be expressed at the population level in both bloodstream- and metacyclic-form parasites. Further analysis of the dynamics of metacyclic VSG expression in spontaneous trypanosome infections may identify constitutively expressed or metacyclic-specific VSG genes that could serve as potential targets for vaccine development. Moreover, the discovery of 152 novel putative proteins with differential expression in mouthpart parasites (Table 4.3) suggests the existence of additional undiscovered *Trypanosome* gene functionalities (Pereira et al., 2022).

In a separate study, Peylhard et al. (2023) aimed to identify genes that are differentially expressed in five West African cattle breeds during experimental infection with *Tr. congolense*, along with their biological activities, to gain a better understanding of the biological processes involved in trypanotolerance versus trypanosusceptibility. They employed RNA sequencing to characterise the whole blood genome-wide transcriptome of four different breeds. Regardless of the breed, infection significantly influenced the transcriptome of cattle blood, as anticipated.

4.3 TRANSCRIPTOMIC PROFILING OF HELMINTHS

With the absence of commercial vaccinations against the majority of helminth infections, anthelmintic therapy remains the primary treatment for helminth-related infections in animals. However, in endemic areas, hosts may experience reinfection due to a lack of acquired immunity and the emergence of medication resistance. Thus, there is an urgent need for innovative approaches to combat drug-resistant diseases in humans and manage helminth infections in animals (Kaplan and Vidyashankar, 2012).

The "immuno-omic approach" has played a pivotal role in identifying potential vaccine and diagnostic candidates by leveraging insights into parasite biology gained through systematic comparisons across developmental stages and related parasites (Bennuru et al., 2016). Consequently, the information derived from transcriptome studies of helminths holds promise for the development of novel therapeutic or diagnostic strategies aimed at halting the proliferation and transmission of helminths.

4.3.1 TREMATODES

Recent advancements in various high-throughput omics technologies have facilitated the identification of novel drug and vaccine targets, as well as crucial biomolecules essential to parasite transmission mechanisms. Two high-throughput omics approaches, namely next-generation sequencing (NGS) for gene identification at the nucleotide level and liquid chromatography-mass spectrometry (LC-MS) for protein identification at the peptide level (Figure 4.1), serve as key tools in characterising the characteristic profile of each parasite (Haçarız and Sayers, 2016). Socioeconomically significant fluke species have benefited from a wealth of omics data. For instance, comprehensive insights into transcriptional and genomic diversity have been achieved by combining transcriptomic analyses with genome sequencing and assembly for *S. japonicum* (Liu et al., 2006; Hokke et al., 2007). These datasets, when integrated with omics techniques, enable large-scale screenings of the transcriptome and proteome of *S. japonicum* (Hokke et al., 2007).

Peptidases, a group of enzymes that have undergone significant differentiation within trematodes (McNulty et al., 2017), play crucial roles in various defence and homeostatic mechanisms, including protein metabolism, folding, activation or degradation, tissue remodelling, intracellular signalling, migration, and evasion of immune responses (Kašný et al., 2009; Yang et al., 2015). Previous studies on closely related *Schistosoma* species have revealed that a majority of the proteins produced by their eggs are involved in catalytic activities, particularly proteolysis (Carson et al., 2020). Of note, cysteine peptidases such as cathepsin L, cathepsin B, and legumain have undergone remarkable sequence and functional diversification (Cwiklinski et al., 2015).

Ilgová et al. (2022) conducted a comprehensive investigation into the cysteine cathepsin isoforms present in the transcriptome and proteome of *F. hepatica* eggs. Among the RNA-seq data, 16 out of 17 cysteine cathepsin isoforms were identified. The most highly expressed peptidase transcripts included one isoform of cathepsin B (CB9) and two isoforms of cathepsin L (CL0 and CL1_3a). Across the three embryonic stages of the eggs, RNA-seq analysis revealed the transcription of ten cathepsin L isoforms, five cathepsin B isoforms, and one cathepsin F isoform, as detailed in Table 4.4.

A neglected zoonotic parasite that affects humans, animals, and poultry's gallbladder and bile duct is called *Metorchis (M.) orientalis*. There have been numerous reports of it in Asian countries, such as China, Japan, and Korea, where there may

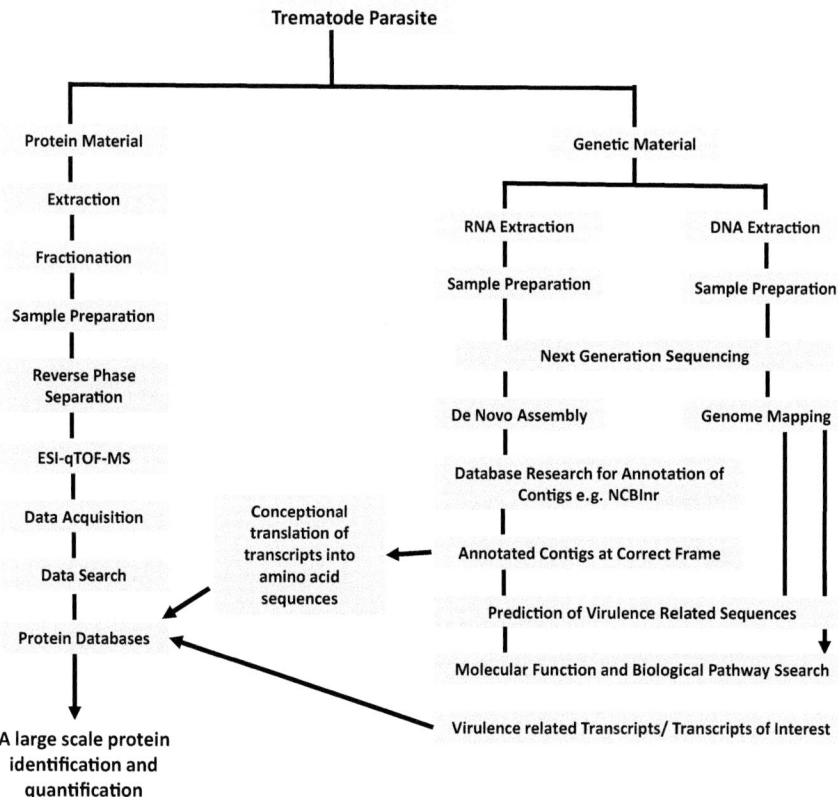

FIGURE 4.1 Flowchart representing the liquid chromatography-mass spectrometry and next-generation sequencing in trematodes.

be a health risk (Saijuntha et al., 2021). There are not many published transcriptome and proteomics data accessible, despite its importance as a pathogen for both humans and animals. In order to examine the gene and protein expression of adult and metacercariae stages of *M. orientalis*, transcriptome Illumina RNA sequencing and label-free protein quantification were used by Gao et al. (2021). Comparative analyses of the transcriptome and proteome revealed that many up-regulated genes in the adult stage were primarily enriched in the actin filament capping, spectrin, and glucose metabolic processes. Whereas, the up-regulated genes in the metacercariae stage were primarily associated with motile cilia, cilium assembly, and cilium movement (Table 4.5).

4.3.2 Nematodes

The phylum nematoda consists of a wide variety of organisms ranging from free-living to parasitic forms. The GI nematodes are the main parasites of veterinary and public health significance (Hotez et al., 2016). It is not easy to say that to cope

TABLE 4.4
Transcriptomics Data of Peptidases Genes Identified at Different Time Points of *Fasciola hepatica* Eggs

Sr. #	Gene ID (TPM)	Expression Level at Time Point
1	Secreted cathepsin L (CL1_3a) (191.84)	T0
2	Signalase 2A (255.07)	
3	**Cathepsin D** (3846.41)	
4	Cathepsin B (CB9) (202.27)	
5	**Cathepsin L (*CL0*)** (1157.89)	
6	Peptidase S1 domain-containing protein (213.41)	
7	**Signalase subunit** (413.73)	
8	Cercarial peptidase (227.85)	
9	**Furin** (265.74)	
10	Ubiquitin carboxyl terminal hydrolase (265.14)	
1	Putative signalase (209.55)	T5
2	**Cathepsin D** (3387.20)	
3	Proteasome subunit α_1 (218.11)	
4	**Cathepsin L (*CL0*)** (963.85)	
5	Furin_1 (232.23)	
6	**Cathepsin B (CB9)** (585.06)	
7	Mov34/MPN/PAD-1 family protein (239.47)	
8	**Signalase subunit** (370.72)	
9	Ubiquitin carboxyl terminal hydrolase (247.31)	
10	**Proteasome subunit β_1** (282.88)	
1	Proteasome subunit β_4 (216.17)	T10
2	**Cathepsin D** (2406.63)	
3	Proteasome subunit α_1 (266.31)	
4	**Cathepsin L (CL0)** (712.57)	
5	Proteasome subunit β_3 (271.71)	
6	**Signalase subunit** (449.44)	
7	Proteasome subunit β_2 (290.20)	
8	**Cathepsin B (*CB9*)** (438.60)	
9	Mov34/MPN/PAD-1 family protein ()	
10	**Proteasome subunit β_1** (349.47)	

*The genes in bold had higher expression at different time points i.e. T0, T5 and T10

with the development of anthelmintic resistance, new drugs against helminths will be developed at an equivalent pace (Geary et al., 2004). Therefore, studies are being focused on the development of vaccines for the persistent mitigation of GI nematodes in humans and livestock populations (Hotez et al., 2016). Analyses of transcriptomic profiling of different nematodes, including *H. contortus*, *Radopholus similis*, and

TABLE 4.5

Transcriptomic Analyses of Adult and Metacercariae Stages of *Metorchis orientalis*

Differentially Expressed Genes	Expression Level	Parasite Life Cycle Stage
Phosphoglycerate mutase	up-regulated	adult stage
Translation initiation factor 3 subunit B	up-regulated	adult stage
Cathepsin F precursor	up-regulated	adult stage
Cytoplasmic 1	up-regulated	metacercariae stage
Serpin	up-regulated	metacercariae stage
Glutamine synthetase	up-regulated	metacercariae stage
Elongation factor 1-gamma	up-regulated	metacercariae stage
Lactate dehydrogenase	up-regulated	metacercariae stage

Ascaris suum, by various technologies result in better knowledge of molecular as well as biochemical pathways associated with the replication, growth, and parasite–host relationship of these nematodes (Jacob et al., 2008; Wang, 2021; Reyes-Guerrero et al., 2023).

Either immunisation through vaccines or in combination with anthelmintic administration may help in minimising the drug resistance development (Lee et al., 2011). However, there are challenges faced in developing vaccines against nematodes, including immunoregulatory capability and complex antigenic variations of these parasites (Hewitson and Maizels, 2014). Barbervax® and Bovilis huskvac® are the only two vaccines available commercially for nematodes *Haemonchus (H.) contortus* (Barber pole worm) and *Dictyocaulus viviparus* (cattle lungworm), respectively. The latter vaccine consists of an irradiated larval form while Barbervax® consists of two protease fractions (H11 and H-gal-GP), gut membrane glycoproteins (Kearney et al., 2016; McKeand, 2000).

As the available vaccine (Barbervax®, registered in Australia) against *H. contortus* nematodes consists of a limited number of protein fractions, the selection of nematodes with alternate sequences or expression of the vaccine candidates is desirable. Sallé et al. (2018) performed a comparison of the transcriptomes of *H. contortus* in two groups of sheep, one as control and the other vaccinated with the Barbervax® vaccine. They found that genes encoding the vaccine antigens showed no change in their expressions procured from vaccinated sheep, while up regulation of other genes encoding lysosome trafficking stimulators and other proteases was observed. In addition, increased expression of lipid deposition was also identified. These factors may compromise the efficiency of the vaccine. Further results of transcriptional analysis of *H. contortus* in response to host vaccination conducted by Sallé et al. (2018) have been summarised in Table 4.6.

Laing et al. (2013) conducted a comprehensive investigation of the draft genome assemblage and massive transcriptomic data for GI nematode, *H. contortus*. This was the first study which reported the genome of *H. contortus* and the massive

TABLE 4.6

Transcriptional Analysis of *Haemonchus contortus* in Response to Host Vaccination

Gene Encoding	Expression Level	Experimental Group
Glycoside hydrolase domain-containing protein	Down-regulated	Adult worms survived post vaccination
Gamma IFN-inducible lysosomal thiol reductase	Down-regulated	Adult worms survived post vaccination
Proteins containing peptidase domains	Up-regulated	Adult worms survived post vaccination
Eptidase inhibitor I4 domain	Up-regulated	Adult worms survived post vaccination
Lys-8 encoding gene	Up-regulated	Adult worms survived post vaccination
Antimicrobial peptide theromacin	Up-regulated	Adult worms survived post vaccination
Proteinase inhibitor	Up-regulated	Adult worms survived post vaccination
Prolyl-carboxypeptidase	Up-regulated	Adult worms survived post vaccination
Genes encoding Barbervax® antigens	No change	Adult worms survived post vaccination

transcriptomic data for this parasite. The genes associated with biochemical and molecular processes related to drug metabolism, blood-sucking, and neurophysiology in nematodes were identified. The whole genome library for known drug candidates was particularly defined, thereby elucidating the mode of action of various drugs against helminths. The transcriptional analysis of *H. contortus* in its different life cycle stages and intestine is given in Table 4.7.

Parkinson et al. (2004) used 265,494 expressed-sequence tag sequences from 30 species, including 28 parasitic organisms, which correspond to 93,645 potential genes, to examine the genome of the phylum nematoda. Proteins from *Caenorhabditis elegans*, which is the model nematode, shared considerable similarities with the identified genes ranging from 35 to 70% in each species, as given in Figure 4.2.

4.3.3 Cestodes

Numerous parasitic flatworms exhibit complex life cycles, characterised by distinct developmental stages finely tuned to their respective hosts. Their genomes encode the genetic information necessary for the formation and maintenance of these diverse life forms, as well as for their metabolic and immune interactions with specific hosts (Martínez-González et al., 2022). Most genera of cestodes have hermaphroditic

TABLE 4.7

Transcriptional Analysis of *Haemonchus contortus* in Its Different Life Cycle Stages and Intestine

Life Cycle Stage/ Intestine	No. of Up-Regulated Genes	Up-Regulated Genes description	No. of Down-Regulated Genes	Down-Regulated Genes Description
Egg	2604	genes encoding: • chromosome organisation • apoptosis • DNA replication • larval and embryo development • oxidoreductase activity • body morphogenesis and development	1295	not reported
L1	1779	Same as observed in eggs	1264	not reported
L2	829	Same as observed in eggs	1584	not reported
L3	2613	genes linked with: • binding of cobalamin (vitamin B12) • heme-binding • acetyl-CoA metabolic process • oxygen transport • cytochrome P450 activity	1121	genes encoding: • motor activity • variety of metabolic processes • myosin complex
L4	1227	genes linked with: • body morphogenesis • myosin complex • variety of metabolic processes • locomotion • response to oxidative stress • collagen development • cuticle development • motor activity • heme-binding genes	3942	heme-binding genes

(Continued)

TABLE 4.7 (CONTINUED)
Transcriptional Analysis of *Haemonchus contortus* in Its Different Life Cycle Stages and Intestine

Life Cycle Stage/ Intestine	No. of Up-Regulated Genes	Up-Regulated Genes description	No. of Down-Regulated Genes	Down-Regulated Genes Description
Adult male	2847	sperm protein genes	1505	genes associated with: • moulting • cuticle development • heme-binding • body morphogenesis • oxidoreductase activity • response to oxidative stress • collagen development
Adult female	1658	genes associated with: • oogenesis • vulval development • germ-line cell cycle switching • genitalia development • embryo development • ovulation • gender-specific development • meiosis regulation	1460	not reported
Gut	654	genes associated with: • cysteine-type peptidase • sugar binding • cobalamin binding • transport of cations • cysteine-type peptidase inhibitor • transport of anions • transport of oligopeptides • oxidoreductase activity • protein kinase	4493	not reported

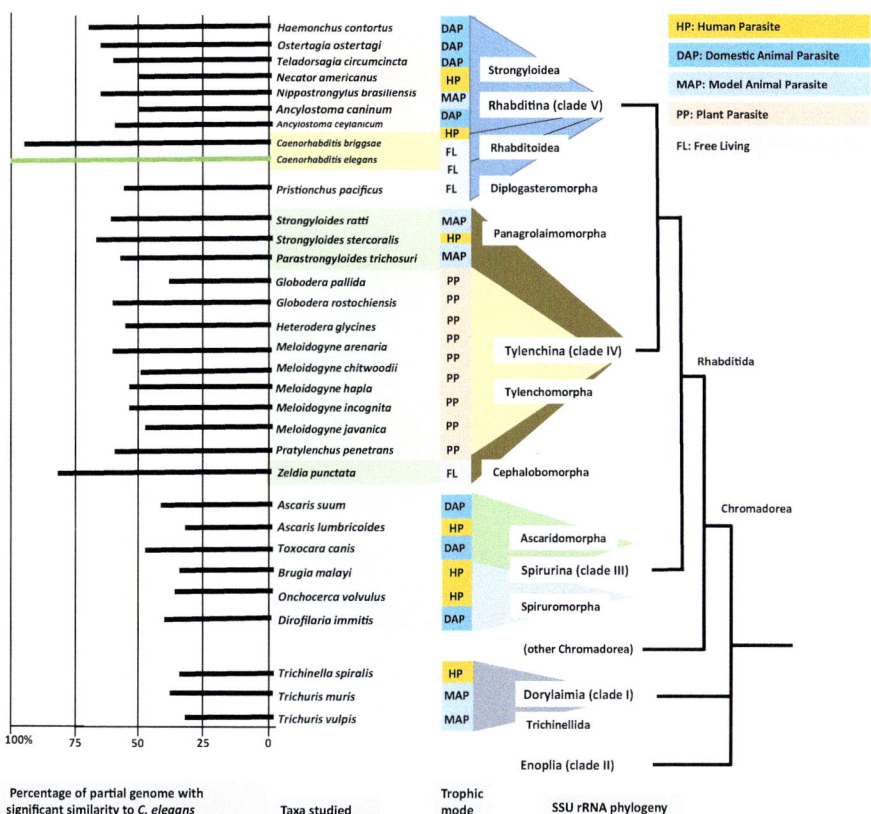

FIGURE 4.2 Expressed-sequence tag sequence representing the phylum nematoda.

adult stages that parasitise the gastrointestinal tract of vertebrate hosts (Benesh et al., 2021).

Zoonotic infections like *Taenia solium*, *Echinococcus multilocularis*, and *Echinococcus granulosus* affect both livestock and humans. Due to their potential to infect humans and the challenges in maintaining their complete life cycles in laboratory conditions, it is crucial to thoroughly investigate the stage-specific adaptations of these parasitic species (Pérez et al., 2019; Shumuye et al., 2021). Genomic and transcriptomic studies have unveiled the transcriptional modifications of these tapeworms, revealing numerous differentially expressed genes and highlighting variations in gene expression across life cycle stages. These studies have identified a plethora of gene families exhibiting differential expression patterns (Basika et al., 2019). Gene families consist of paralogous copies of genes generated through speciation and duplication events (Lallemand et al., 2020).

However, there has been limited research on the genetic factors controlling crucial developmental stages in cestodes, such as strobilation and larval transformation. Bizarro et al. (2005) employed cDNA library subtraction to identify genes with

TABLE 4.8
Transcriptomic Analysis of *Hymenolepis microstoma*

Phase of Life Cycle	Host Type	No. of Genes Expressed (out of 12,371)	No. of Genes Up-Regulated (out of 12,371)	Characterisation of Development
Larval forms	*Tribolium* spp. (beetle)	10,257	2266	differentiation of the principal axis of the body, and nascent nerve muscle formation in cyst forms
Complete adult form	*Mus musculus* (mouse)	10,139	3087	as mentioned in individual regions of the body
Anterior part of body (scolex & neck regions)	*Mus musculus* (mouse)	9564	1052	proliferation of growing segments and proglottids along with nerve, muscle, and excretory systems
Middle region of body	*Mus musculus* (mouse)	10,170	2066	development of the female system and fertilisation
Posterior region of body	*Mus musculus* (mouse)	10,095	1440	embryogenesis as well as ageing of body segments

differential expression in tetrathyridia and adults of *Mesocestoides corti*, predating the development of whole-genome sequencing techniques. Despite the functional characterisation of these transcripts revealing significant variations across samples in various cellular functions, NGS approaches could only uncover a limited number of variables. Olson et al. (2018) identified differentially expressed genes in larval and mature forms, as well as in the anterior, middle, and posterior regions of the strobilar cestode, which roughly correspond to the major developmental stages in the typical cestode life cycle, using whole-genome transcriptome profiling of *Hymenolepis microstoma* (Table 4.8).

4.4 TRANSCRIPTOMIC PROFILING OF ARTHROPODS

Among the arthropods, fleas are blood-feeding insects that act as carriers for a number of microorganisms, i.e. *Yersinia (Y.) pestis*, *Rickettsia (R.) typhi*, *R. felis*, and *Bartonella* spp. (Eisen and Gage, 2012). Fleas play an important role in the spread of the plague-causing pathogen, *Y. pestis*. This pathogen attains a replicative niche in the digestive tract of the flea after ingestion and creates a biofilm that boosts its colonisation and spread. Fleas can naturally control the infection of this pathogen, but the mechanisms involved in this defence are not clearly known. To understand the mechanism involved in fleas in clearing themselves of this pathogen, a study was performed on the transcriptomic profiling of the gut of *Xenopsylla (X.) cheopis*,which were divided into three groups: one which received sterile blood, a second which ingested *Y. pestis* infected blood and third that was fed no blood for five days. On analysis of the transcripts, 11 unknown and 23 annotated transcripts were identified, which were correlated with the response of the *X. cheopis* digestive tract to the *Y. pestis* infection. It was found that the initial immune response of the rat flea was based on the synthesis of antimicrobial peptides adjusted by the immune-deficiency pathway. The rest of the transcripts observed in response to infection were not linked to immune response and were associated with physiological operations including the synthesis of chitin-binding proteins, alteration of digestion, and modification in response to chemical stimuli and digestive tract peristalsis (Bland et al., 2020).

Myiasis is the condition developed due to the infestation of fly larvae on the live human or animal host (Francesconi and Lupi, 2012). *Wohlfahrtia (W.) magnifica* is an obligatory parasite that belongs to order Diptera and family Sarcophagidae. It causes myiasis in mammals in many Asian, African, and European countries (Gaglio et al., 2011). Adult female flies lay larvae (first stage) on the open wounds or natural orifices in the body of the host, and from this point, these larvae settle on the tissues of the host and obtain nutrition for their growth and development. This traumatic myiasis may result in serious health concerns, welfare issues, and heavy financial losses. To present, available knowledge about the molecular processes responsible for myiasis due to *W. magnifica* is very limited (Liu et al., 2022).

A study was conducted on myiasis due to *W. magnifica* in Bactrian camels to investigate the transcriptomic profiling of various life cycle stages of the flies with a particular focus on identifying the gene families involved in causing myiasis in wounds. Almost 2049 excretory/secretory (ES) proteins were found to be linked with metabolic mechanisms, defensive response, peptidase activity, and cuticle formation. During first-stage larvae, it was observed that genes related to RNA transcription and translation, peptidase activity, and cuticle formation were up-regulated. In addition, genes related to nutrient reservoir activity and peptidase inhibition were up-regulated during third-stage larvae, while in adult flies up-regulated genes were related to adult behaviour and light sensitivity. Analysis of myiasis-related genes in larvae procured from the wounds showed that among the up-regulated genes, heat shock protein genes, cuticle protein genes, and peptidase genes were 21, 110, and 88 genes, respectively. Furthermore, in the parasitic fly larvae, diptericin and defensin genes among two antimicrobial peptide genes were also found to be up-regulated (Jia et al., 2024).

Forensic entomology has crucial significance in evaluating the minimal post-mortem interval in criminal inquiries. For an accurate assessment of the minimal postmortem interval, it is mandatory to recognise the species and life cycle stage of insects in dead animals (Brown et al., 2015). Some of the flies belonging to the order Diptera are lured towards the corpses of animals. *Sarcophaga (Sa.) peregrina* has been found at various death scenes and in insect studies (Wang et al., 2017).

The genome data of *Sa. peregrina* have not been extensively defined, despite its significance for forensic purposes. Thus, in order to better understand the *Sa. peregrina* transcriptome, RNA sequencing was used in a study to create an extensive gene expression dataset and then perform *de novo* assembly. Two different methods were used to obtain accurate sequencing data for RNA transcripts. Consequently, the Illumina MiSeq and PacBio RS II Iso-seq sequencing applications yielded 26,580,352 and 83,221 raw reads, respectively. About 55,730 contigs have been accurately annotated from these readings. The resulting *Sa. peregrina* genome information is presented in this work (Kim et al., 2018).

Ticks are blood-sucking arthropods having great veterinary and public health significance (de La Fuente et al., 2008). Ticks act as vectors of various deadly pathogens, including protozoans, bacteria, and viruses (Brites-Neto et al., 2015). Tick-borne infections have increased in prevalence over the last few years due to the new establishment of tick habitats because of climate change and anthropogenic activities like urbanisation, international animal migration, and deforestation, etc. (Gray et al., 2009). The ixodid ticks strongly stick to their hosts due to their chelicerae, which is inserted deep into the skin to aid in feeding through hypostomes (Pham et al., 2021). This activity of ticks leads to the rupturing of small vessels causing haemorrhagic lesions (Aounallah et al., 2020).

Ticks protect themselves from the host's hemostatic, immunological, and inflammatory reactions with the help of salivary gland substances (Pham et al., 2021). Additionally, the tick midgut is essential to hematophagy. It also plays a role in controlling the storage and digestion of blood meals as well as guarding against diseases from pathogens and host immunity (Oleaga et al., 2017). The complex nature of tick mialomes (midgut transcriptomes) and tick sialomes (salivary gland transcriptomes), which encode for disintegrins, histamine-binding proteins, protease inhibitors, and a number of other proteins related to ticks, was discovered by earlier transcriptomic investigations (Kotsyfakis et al., 2015; Chmelař et al., 2016). It has been shown in numerous studies that mammals that are repeatedly bitten by ticks develop immunity to tick bites. Therefore, it is crucial to understand how tick mialomes and sialomes react to resistant hosts since this information might be used to create new tick control tactics and applications.

In a study, the variations in gene expression in the midguts and the salivary glands of mature female ticks were observed following the recurrent natural tick bites in a lab environment. The rabbits underwent two infestations: a first infestation (where they fed on an unsuspecting host) and a subsequent infestation where the subjects were introduced to different ticks. To lessen genetic heterogeneity between individual ticks, single salivary glands and midguts dissected from adult pathogen-free female *Ixodes (I.) ricinus* siblings were used. Through thorough examination of 88 RNA-seq datasets, excellent annotations of sialomes and mialomes from individual ticks were performed. Based on the data, up to 3000 potential differentially expressed genes were found (Medina et al., 2022).

With the passage of time, resistance against the acaricides, the resistance has emerged through metabolic detoxification in ticks due to the excessive use of these acaricides to control ticks (Vudriko et al., 2018). Therefore, recognition of the genes responsible for metabolic detoxification is very necessary to mark the precise drug targets and to devise effective tick control strategies. In a study, using RNA sequencing, detoxifying genes were identified which were expressed as a result of being exposed to acaricide in both amitraz-treated and untreated *Rhipicephalus* (*Boophilus*) *annulatus*. The data were subsequently assembled into contigs and clustered into 50,591 and 71,711 uni-gene sequences, respectively. In *Rhipicephalus* (*Boophilus*) *annulatus*, the detoxification gene expression levels were found to be elevated (16,635 transcripts) and down-regulated (15,539 transcripts) at distinct stages of development. Seventy detoxification genes were found to be significantly expressed in response to the amitraz therapy, according to the annotations of the differentially expressed genes expressed differentially (Achuthkumar et al., 2023).

4.5 CONCLUSION

Transcriptomic profiling has revolutionised our understanding of parasitology by providing invaluable insights into the molecular and biochemical pathways governing the replication, growth, and interactions between parasites and their hosts. Through the analysis of transcriptomic data from various protozoa, helminths, and arthropods, significant progress has been made in unravelling the complexities of parasite biology. Studies on protozoa such as *Eimeria brunetti* and *Leishmania donovani* have shed light on the mechanisms underlying parasite replication and host interaction. Similarly, investigations into helminths like *Haemonchus contortus* and *Ascaris suum* have elucidated crucial molecular pathways involved in parasite growth and survival. Transcriptomic profiling of trematodes including *Clonorchis sinensis*, *Schistosoma mansoni*, and *Schistosoma japonicum* has provided valuable insights into the host-parasite relationship and pathogenesis of parasitic infections. Furthermore, model systems like *Rhipicephalus* (*Boophilus*) *annulatus* and *Xenopsylla (X.) cheopis* have been instrumental in establishing genomic resources and techniques for studying gene expression in arthropods. These studies have expanded our understanding of the fundamental biology of parasites and their intricate interactions with hosts. Overall, transcriptomic profiling has emerged as a powerful tool in parasitology, offering new perspectives on previously challenging questions and advancing our knowledge of protozoans, helminths, and arthropods. By deciphering the complex interplay between parasites and their hosts at the molecular level, transcriptomic studies pave the way for developing innovative therapeutic strategies and interventions to combat parasitic diseases effectively.

REFERENCES

Aarthi, S., Raj, G.D., Raman, M., Blake, D., Subramaniam, C. *et al.* (2011) Expressed sequence tags from *Eimeria brunetti*—preliminary analysis and functional annotation. *Parasitology Research*, 108, 1059–1062.

Achuthkumar, A., Uchamballi, S., Arvind, K., Vasu, D.A., Varghese, S. *et al.* (2023) Transcriptome profiling of *Rhipicephalus annulatus* reveals differential gene expression of metabolic detoxifying enzymes in response to acaricide treatment. *Biomedicines*, 11(5), 1369.

Akoniyon, O.P., Adewumi, T.S., Maharaj, L., Oyegoke, O.O., Roux, A. *et al.* (2022) Whole genome sequencing contributions and challenges in disease reduction focused on malaria. *Biology*, 11(4), 587.

Ankarklev, J., Franzén, O., Peirasmaki, D., Jerlström-Hultqvist, J., Lebbad, M. *et al.* (2015) Comparative genomic analyses of freshly isolated *Giardia* intestinalis assemblage A isolates. *BMC Genomics*, 16, 697.

Aounallah, H., Bensaoud, C., M'ghirbi, Y., Faria, F., Chmelař, J. *et al.* (2020) Tick salivary compounds for targeted immunomodulatory therapy. *Frontiers in Immunology*, 11, 583845.

Barash, N.R., Nosala, C., Pham, J.K., McInally, S.G., Gourguechon, S. *et al.* (2017) *Giardia* colonizes and encysts in high-density foci in the murine small intestine. *MSphere*, 2(3), 10–1128.

Basika, T., Paludo, G.P., Araujo, F.M., Salim, A.C., Pais, F. *et al.* (2019) Transcriptomic profile of two developmental stages of the cestode parasite *Mesocestoides corti*. *Molecular and Biochemical Parasitology*, 229, 35–46.

Benesh, D.P., Parker, G. and Chubb, J.C. (2021) Life-cycle complexity in helminths: what are the benefits?. *Evolution*, 75(8), 1936–1952.

Bengaly, Z., Sidibé, I., Ganaba, R., Desquesnes, M., Boly, H. *et al.* (2002) Comparative pathogenicity of three genetically distinct types of *Trypanosoma congolense* in cattle: clinical observations and haematological changes. *Veterinary Parasitology*, 108(1), 1–19.

Bennuru, S., Cotton, J.A., Ribeiro, J.M., Grote, A., Harsha, B. *et al.* (2016) Stage-specific transcriptome and proteome analyses of the filarial parasite *Onchocerca volvulus* and its Wolbachia endosymbiont. *mBio* 7, e02028-16.

Bizarro, C.V., Bengtson, M.H., Ricachenevsky, F.K., Zaha, A., Sogayar, M.C. and Ferreira, H.B. (2005) Differentially expressed sequences from acestode parasite reveals conserved developmental genes in platyhelminthes. *Molecular Biochemistry in Parasitology*, 144(1), 114–118.

Bland, D.M., Martens, C.A., Virtaneva, K., Kanakabandi, K., Long, D. *et al.* (2020) Transcriptomic profiling of the digestive tract of the rat flea, *Xenopsylla cheopis*, following blood feeding and infection with *Yersinia pestis*. *PLoS Neglected Tropical Diseases*, 14(9), e0008688.

Brites-Neto, J., Duarte, K.M.R. and Martins, T.F. (2015) Tick-borne infections in human and animal population worldwide. *Veterinary World*, 8, 301.

Brown, K., Thorne, A. and Harvey, M. (2015) *Calliphora vicina* (Diptera: Calliphoridae) pupae: a timeline of external morphological development and a new age and PMI estimation tool. *International Journal of Legal Medicine*, 129, 835–850.

Carson, J.P., Robinson, M.W., Hsieh, M.H., Cody, J., Le, L., You, H., McManus, D.P., Gobert, G.N. (2020) A comparative proteomics analysis of the egg secretions of three major schistosome species. *Molecular and Biochemical Parasitology*, 240, 111322.

Chelomina, G.N. (2017) Genomics and transcriptomics of the Chinese liver fluke *Clonorchis sinensis* (Opisthorchiidae, Trematoda). *Molecular Biology*, 51, 184–193.

Chmelař, J., Kotál, J., Karim, S., Kopacek, P. and Francischetti, I.M. (2016) Sialomes and mialomes: a systems-biology view of tick tissues and tick–host interactions. *Trends in Parasitology*, 32(3), 242–254.

Christiansen, C. (2022). *A novel in vitro model for mature Toxoplasma gondii tissue cysts allows functional characterization of bradyzoite biology.* Humboldt Universitaet zu Berlin (Germany).

Chung, M., Bruno, V.M., Rasko, D.A., Cuomo, C.A., Muñoz, J.F. *et al.* (2021) Best practices on the differential expression analysis of multi-species RNA-seq. *Genome Biology*, 22(1), 1–23.

Coghlan, A., Tyagi, R., Cotton, J.A., Holroyd, N., Rosa, B.A. *et al.* (2019) Comparative genomics of the major parasitic worms. *Nature Genetics*, 51, 163–174.

Cwiklinski, K., Dalton, J.P., Dufresne, P.J., La Course, J., Williams, D.J. *et al.* (2015) The *Fasciola hepatica* genome: gene duplication and polymorphism reveals adaptation to the host environment and the capacity for rapid evolution. *Genome Biology*, 16, 1–13.

Davies, A.P. and Chalmers, R.M. (2009) Cryptosporidiosis. *BMJ*, 339, b4168.

de La Fuente, J., Estrada-Pena, A., Venzal, J.M., Kocan, K.M. and Sonenshine, D.E. (2008) Overview: Ticks as vectors of pathogens that cause disease in humans and animals. *Frontiers in Bioscience,* 13, 6938–6946.

Deitsch, K.W., Lukehart, S.A. and Stringer, J.R. (2009) Common strategies for antigenic variation by bacterial, fungal and protozoan pathogens. *Nature Reviews Microbiology*, 7(7), 493–503.

Dubey, J.P. (2020) The history and life cycle of *Toxoplasma gondii*. In *Toxoplasma gondii* (pp. 1–19). Academic Press.

Ebneter, J.A., Heusser, S.D., Schraner, E.M., Hehl, A.B. and Faso, C. (2016) Cyst-wall-protein-1 is fundamental for Golgi-like organelle neogenesis and cyst-wall biosynthesis in *Giardia lamblia*. *Nature Communication*, 15(7), 13859.

Eisen, R.J. and Gage, K.L. (2012) Transmission of flea-borne zoonotic agents. *Annual Review of Entomology*, 57, 61–82.

Fink, M.Y., Shapiro, D. and Singer, S.M. (2020) *Giardia lamblia*: laboratory maintenance, lifecycle induction, and infection of murine models. *Current Protocols in Microbiology*, 57(1), e102.

Francesconi, F. and Lupi, O. (2012) Myiasis. *Clinical Microbioliology Reviews,* 25(1), 79–105.

Gaglio, G., Brianti, E., Abbene, S. and Giannetto, S. (2011) Genital myiasis by *Wohlfahrtia magnifica* (Diptera, Sarcophagidae) in Sicily (Italy). *Parasitology Research,* 109, 1471–1474.

Gao, J.F., Lv, Q.B., Mao, R.F., Sun, Y.Y., Chen, Y.Y. *et al.* (2021) Integrative transcriptomics and proteomics analyses to reveal the developmental regulation of *Metorchis orientalis*: a neglected trematode with potential carcinogenic implications. *Frontiers in Cell Infection and Microbiology*, 11, 783662.

Geary, T.G., Conder, G.A. and Bishop, B. (2004) The changing landscape of antiparasitic drug discovery for veterinary medicine. *Trends in Parasitology*, 20(10), 449–455.

Gray, J.S., Dautel, H., Estrada-Peña, A., Kahl, O. and Lindgren, E. (2009) Effects of climate change on ticks and tick-borne diseases in Europe. *Interdisciplinary Perspectives on Infectious Diseases*, 2009, 593232.

Gupta, N. and Verma, V.K. (2019) Next-generation sequencing and its application: empowering in public health beyond reality. *Microbial Technology for the Welfare of Society*, 313–341.

Haçarız, O. and Sayers, G.P. (2016) The omic approach to parasitic trematode research—a review of techniques and developments within the past 5 years. *Parasitology Research,* 115, 2523–2543.

Hakimi, M.A., Olias, P. and Sibley, L.D. (2017) *Toxoplasma* effectors targeting host signaling and transcription. *Clinical Microbiology Reviews*, 30(3), 615–645.

He, H., Brenier-Pinchart, M.P., Braun, L., Kraut, A., Touquet, B. *et al.* (2018) Characterization of a *Toxoplasma* effector uncovers an alternative GSK3/β-catenin-regulatory pathway of inflammation. *Elife*, 7, e39887.

Hehl, A.B., Basso, W.U., Lippuner, C., Ramakrishnan, C., Okoniewski, M. *et al.* (2015) Asexual expansion of *Toxoplasma gondii* merozoites is distinct from tachyzoites and entails expression of non-overlapping gene families to attach, invade, and replicate within feline enterocytes. *BMC Genomics*, 16(1), 1–16.

Hewitson, J.P. and Maizels, R.M. (2014) Vaccination against helminth parasite infections. *Expert Review of Vaccines*, 13(4), 473–487.

Hokke, C.H., Fitzpatrick, J.M. and Hoffmann, K.F. (2007) Integrating transcriptome, proteome and glycome analyses of *Schistosoma* biology. *Trends in Parasitology*, 23(4), 165–174.

Hotez, P.J., Strych, U., Lustigman, S. and Bottazzi, M.E. (2016) Human anthelminthic vaccines: rationale and challenges. *Vaccine*, 34(30), 3549–3555.

Hu, R.S., He, J.J., Elsheikha, H.M., Zou, Y., Ehsan, M. *et al.* (2020) Transcriptomic profiling of mouse brain during acute and chronic infections by *Toxoplasma gondii* oocysts. *Frontiers in Microbiology*, 11, 570903.

Ilgová, J., Vorel, J., Roudnický, P., Škorpíková, L., Horn, M. and Kašný, M. (2022) Transcriptomic and proteomic profiling of peptidase expression in *Fasciola hepatica* eggs developing at host's body temperature. *Scientific Reports*, 12(1), 10308.

Jacob, J., Mitreva, M., Vanholme, B. and Gheysen, G. (2008) Exploring the transcriptome of the burrowing nematode *Radopholus similis*. *Molecular Genetics and Genomics*, 280, 1–17.

Jenkins, M.B., Eaglesham, B.S., Anthony, L.C., Kachlany, S.C., Bowman, D.D. *et al.* (2010) Significance of wall structure, macromolecular composition, and surface polymers to the survival and transport of *Cryptosporidium parvum* oocysts. *Applied and Environmental Microbiology*, 76(6), 1926–1934.

Jia, Z., Hasi, S., Zhan, D., Vogl, C. and Burger, P.A. (2024) Transcriptomic profiling of different developmental stages reveals parasitic strategies of *Wohlfahrtia magnifica*, a myiasis-causing flesh fly. *BMC Genomics*, 25(1), 111.

Kaplan, R.M. and Vidyashankar, A.N. (2012) An inconvenient truth: global worming and anthelmintic resistance. *Veterinary Parasitology*, 186(1–2), 70–78.

Kašný, M., Mikeš, L., Hampl, V., Dvořák, J., Caffrey, C.R. *et al.* (2009) Peptidases of trematodes. *Advances in Parasitology*, 69, 205–297.

Kearney, P.E., Murray, P.J., Hoy, J.M., Hohenhaus, M. and Kotze, A. (2016) The 'Toolbox'of strategies for managing *Haemonchus contortus* in goats: what's in and what's out. *Veterinary Parasitology*, 220, 93–107.

Kim, J.Y., Lim, H.Y., Shin, S.E., Cha, H.K., Seo, J.H. *et al.* (2018) Comprehensive transcriptome analysis of *Sarcophaga peregrina*, a forensically important fly species. *Scientific Data*, 5, 180220.

Kim, J.Y. and Park, S.J. (2019) Role of gamma-giardin in ventral disc formation of *Giardia lamblia*. *Parasites Vectors*, 12, 227.

Kotsyfakis, M., Schwarz, A., Erhart, J. and Ribeiro, J.M. (2015) Tissue-and time-dependent transcription in *Ixodes ricinus* salivary glands and midguts when blood feeding on the vertebrate host. *Scientific Reports*, 5(1), 9103.

Krücken, J., Fraundorfer, K., Mugisha, J.C., Ramünke, S., Sifft, K.C. *et al.* (2017) Reduced efficacy of albendazole against Ascaris lumbricoides in Rwandan schoolchildren. *International Journal for Parasitology: Drugs and Drug Resistance*, 7(3), 262–271.

Kulski, J.K. (2016) Next-generation sequencing—an overview of the history, tools, and "Omic" applications. *Next Generation Sequencing-Advances, Applications and Challenges*, 10, 61964.

Laing, R., Kikuchi, T., Martinelli, A., Tsai, I.J., Beech, R.N. *et al.* (2013) The genome and transcriptome of *Haemonchus contortus*, a key model parasite for drug and vaccine discovery. *Genome Biology,* 14, R88.

Lallemand, T., Leduc, M., Landès, C., Rizzon, C. and Lerat, E. (2020) An overview of duplicated gene detection methods: why the duplication mechanism has to be accounted for in their choice. *Genes*, 11(9), 1046.

Lee, B.Y., Bacon, K.M., Bailey, R., Wiringa, A.E. and Smith K.J. (2011) The potential economic value of a hookworm vaccine. *Vaccine*, 29(6), 1201–1210.

Lin, R., Lü, G., Wang, J., Zhang, C., Xie, W. *et al.* (2011) Time course of gene expression profiling in the liver of experimental mice infected with *Echinococcus multilocularis*. *PloS One*, 6(1), e14557.

Liu, F., Lu, J., Hu, W., Wang, S.Y., Cui, S.J. *et al.* (2006) New perspectives on host-parasite interplay by comparative transcriptomic and proteomic analyses of *Schistosoma japonicum*. *PLoS Pathogens*, 2(4), e29.

Liu, J., Hou, B., Wuen, J., Jiang, N. and Gao, T. (2022) Epidemiological investigation on genital myiasis of bactrian camels in parts of Inner Mongolia, China. *Journal of Camel Practice and Research,* 29, 229–235.

Martínez-González, J.D.J., Guevara-Flores, A. and del Arenal Mena, I.P. (2022) Evolutionary adaptations of parasitic flatworms to different oxygen tensions. *Antioxidants*, 11(6), 1102.

McKeand, J.B. (2000) Vaccine development and diagnostics of *Dictyocaulus viviparus*. *Parasitology*, 120(7), 17–23.

McKellar, Q.A. and Jackson, F. (2004) Veterinary anthelmintics: old and new. *Trends in Parasitology*, 20(10), 456–461.

McNulty, S.N., Tort, J.F., Rinaldi, G., Fischer, K., Rosa, B.A. *et al.* (2017) Genomes of Fasciola hepatica from the Americas reveal colonization with *Neorickettsia endobacteria* related to the agents of Potomac horse and human Sennetsu fevers. *PLoS Genetics*, 13(1), e1006537.

Medina, J.M., Jmel, M.A., Cuveele, B., Gómez-Martín, C., Aparicio-Puerta, E. *et al.* (2022) Transcriptomic analysis of the tick midgut and salivary gland responses upon repeated blood-feeding on a vertebrate host. *Frontier Cell Infection and Microbiology*, 12, 919786.

Menard, K.L., Haskins, B.E. and Denkers, E.Y. (2019) Impact of *Toxoplasma gondii* infection on host non-coding RNA responses. *Frontiers in Cellular and Infection Microbiology*, 9, 132.

Nagaraj, S.H., Deshpande, N., Gasser, R.B. and Ranganathan, S. (2007) ESTExplorer: an expressed sequence tag (EST) assembly and annotation platform. *Nucleic Acids Research*, 35, 143–147.

Nosala, C. and Dawson, S.C. (2015) The critical role of the cytoskeleton in the pathogenesis of giardia. *Current Clinical Microbiology Reports*, 2, 155–162.

O'connor, R.M., Shaffie, R., Kang, G. and Ward, H.D. (2011) Cryptosporidiosis in patients with HIV/AIDS. *Aids*, 25(5), 549–560.

Oleaga, A., Obolo-Mvoulouga, P., Manzano-Román, R. and Pérez-Sánchez, R. (2017) Functional annotation and analysis of the *Ornithodoros moubata* midgut genes differentially expressed after blood feeding. *Ticks and Tick-borne Diseases*, 8(5), 693–708.

Olson, P.D., Zarowiecki, M., James, K., Baillie, A., Bartl, G., Burchell, P., Chellappoo, A., Jarero, F., Tan, L.Y., Holroyd, N. and Berriman, M. (2018) Genome-wide transcriptome profiling and spatial expression analyses identify signals and switches of development in tapeworms. *EvoDevo*, 9, 1–29.

Parkinson, J., Mitreva, M., Whitton, C., Thomson, M., Daub, J. *et al.* (2004) A transcriptomic analysis of the phylum Nematoda. *Nature Genetics*, 36(12), 1259–1267.

Pereira, S.S., Heap, J., Jones, A.R. and Jackson, A.P. (2019) VAPPER: High-throughput variant antigen profiling in African trypanosomes of livestock. *Gigascience*, 8(9), giz091.

Pereira, S.S., Jackson, A.P. and Figueiredo, L.M. (2022) Evolution of the variant surface glycoprotein family in African trypanosomes. *Trends in Parasitology*, 38(1), 23–36.

Pérez, M.G., Spiliotis, M., Rego, N., Macchiaroli, N., Kamenetzky, L. *et al.* (2019) Deciphering the role of miR-71 in *Echinococcus multilocularis* early development in vitro. *PLoS Neglected Tropical Diseases*, 13(12), e0007932.

Peylhard, M., Berthier, D., Dayo, G.K., Chantal, I., Sylla, S. *et al.* (2023) Whole blood transcriptome profiles of trypanotolerant and trypanosusceptible cattle highlight a differential modulation of metabolism and immune response during infection by *Trypanosoma congolense*. *Peer Community Journal*, 3, e17.

Pham, J.K., Nosala, C., Scott, E.Y., Nguyen, K.F., Hagen, K.D. *et al.* (2017) Transcriptomic profiling of high-density *Giardia foci* encysting in the murine proximal intestine. *Frontiers in Cellular and Infection Microbiology*, 7, 227.

Pham, M., Underwood, J. and Oliva Chávez, A.S. (2021) Changing the recipe: pathogen directed changes in tick saliva components. *International Journal of Environmental Research and Public Health*, 18(4), 1806.

Poran, A., Nötzel, C., Aly, O., Mencia-Trinchant, N., Harris, C.T. *et al.* (2017) Single-cell RNA sequencing reveals a signature of sexual commitment in malaria parasites. *Nature*, 551(7678), 95–99.

Raetz, M., Kibardin, A., Sturge, C.R., Pifer, R., Li, H. *et al.* (2013) Cooperation of TLR12 and TLR11 in the IRF8-dependent IL-12 response to *Toxoplasma gondii* profilin. *Journal Immunology,* 191, 4818–4827.

Reid, A.J., Talman, A.M., Bennett, H.M., Gomes, A.R., Sanders, M.J. *et al.* (2018) Single-cell RNA-seq reveals hidden transcriptional variation in malaria parasites. *Elife*, 7, e33105.

Reyes-Guerrero, D.E., Jiménez-Jacinto, V., Alonso-Morales, R.A., Alonso-Díaz, M.Á., Maza-Lopez, J. *et al.* (2023) Assembly and analysis of *Haemonchus contortus* transcriptome as a tool for the knowledge of ivermectin resistance mechanisms. *Pathogens*, 12(3), 499.

Rider Jr, S.D. and Zhu, G. (2010) Cryptosporidium: genomic and biochemical features. *Experimental Parasitology*, 124(1), pp. 2–9.

Robertson, L.J. and Gjerde, B.K. (2007) *Cryptosporidium* oocysts: challenging adversaries?. *Trends in Parasitology*, 23(8), 344–347.

Rosowski, E.E., Lu, D., Julien, L., Rodda, L., Gaiser, R.A. *et al.* (2011) Strain-specific activation of the NF-κB pathway by GRA15, a novel *Toxoplasma gondii* dense granule protein. *Journal of Experimental Medicine*, 208(1), 195–212.

Saijuntha, W., Sithithaworn, P., Petney, T.N. and Andrews, R.H. (2021) Foodborne zoonotic parasites of the family Opisthorchiidae. *Research in Veterinary Science,* 135, 404–411.

Sallé, G., Laing, R., Cotton, J.A., Maitland, K., Martinelli, A. *et al.* (2018) Transcriptomic profiling of nematode parasites surviving vaccine exposure. *International Journal for Parasitology*, 48(5), 395–402.

Sasai, M., Pradipta, A. and Yamamoto, M. (2018) Host immune responses to *Toxoplasma gondii*. *International Immunology,* 30, 113–119.

Shendure, J. and Ji, H. (2008) Next-generation DNA sequencing. *Nature Biotechnology*, 26, 1135–1145.

Shumuye, N.A., Ohiolei, J.A., Gebremedhin, M.B., Yan, H.B., Li, L. *et al.* (2021) A systematic review and meta-analysis on prevalence and distribution of *Taenia* and *Echinococcus* infections in Ethiopia. *Parasites & Vectors*, 14, 1–22.

Stacer, A.C., Nyati, S., Moudgil, P., Iyengar, R., Luker, K.E. *et al.* (2013) NanoLuc reporter for dual luciferase imaging in living animals. *Molecular Imaging,* 12, 1–13.

Svensson, V., Natarajan, K.N., Ly, L.H., Miragaia, R.J., Labalette, C. *et al.* (2017) Power analysis of single-cell RNA-sequencing experiments. *Nature Methods*, 14(4), 381–387.

Svensson, V., Vento-Tormo, R. and Teichmann, S.A. (2018) Exponential scaling of single-cell RNA-seq in the past decade. *Nature Protocols*, 13(4), 599–604.

Thompson, R.A., Olson, M.E., Zhu, G., Enomoto, S., Abrahamsen, M.S. *et al.* (2005) *Cryptosporidium* and cryptosporidiosis. *Advances in Parasitology*, 59, 77–158.

Tong, W.H., Pavey, C., O'Handley, R. and Vyas, A. (2021) Behavioral biology of *Toxoplasma gondii* infection. *Parasites & Vectors,* 14, 1–6.

Vudriko, P., Okwee-Acai, J., Byaruhanga, J., Tayebwa, D.S., Omara, R., Muhindo, J.B., Lagu, C., Umemiya-Shirafuji, R., Xuan, X., Suzuki, H. (2018) Evidence-based tick acaricide resistance intervention strategy in Uganda: Concept and feedback of farmers and stakeholders. *Ticks and Tick-borne Diseases*, 9(2), 254–265.

Wang, J. (2021) Genomics of the parasitic nematode Ascaris and its relatives. *Genes*, 12(4), 493.

Wang, Y., Ma, M.Y., Jiang, X.Y., Wang, J.F., Li, L. *et al.* (2017) Insect succession on remains of human and animals in Shenzhen, China. *Forensic Science International*, 271, 75–86.

Witmer, K., Dahalan, F.A., Metcalf, T., Talman, A.M. and Howick, V.M. (2021) Using scRNA-seq to identify transcriptional variation in the malaria parasite ookinete stage. *Frontier in Cell Infection and Microbiology*, 11, 604129.

Yang, Y., jun Wen, Y., Cai, Y.N., Vallée, I., Boireau, P. *et al.* (2015) Serine proteases of parasitic helminths. *The Korean Journal of Parasitology*, 53(1), 1.

Yarovinsky, F. (2014) Innate immunity to *Toxoplasma gondii* infection. *Nature Reviews Immunology,* 14, 109–121.

Zhang, H., Guo, F., Zhou, H. and Zhu, G. (2012) Transcriptome analysis reveals unique metabolic features in the *Cryptosporidium parvum* Oocysts associated with environmental survival and stresses. *BMC Genomics,* 13, 1–15.

Ziegenhain, C., Vieth, B., Parekh, S., Reinius, B., Guillaumet-Adkins, A. *et al.* (2017) Comparative analysis of single-cell RNA sequencing methods. *Molecular Cell*, 65(4), 631–643.

5 Proteomics and Metabolomics in Parasitic Research

Mahvish Maqbool[1,2], Muhammad Usman Mazhar[3], Saadiya Zia[4], Hizqeel Ahmed Muzaffar[5], and Asim Shamim[6]

[1]Department of Parasitology, Faculty of Veterinary Science, University of Agriculture, Faisalabad, Pakistan

[2]College of Agricultural and Life Sciences, Virginia Tech, Blacksburg, Virginia, USA

[3]Senior Scientist, Animal Sciences Division, National Institute of Animal Biotechnology, Faisalabad, Pakistan

[4]Department of Biochemistry, University of Agriculture, Faisalabad, Pakistan

[5]Faculty of Veterinary Sciences, KBCMA College of Veterinary and Animal Sciences, Narowal, Sub-campus University of Veterinary and Animal Sciences, Lahore, Pakistan

[6]Department Veterinary Parasitology, Faculty of Veterinary and Animal Sciences, University of the Poonch Rawalakot, Azad Kashmir, Pakistan

5.1 INTRODUCTION

Parasitic diseases pose a significant global health challenge, affecting billions of people and animals worldwide. Parasitic diseases have a significant impact on human health and the livestock sector, leading to a reduction in productivity and increased mortality (Nahed-Toral et al., 2003; Ekong et al., 2012). Livestock parasitism also causes economic loss and hinders the efficiency of the agricultural sector (Hesterberg et al., 2007). The estimated loss caused by parasites is reported to be $7107.97 million (Grisi et al., 2014). Extensive use of anthelmintic drugs has raised concerns related to environmental contamination and resistance (Lin et al., 2020). Globally about 3.5 billion people are infected by parasites, resulting in 450 million morbidities (Abdullah et al., 2016; Isaac et al., 2019). Prevention and control of parasitic diseases are important for the well-being and socio-economic development of affected communities. Current

DOI: 10.1201/9781032651071-5

control methods include the use of drugs, which in turn causes concerns of resistance emergence, negative impacts on the environment, and effects on non-target species (Khan et al., 2017). To overcome these issues, there is a need to adopt an "omics" approach, integrating proteomics, genomics, metabolomics, and transcriptomics, for a deeper understanding of parasite biology and parasite–host interaction (Deng et al., 2023). Understanding the molecular mechanisms underlying host–parasite interactions is crucial for developing effective therapeutic strategies and control measures. In this context, the fields of proteomics and metabolomics play pivotal roles in unravelling the intricate dynamics of parasitic infections (Biron et al., 2011).

Proteomics involves the large-scale study of proteins, their structures, functions, and interactions within a biological system (Al-Amrani et al., 2021). In parasitology research, proteomics provides a comprehensive view of the proteome, allowing researchers to identify, quantify, and characterise proteins involved in the complex interplay between host and parasite. It enables identification of specific parasite proteins involved in host invasion, evasion, and pathogenesis (Stryiński et al., 2020). It also helps in this regard by shedding light on the molecular mechanisms involved in infection and host response to those mechanisms (Biron et al., 2011). Proteomics also helps to identify potential drug targets for therapeutic intervention (Cooper and Carucci, 2004).

Metabolomics approaches are used in parasitology research to understand metabolic adaptations in the host and parasite during infection. They enable complete profiling of metabolites and provide a snapshot of metabolic activity in parasites, offering information on nutritional requirements and metabolic pathways involved in parasite survival (Olson et al., 2020). Metabolomics approaches help identify changes in the host metabolic profile during parasitic infection, enhancing the understanding of host defence mechanisms (Olszewski et al., 2009; Kloehn et al., 2016). Metabolic markers related to parasitic diseases are being discovered using metabolomic approaches (Tounta et al., 2021). Metabolic pathways targeted by anti-parasitic drugs are being identified using this approach, as well as in understanding mechanisms involved in drug resistance (Mukherjee et al., 2016; Tounta et al., 2021).

5.2 METHODS INVOLVED IN PROTEOMIC APPROACHES IN PARASITES

Parasite proteomics is mainly focused on the characterisation of entire protein sets expressed by parasites under different conditions to provide information on parasite–host interactions, parasite biology, and potential drug targets (Stryiński et al., 2020). The most important techniques involved in proteomic approaches include the following.

5.2.1 Two-Dimensional Gel Electrophoresis

Electrophoresis can separate proteins based on molecular weight and isoelectric point. Separated proteins can be further processed and quantified for comparison within the same parasite at different stages or in response to different treatments.

This method consists of two main steps, isoelectric focussing and sodium dodecyl-sulphate–polyacrylamide gel electrophoresis (SDS-PAGE). In the first step, proteins are separated based on their isoelectric points in a pH gradient gel; an electric current causes proteins to migrate to their respective isoelectric points. In the second step, focused proteins are further separated based on molecular weight on a polyacrylamide gel according to their charge and size (Pergande and Cologna, 2017; Molina-Mora et al., 2020).

This method provides high resolution and separation of complex proteins in a mixture in a single experiment. It enables simultaneous and comprehensive protein profiling of a biological sample. It also helps identify post-translational modifications such as glycosylation (Kim and Kim, 2007). This method also assists in the comparative analysis of protein expression at different developmental stages of a parasite or different treatment levels (Ashrafmansouri et al., 2019).

Examples of the utility of two-dimensional gel electrophoresis (2-DE) in parasitology research include detection of 20 proteins in *Leishmania braziliensis* classified into 15 groups; 40% of these proteins were not reported previously in the proteomic map of *Leishmania* (Cuervo et al., 2007). Proteomic profiles of *Toxoplasma gondii* genotypes were obtained using 2-DE along with matrix-assisted laser desorption/ionisation (MALDI-TOF) mass spectrometry (Cohen et al., 2002; Zhou et al., 2014). Immunoreactive proteins of *Trichinella spiralis* and *T. britovi* were identified through 2-DE along with mass spectrometry and immunoblot (Grzelak et al., 2021). In filariae, 2-DE and MALDI mass spectrometry were used to identify different proteins expressed after the inhibition of prolyl oligopeptidase (Wadhawan et al., 2022).

5.2.2 Mass Spectrometry

Mass spectrometry, a crucial aspect of proteomic analysis, utilises techniques like electrospray ionisation (ESI) and MALDI-TOF for protein quantification. Mass spectrometry (MS) identifies and quantifies molecules based on the mass-to-charge ratio. Tandem mass spectrometry sequences peptides and identifies associated proteins (Han et al., 2008). The basic steps involved are ionisation, mass analysis, ion detection, and database search. Briefly, the sample is ionised using ESI or MALDI, and molecules are converted into ions which are accelerated using an electric or magnetic field and separated based on the charge-to-mass ratio (Urban, 2016). Resulting spectra provide information on the abundance and mass of the ions. Detected ions and their mass spectra are compared with previous submissions to databases to identify the proteins (Le et al., 2021). This method provides highly sensitive and specific data that allow identification and quantification of molecules. Mass spectrometry can also identify post-translational modifications in proteins (Doll and Burlingame, 2015).

The mass spectrometry-based technique MALDI-TOF is used to identify parasite proteins, exemplified by the identification of tick species and mosquito species (Sánchez-Juanes et al., 2022). Mass spectrometry-based proteomic analysis of *Babesia canis* has been reported, and 51–52 kDa protein fragment was procured from blood samples of infected dogs (Adaszek et al., 2014). Spectra of 408 samples from lice in the genera *Bovicola, Menacanthus, Linognathus, Chelopistes, Lipeurus,*

Goniocotes, Menopon, and the species *Pediculus humanus corporis* were obtained by MALDI-TOF (Ouarti et al., 2020). Proteomic profiling of *Taenia crassiceps* larval stages was performed after 2DE (Jiménez et al., 2023). MALDI-TOF mass spectrometry was performed to check the response of T helper cells during cysticercosis (Díaz-Zaragoza et al., 2020).

Recently, MALDI-TOF was used to identify adult cestodes (*Taenia saginata*) proglottids (Wendel et al., 2021). The proteomics used for identification, characterisation, and detection of species-specific peptide biomarkers for food-borne parasites are given in Figure 5.1. In the case of nematodes, two closely related species, *Cylicostephanus minutus* and C. *longibursatus*, were identified by MS analysis (Bredtmann et al., 2019). Nagorny et al. (2022) reported the identification of *Dirofilaria repens* from a human and *D. immitis* from dogs with 100% and 70% concordance rates, respectively.

5.2.3 Shotgun Proteomics

In this procedure, proteins are digested using proteases, and peptides are then processed using MS. The shotgun method has high throughput compared to 2-DE and can identify multiple proteins in a mixture (McDonald and Yates, 2002). During this process, extracted proteins from a biological sample are digested with trypsin

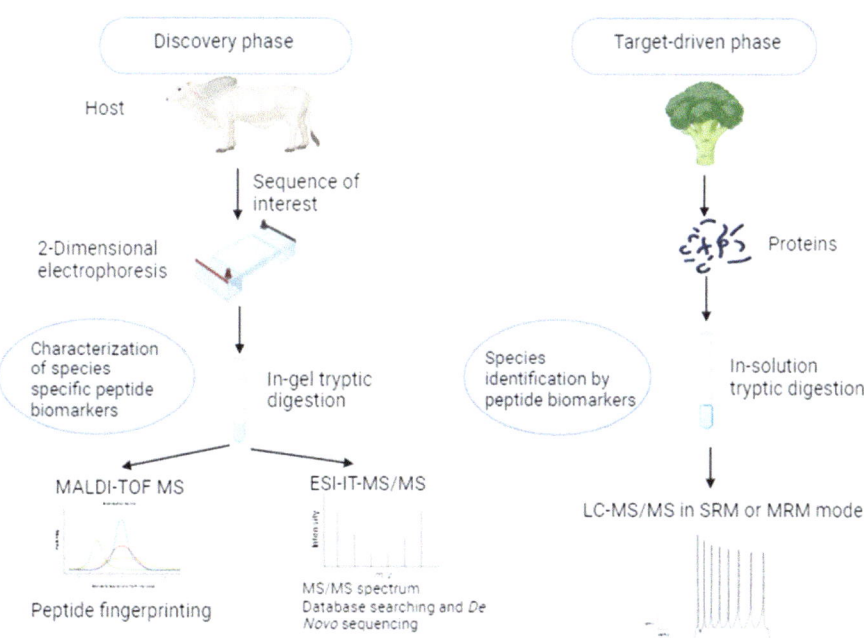

FIGURE 5.1   The proteomics used for identification, characterisation, and detection of species-specific peptide biomarkers for food-borne parasites.

or other proteases into peptides which are separated using liquid chromatography and subjected to MS for identification. Spectra are compared with protein databases (Gilmore and Washburn, 2010). The shotgun approach has high sensitivity and can detect low-abundance proteins. It can also identify post-translational modifications on proteins, helping to understand their function and regulation. It allows quantification by incorporating stable isotopes (Gao and Yates, 2019).

Shotgun analysis was used for proteomic profiling of *Schistosoma mansoni* (Campos et al., 2017) and to identify candidates for the immunodiagnosis of human strongyloidiasis. *Strongyloides venezuelensis* is an alternative antigen source for human strongyloidiasis diagnosis; 877 proteins were identified using shotgun analysis of third stage larvae (Fonseca et al., 2020). Shotgun analysis was used to generate a molecular profile of *Leishmania infantum*; 102 proteins were identified and bioinformatic analysis indicated that 60% were secreted, with 85% into the extracellular environment (Braga et al., 2014).

5.2.4 STABLE ISOTOPE LABELING

This technique includes Isotope-Coded Affinity Tags (ICAT) and Isobaric Tags for Relative and Absolute Quantification (ITRAQ) methods used for quantitative comparison of expression levels of proteins. This technique helps to understand changes in parasite proteomes (Chokkathukalam et al., 2014). This technique involves incorporation of stable isotopes into proteins and allows comparison of abundant proteins among different conditions. Two approaches are commonly us: metallic labelling and chemical labelling (DeArmond et al., 2011). In metallic labelling, organisms are cultured in media that contain stable isotopes as part of essential nutrients. A cell incorporates these isotopes into its proteins and labelled and unlabelled proteins can be easily distinguished by MS. In the case of chemical labelling, proteins are chemically modified with stable isotopes. Isotope labelling helps quantify proteins and allows simultaneous quantification of multiple samples, reducing experimental variation, and enabling high-throughput analysis (Creek et al., 2012).

Stable isotopes were employed to determine the discrimination factor among 13 parasite-host pairings of helminths and fish (Riekenberg et al., 2021). Quantitative proteomics enabled the whole proteomic characterisation at different lifecycle stages of the parasite, with stable isotope labelling used to determine *Trypanosoma brucei* proteomic characterisation through stable isotope-enriched culture media (Cirovic and Ochsenreiter, 2014). In a recent study, stable isotope labelling and MS were combined to assess diglycerides and triglycerides during the ovarian previtellogenic stage of Aedes aegypti (Tose et al., 2022).

5.2.5 PROTEIN MICROARRAYS

Microarrays involve immobilisation of proteins on a solid surface, enabling screening of how they interact with other ligands, including other proteins (Templin et al., 2002). The main steps involved in this process include attachment of purified proteins on solid surfaces in an array format in which non-specific binding sites are blocked. The microarray is then exposed to a sample that contains non-labelled or labelled ligands such as antibodies, cell lysate, and serum (Duncan et al., 2004). After incubation, interactions among immobilised proteins and ligands are checked. Protein microarrays can analyse protein–protein interactions and can assist in drug target identification (Berrade et al., 2011). As a high throughput technique, it can detect a large number of interactions of proteins with other proteins, nucleic acids, and other small molecules. It can be used for antibody profiling in a serum sample and help identify potential vaccine antigens and diagnostic markers (Boothroyd et al., 2003).

Protein microarrays have been used for the simultaneous detection of multiple food-borne helminthiases by using antigens from five parasite species (*Trichinella spiralis*, *Cysticercus cellulosae*, *Spirometra* sp., *Paragonimus westermani*, and *Angiostrongylus cantonensis*) (Chen et al., 2012). Novel vaccine candidates for *S. japonicum* were discovered using a protein microarray to characterise local antibody responses (McWilliam et al., 2014). B-cell epitopes of *S. haematobium* and *S. mansoni* with diagnostic potential were identified using peptide microarray technology (Vengesai et al., 2023). A protein microarray was used to identify antigens of *Cryptosporidium* that are associated with reinfection immunity in Bangladesh, and 1716 antigens of *C. meleagridis*, *C. parvum*, and *C. hominis* were analysed; seven antigens were linked to reinfection immunity (Gilchrist et al., 2023).

5.2.6 BOTTOM-UP PROTEOMICS

In this technique, proteins are digested by proteases to enable peptide-centric proteomics (Chait, 2006). The main steps are the extraction of proteins from biological samples, followed by protease digestion and separation of peptides using liquid chromatography based on their hydrophobicity. Separated peptides are further processed for MS, and spectra are compared with protein sequence databases (Tolmachev et al., 2008). This technique is very sensitive, high-throughput, and enables the detection of low-abundance proteins. The bottom-up technique is useful for the detection of post-translational modifications and allows quantification of peptides (Robinson and Cwiklinski, 2021).

The bottom-up proteomic approach was used to analyse the proteome profile of cercariae of *S. mansoni* (Perera et al., 2020). Hookworm–host interactions between dogs and *Ancylostoma caninum* were studied using bottom-up proteomics, which identified three times more proteins compared to a previous study (Morante et al., 2017). Proteomic profiling of *Teladorsagia circumcincta* using bottom-up approaches identified 17 proteins (Price et al., 2019).

5.2.7 TOP-DOWN PROTEOMICS

In this technique, intact proteins are analysed. Proteins are extracted from a biological sample and subjected to separation through liquid chromatography. Intact proteins are then analysed by MS, and obtained spectra are analysed (Catherman et al., 2014). This method is used to characterise proteins and identify post-transcriptional changes. Top-down proteomics also allows the identification of complex isoforms of proteins (Sánchez-Ovejero et al., 2016). Top-down proteomics was used to check the mature proteoforms expressed in *Echinococcus granulosus* subcellular fractions. Cytosolic and nuclear extracts were used, and proteins were analysed. Through top-down analysis, 186 proteins were identified along with 207 proteoforms (Lorenzatto et al., 2015).

5.3   METHODS INVOLVED IN METABOLOMICS APPROACHES IN PARASITES

In the metabolomics approaches, we mainly discuss the metabolic pathways of different parasites. The most important techniques involved in metabolomics approaches are as follows:

5.3.1   METABOLOME-WIDE ASSOCIATION STUDY

A metabolome-wide association study (MWAS) identifies the changes in non-infected and parasite-infected cultures at various time intervals. In metabolomics, MWAS is used to find relationships between metabolite levels and particular features or disorders (Tounta et al., 2021). In contrast to other omics techniques, such as proteomics or genomics, which concentrate on genes or proteins, MWAS looks at the whole array of tiny molecules (metabolites) in a biological sample (Pinu et al., 2019). Researchers can find metabolites that are strongly linked to the characteristic or condition they are studying by comparing the metabolite profiles of various samples, such as individuals with and without a certain disease. Personalised therapy, biomarker development, and disease mechanisms can all benefit from the insights that MWAS can offer (Gowda et al., 2008). It also describes the magnitude of changes and allows us to identify significant data points (metabolites) that display large change in their magnitudes (Park et al., 2015).

5.3.2   MASS SPECTROMETRY

Mass spectrometry is an important tool to study metabolomics of parasites. In this technique, cells are grown in cultures because animals are not preferred for their growth due to a high level of biological variation. Then specific drugs are added, and cell extracts are then analysed using mass spectrometry, which then records the level of each metabolite (Vincent and Barrett, 2015). Mass spectrometry is a promising approach because it allows us to detect hundreds and thousands of compounds in a single sample and is highly sensitive. Mass spectrometers require chromatography for proper functioning (Dunn et al., 2011). Furthermore, different techniques have been developed using mass spectrometry, including liquid chromatography-mass spectrometry, gas chromatography-mass spectrometry, and capillary electrophoresis-mass spectrometry. All of these techniques detect metabolites efficiently (Wangchuk et al., 2023). Mass spectrometry-based metabolomics have quantified the metabolites of a variety of parasites like *Toxocara canis*, *Ascaris lumbricoides*, *Trichuris muris*, *Ancylostoma caninum*, *Nippostrongylus brasiliensis*, *Onchocerca volvulus*, *Opisthorcis felis*, and *Schistosoma* spp. (Whitman et al., 2021).

5.3.3 NUCLEAR MAGNETIC RESONANCE

Nuclear magnetic resonance (NMR) detectors are one of the most commonly used instruments for metabolite detection. The NMR detects metabolites depending on the vibrational energy of bonds. This technique gives information about the chemical structure of metabolites and is a quantitative technique that leads to identification of metabolites (Emwas et al., 2019). Although less sensitive compared to mass spectrometry, nuclear magnetic resonance (NMR) spectroscopy still plays a significant role in metabolite detection. It can be used in combination with mass spectrometry to enhance metabolomic analysis (Summer et al., 2007). Untargeted metabolomics offers the advantage of identifying both known and unknown metabolites associated with phenotypic changes. Each signal detected by analytical instruments undergoes statistical analysis to determine its potential biological relevance. Metabolites showing high correlation are further investigated through techniques such as database searches, MS/MS, and 2D NMR experiments (Jousse et al., 2020). This approach is suitable for both quantitative and qualitative analysis of metabolites in complex mixtures without the need for prior extraction (Guidi et al., 2020). NMR has been utilised to study various metabolic pathways in parasites, including ammonia recycling, betaine, methionine, glycine, serine, threonine, arginine, proline, aspartate, alanine, and tyrosine metabolism (Tabrizi et al., 2021).

5.3.4 MULTIPLE REACTION MONITORING

In Multiple Reaction Monitoring (MRM), several target ions are isolated and fragmented to identify metabolites (Yannell et al., 2018). Unlike untargeted methods that analyse the abundance of each mass peak to identify metabolites post-data collection and filtering, targeted approaches like MRM provide definitive metabolite identifications. After collecting raw data, it's essential to choose, align, and filter the peaks corresponding to authentic metabolites before conducting statistical comparisons (Creek et al., 2011).

5.4 METABOLIC PATHWAYS AND PROTEINS INVOLVED IN PARASITE SURVIVAL AND PATHOGENESIS

Parasites use different pathways to interact with host metabolic pathways to acquire nutrients for survival and pathogenesis (Figure 5.2). The main energy metabolism pathway for parasite survival is glycolysis (Parab and McCall, 2021). Most protozoa, e.g. *Plasmodium* spp., completely depend on glycolysis for energy production (Olszewski and Llinás, 2011). The Krebs cycle is utilised by a variety of parasites

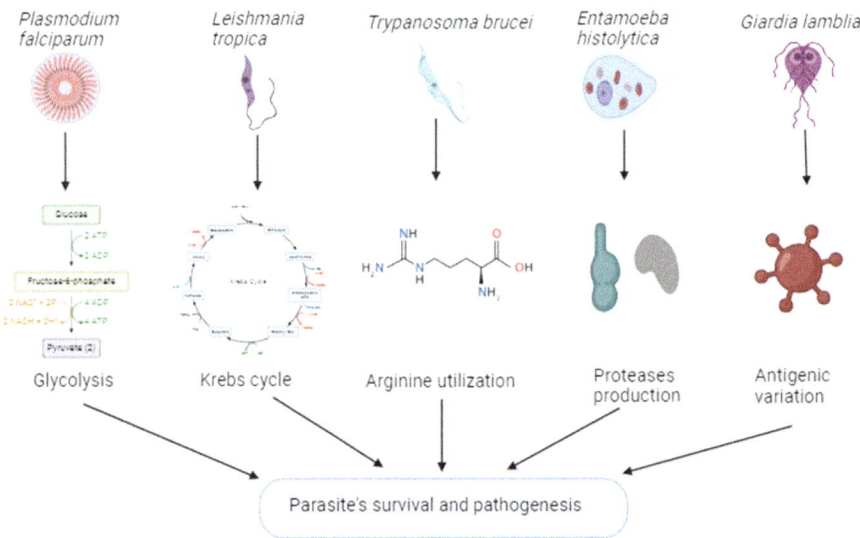

FIGURE 5.2 Different metabolic approaches used by parasites for their survival and pathogenesis.

for energy production; *Leishmania* spp. use the Krebs cycle for energy production, which in turn helps adaptation to the host environment (McConville and Naderer, 2011). Some parasites evade the host immune system by consuming large amounts of arginine, e.g. *Trypanosoma brucei* (Holzmuller et al., 2018). Some parasites produce cysteine proteases that help in invasion, e.g. *Entamoeba histolytica* (Que X and Reed, 2000). Parasites often have specialised pathways for nucleotide synthesis by using purines and pyrimidines acquired from the host (Krishnan and Soldati-Favre, 2021). Parasites can also use protein modification processes, e.g. glycosylation and protein export, for survival and evade the host immune system, as for *Trypanosoma cruzi* and *P. falciparum* (Cardoso et al., 2016; Wang et al., 2021). Parasites evade the host immune system through antigenic variation by changing their surface proteins and by the production and release of immunomodulatory proteins. A complete understanding of these pathways is important for designing strategies to control parasitic infections (Schmid-Hempel, 2009). Targeting these specific metabolic pathways provides potential target sites for new parasitic drug development (Parab and McCall, 2021).

5.5   PROTEOMICS AND METABOLOMICS SIGNATURES OF PARASITE DEVELOPMENT AND LIFE CYCLE

Proteomics and metabolomics have enabled researchers to study the expression of proteins and metabolites. In parasitology, these techniques provide information regarding molecular mechanisms in parasites, drug targets in parasites, and host–parasite interactions (Biron et al., 2011; Denery et al., 2010). Integrating both metabolomics and proteomics can lead to a holistic understanding of all the molecular events occurring during parasite development (Antunes et al., 2013).

5.5.1 PROTEOMICS SIGNATURES

Proteomics can be used to investigate the signatures of parasite development and lifecycles in the following ways:

a) *Protein expression profiling*
Changes in protein expression among different parasite life cycle stages can be determined using comparative proteomics. This approach is used to identify proteins involved in reproduction, host invasion, and immune system evasion (Bertin et al., 2013; Jia et al., 2024).

b) *Post-translational modification*
Post-translational modification processes such as acetylation, phosphorylation, and glycosylation highlight regulatory mechanisms that affect protein functions necessary for parasite development (Doerig et al., 2015; Manzano-Román and Fuentes, 2020; Rex et al., 2022).

c) *Protein–protein interactions*
Analysis of protein–protein interactions among protein networks across parasite life cycle stages can uncover signalling pathways and potential drug targets. Identification of stage-specific protein biomarkers aids in therapeutic and diagnostic development (Cuesta-Astroz and Oliveira, 2018; Lin et al., 2020).

5.5.2 METABOLOMICS SIGNATURES

a) *Metabolite profiling*
Metabolic profiling is important because it allows the simultaneous quantification of small molecules and metabolic changes associated with different stages of the parasite life cycle (Bennuru et al., 2017; Olson et al., 2020).

b) *Metabolic pathway analysis*
Metabolic pathways mapping provides information on metabolic adaptations and nutrient and energy requirements of parasites during development and also highlights potential drug target sites (Denery et al., 2010).

c) *Host–parasite metabolic interactions*
Host-parasite interactions provide information on metabolites produced by the host in response to infection, which can unravel the crosstalk between parasites and the host (Kafsack and Llinás, 2010; Kloehn et al., 2016).

5.6 HOST–PARASITE INTERACTIONS AT THE PROTEOMICS AND METABOLOMICS LEVEL

Host–parasite interactions underlie parasitic disease and involve various biochemical and chemical processes at proteomic and metabolomic levels (Biron et al., 2011).

A proper understanding of host–parasite interaction provides information on infection mechanisms, host defence systems against parasites, and potential therapeutic target sites (Kloehn et al., 2016).

Parasites on entry can manipulate the host cell machinery to enhance their survival in the host. Through proteomic analysis, this change can be identified at the level of protein expression and post-translational modifications. Changes in host signalling pathways and metabolic processes can also be highlighted through proteomic analysis (Negrao et al., 2019). During infection, proteomic analysis of host proteins provides information regarding immune responses and changes in the expression of immune-related proteins like chemokines and cytokines and the identification of parasite antigens (Li et al., 2021). Post-translational modifications in host proteins are also revealed by proteomics for a better understanding of the dynamic nature of host-parasite interactions (Goncalves-Silva et al., 2022). A comprehensive understanding of the parasite proteome is essential to identify potential drug targets. Proteomics helps characterise parasite-specific proteins involved in biological processes and host evasion mechanisms. These proteins also facilitate host environment adaptation. Proteomics also highlights post-translational modifications in parasite proteins during infection (González-Miguel et al., 2020; Deng et al., 2023).

Parasites induce metabolic changes in host cells to ensure survival. Metabolomics can identify these alterations. Understanding parasite metabolic pathways aids in identifying potential therapeutic targets (Zhao et al., 2022; Ewald et al., 2024). Metabolomic analysis of parasites provides information regarding the energy and nutrient requirements of the parasite along with the waste elimination process. Parasite-specific metabolomics can provide new targets for diagnosis and potential drug targets (Olszewski et al., 2009; Olson et al., 2020). Through metabolomics, we can explore the interaction between host and parasite and their competition for nutrients and immunomodulatory properties around metabolite production. Metabolomic profiling also provides information regarding the environmental adaptations of parasites in the host (Hossain et al., 2020; Beri et al., 2023).

5.7 INTEGRATION OF PROTEOMICS AND METABOLOMICS DATA WITH OTHER OMICS APPROACHES

Proteomic and metabolomic integration with other omics approaches, such as transcriptomics and genomics, is a powerful strategy in systems biology. This integration provides a detailed understanding of biological systems and requires advanced statistical and computational methods along with interdisciplinary interactions (Wanichthanarak et al., 2015; Misra et al., 2019). Integration approaches include (a) analyses that identify correlations among various omics datasets and provide information on potential relationships; however, this analysis does not imply causation; (b) network analysis in which biological networks are constructed that display interactions among proteins, metabolites, and genes; and (c) pathway analysis in which omics data integration with biological pathways is performed, providing information on functional significance (Cambiaghi et al., 2017; Jendoubi, 2021).

Biological systems integration of proteomics and metabolomics with other omics data provides a holistic approach to gain a comprehensive understanding of biological systems through interactions with genes, proteins, transcripts, and metabolites (Figure 5.3). It also identifies complex regulatory pathways and networks in biological systems and aids in the identification of biomarkers and potential therapeutic targets (Krumsiek et al., 2016; Pinu et al., 2019). Different bioinformatics tools and data repositories are involved in proteomic and metabolomic integration with other omics techniques, such as iPathwayGuide, Cytoscape, Human Metabolome Database (HMDB), and Human Proteome Project (HPP), etc. (Wandy and Daly, 2021; Chicco et al., 2023). Biomedical applications of integrative omics approaches are helpful in devising more targeted and effective treatments. This integration is also helpful for personalised medication based on individual genomics, metabolomics, and proteomics profiles (Subramanian et al., 2020; Ivanisevic and Sewduth, 2023).

Integration of various omics techniques faces some challenges: Omics datasets are mostly heterogeneous and their integration requires normalisation and standardisation (Sen and Orešič, 2023). Omics datasets are large, and handling them requires expertise (Yu and Zeng, 2018). Integration requires access to large datasets from various sources, so ethical and privacy considerations are needed (Iii and Elenberg, 2020).

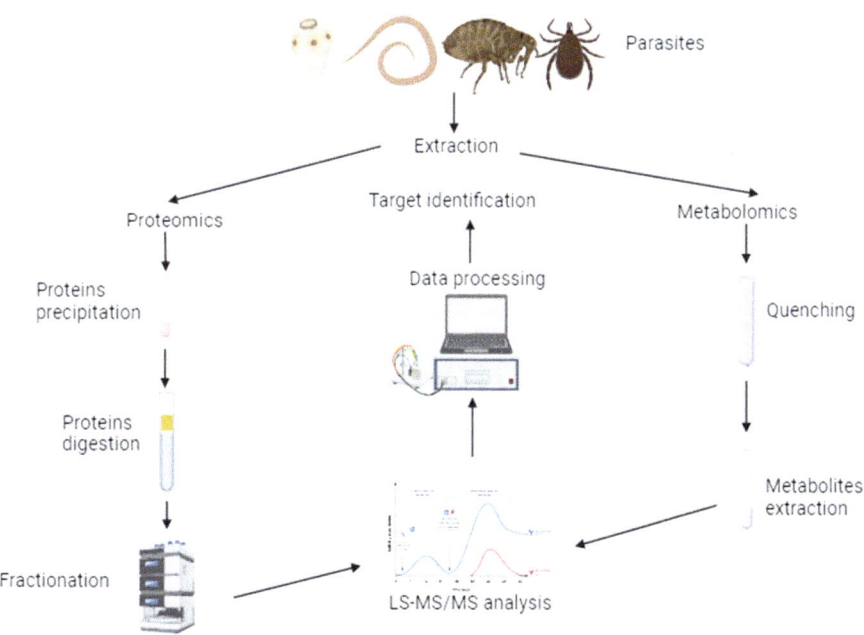

FIGURE 5.3 Flowchart of the integrative multi-omics approaches (metabolomics and proteomics).

5.8   CHALLENGES AND FUTURE PERSPECTIVES IN PROTEOMICS AND METABOLOMICS IN PARASITIC RESEARCH

Generally, omics approaches, specifically metabolomics and proteomics, have played crucial roles in parasitology, including providing unprecedented insights into host–parasite interactions, molecular mechanisms involved in this relationship, disease patterns, and potential drug targets (Prasopdee et al., 2019). However, these approaches face several challenges that need to be explored.

5.9   CHALLENGES

i. Due to the complexity of parasite biology, comprehensive methodologies are needed.
ii. Due to the dynamic nature of host–parasite interactions, the molecular understanding of this interaction is challenging.
iii. Due to the unavailability of metazoan parasites to culture and their low abundance in the host, it becomes difficult to get sufficient amounts of material for some experiments.
iv. Some parasites lack well-annotated genomes, making protein and metabolite identification difficult.
v. Improvements in sequencing technologies and bioinformatics tools are required.
vi. Quantitative precision is also needed in complex biological samples due to preparation variabilities and technical reproducibility.

5.10   FUTURE PERSPECTIVES

i. Advancements in omics integration will provide a comprehensive understanding of molecular mechanisms.
ii. Single-cell omics technologies will help dissect heterogeneity within parasites and host cells.
iii. Continued improvements in MS and nuclear magnetic resonance technologies will enhance the sensitivity and throughput of metabolomics and proteomics analyses.
iv. Continued development of bioinformatics tools will help in the extraction of meaningful biological insights from complex datasets.
v. Identification of potential drug targets through omics integration will facilitate the discovery of new drugs and vaccines.
vi. Will promote global collaborations by sharing data resources and expertise.

REFERENCES

Abdullah, I., Tak, H., Ahmad, F., Gul, N., Nabi, S. and Sofi, T. 2016. Predominance of gastrointestinal protozoan parasites in children: a brief review. *International Journal of Veterinary Sciences and Animal Husbandry*, 1(2):01–06

Adaszek, Ł., Banach, T., Bartnicki, M., Winiarczyk, D., Łyp, P. and Winiarczyk, S. 2014. Application of the mass spectrometry MALDI-TOF technique for detection of *Babesia canis canis* infection in dogs. *Parasitology Research*, 113(11):4293–4295.

Al-Amrani, S., Al-Jabri, Z., Al-Zaabi, A., Alshekaili, J. and Al-Khabori, M. 2021. Proteomics: concepts and applications in human medicine. World *Journal of Biological Chemistry*, 12(5):57–69.

Antunes, L.C.M., Han, J., Pan, J., Moreira, C.J., Azambuja, P., Borchers, C.H. and Carels, N. 2013. Metabolic signatures of triatomine vectors of *Trypanosoma cruzi* unveiled by metabolomics. *PLoS One*, 8(10):e77283.

Ashrafmansouri, M., Sadjjadi, F.S., Seyyedtabaei, S., Haghighi, A., Rezaei-Tavirani, M. and Ahmadi, N. 2019. Comparative two-dimensional gel electrophoresis maps for amastigote-like proteomes of Iranian *Leishmania tropica* and *Leishmania major* isolates. *Galen Medical Journal*, 8:e1520.

Bennuru, S., Lustigman, S., Abraham, D. and Nutman, T.B. 2017. Metabolite profiling of infection-associated metabolic markers of onchocerciasis. *Molecular and Biochemical Parasitology*, 215:58–69.

Beri, D., Singh, M., Rodriguez, M., Goyal, N., Rasquinha, G., Liu, Y., An, X., Yazdanbakhsh, K. and Lobo, C.A. 2023. Global metabolomic profiling of host red blood cells infected with *Babesia divergens* reveals novel antiparasitic target pathways. *Microbiology Spectrum*, 11(2):e04688-22.

Berrade, L., Garcia, A.E. and Camarero, J.A. 2011. Protein microarrays: novel developments and applications. *Pharmacology Research*, 28(7):1480–1499.

Bertin, G.I., Sabbagh, A., Guillonneau, F., Jafari-Guemouri, S., Ezinmegnon, S., Federici, C., Hounkpatin, B., Fievet, N. and Deloron, P. 2013. Differential protein expression profiles between *Plasmodium falciparum* parasites isolated from subjects presenting with pregnancy-associated malaria and uncomplicated malaria in Benin. *Journal of Infectious Diseases*, 208(12):1987–1997.

Biron, D.G., Nedelkov, D., Missé, D. and Holzmuller, P. 2011. Proteomics and host—pathogen interactions: A bright future? In: Tibayrenc, M. (ed.) *Genetics and Evolution of Infectious Disease*. Elsevier, pp. 263–303.

Boothroyd, J.C., Blader, I., Cleary, M. and Singh, U. 2003. DNA microarrays in parasitology: strengths and limitations. *Trends in Parasitology*, 19(10):470–476.

Braga, M.S., Neves, L.X., Campos, J.M., Roatt, B.M., de Oliveira A.S.R.D., Braga, S.L., de Melo, R.D., Reis, A.B. and Castro-Borges, W. 2014. Shotgun proteomics to unravel the complexity of the *Leishmania infantum* exoproteome and the relative abundance of its constituents. *Molecular Biochemistry and Parasitology*, 195(1):43–53.

Bredtmann, C.M., Krücken, J., Murugaiyan, J., Balard, A., Hofer, H., Kuzmina, T.A. and von Samson-Himmelstjerna, G. 2019. Concurrent proteomic fingerprinting and molecular analysis of cyathostomins. *Proteomics*, 19:e1800290.

Cambiaghi, A., Ferrario, M. and Masseroli, M. 2017. Analysis of metabolomic data: tools, current strategies and future challenges for omics data integration. *Briefings in Bioinformatics*, 18(3):498–510.

Campos, J.M., Neves, L.X., de Paiva, N.C.N., de Oliveira, E.C.R.A., Casé, A.H., Carneiro, C.M., Andrade, M.H. and Castro-Borges, W. 2017. Understanding global changes of the liver proteome during murine schistosomiasis using a label-free shotgun approach. *Journal of Proteomics*, 151:193–203.

Cardoso, M.S., Reis-Cunha, J.L. and Bartholomeu, D.C. 2016. Evasion of the immune response by *Trypanosoma cruzi* during acute infection. *Frontier in Immunology*, 6:659.

Catherman, A.D., Skinner, O.S. and Kelleher, N.L. 2014. Top down proteomics: facts and perspectives. *Biochemical and Biophysical Research Communications*, 445(4):683–693.

Chait, B.T. 2006. Chemistry. Mass spectrometry: bottom-up or top-down? *Science*, 314:65–66.

Chen, J.X., Chen, M.X., Ai, L., Chen, J.H., Chen, S.H., Zhang, Y.N., Cai, Y., Zhu, X.Q. and Zhou, X.N. 2012. A protein microarray for the rapid screening of patients suspected of infection with various food-borne helminthiases. *PLoS Neglected Tropical Diseases*, 6(11):e1899.

Chicco, D., Cumbo, F. and Angione, C. 2023. Ten quick tips for avoiding pitfalls in multi-omics data integration analyses. *PLoS Computational Biology*, 19(7):e1011224.

Chokkathukalam, A., Kim, D.H., Barrett, M.P., Breitling, R. and Creek, D.J. 2014. Stable isotope-labeling studies in metabolomics: new insights into structure and dynamics of metabolic networks. *Bioanalysis*, 6(4):511–524.

Cirovic, O. and Ochsenreiter, T. 2014. Whole proteome analysis of the protozoan parasite *Trypanosoma brucei* using stable isotope labeling by amino acids in cell culture and mass spectrometry. *Methods in Molecular Biology*, 1188:47–55.

Cohen, A.M., Rumpel, K., Coombs, G.H. and Wastling, J.M. 2002. Characterisation of global protein expression by two-dimensional electrophoresis and mass spectrometry: proteomics of *Toxoplasma gondii*. *International Journal for Parasitology*, 32(1):39–51.

Cooper, R.A. and Carucci, D.J. 2004. Proteomic approaches to studying drug targets and resistance in *Plasmodium*. *Current Drug Targets – Infectious Disorders*, 4:41–51.

Creek, D.J., Chokkathukalam, A., Jankevics, A., Burgess, K.E.V., Breitling, R. and Barrett, M.P. 2012. Stable isotope-assisted metabolomics for network-wide metabolic pathway elucidation. *Analytical Chemistry*, 84(20):8442–8447.

Creek, D.J., Jankevics, A., Breitling, R., Watson, D.G., Barrett, M.P. and Burgess, K.E. 2011. Toward global metabolomics analysis with hydrophilic interaction liquid chromatography–mass spectrometry: improved metabolite identification by retention time prediction. *Analytical Chemistry*, 83(22):8703–8710.

Cuervo, P., de Jesus, J.B., Junqueira, M., Mendonça-Lima, L., González, L.J., Betancourt, L., Grimaldi Jr, G., Domont, G.B., Fernandes, O. and Cupolillo, E. 2007. Proteome analysis of *Leishmania (Viannia) braziliensis* by two-dimensional gel electrophoresis and mass spectrometry. *Molecular and Biochemical Parasitology*, 154(1):6–21.

Cuesta-Astroz, Y. and Oliveira, G. 2018. Computational and experimental approaches to predict host–parasite protein–protein interactions. *Methods in Molecular Biology*, 1819:153–173.

DeArmond, P.D., West, G.M., Huang, H.T. and Fitzgerald, M.C. 2011. Stable isotope labeling strategy for protein-ligand binding analysis in multi-component protein mixtures. *Journal of the American Society for Mass Spectrometry*, 22(3):418–430.

Denery, J.R., Nunes, A.A., Hixon, M.S., Dickerson, T.J. and Janda, K.D. 2010. Metabolomics-based discovery of diagnostic biomarkers for onchocerciasis. *PLoS Neglected Tropical Diseases*, 4(10):e834.

Deng, B., Vanagas, L., Alonso, A.M. and Angel, S.O. 2023. Proteomics applications in *Toxoplasma gondii*: Unveiling the host–parasite interactions and therapeutic target discovery. *Pathogens*, 13(1):33.

Díaz-Zaragoza, M., Jiménez, L., Hernández, M., Hernández-Ávila, R., Navarro, L., Ochoa-Sánchez, A., Encarnación-Guevara, S., Ostoa-Saloma, P. and Landa, A. 2020. Protein expression profile of *Taenia crassiceps cysticerci* related to Th1- and Th2-type responses in the mouse cysticercosis model. *Acta Tropica*, 212:105696.

Doerig, C., Rayner, J.C., Scherf, A. and Tobin, A.B. 2015. Post-translational protein modifications in malaria parasites. *Nature Reviews Microbiology*, 13(3):160–172.

Doll, S. and Burlingame, A.L. 2015. Mass spectrometry-based detection and assignment of protein posttranslational modifications. *ACS Chemical Biology*, 10(1):63–71.

Duncan, R., Salotra, P., Goyal, N., Akopyants, N., Beverley, S.M. and Nakhasi, H.L. 2004. The application of gene expression microarray technology to kinetoplastid research. *Current Molecular Medicine*, 4:611–621.

Dunn, W.B., Broadhurst, D., Begley, P., Zelena, E., Francis-McIntyre, S., Anderson, N., Brown, M., Knowles, J.D., Halsall, A., Haselden, J.N. and Nicholls, A.W. 2011. Procedures for large-scale metabolic profiling of serum and plasma using gas chromatography and liquid chromatography coupled to mass spectrometry. *Nature Protocols*, 6(7):1060–1083.

Ekong, P.S., Juryit, R., Dika, N.M., Nguku, P. and Musenero, M. 2012. Prevalence and risk factors for zoonotic helminth infection among humans and animals-Jos, Nigeria, 2005-2009. *Pan African Medical Journal*, 12(1):6.

Emwas, A.H., Roy, R., McKay, R.T., Tenori, L., Saccenti, E., Gowda, G.A.N., Raftery, D., Alahmari, F., Jaremko, L., Jaremko, M. and Wishart, D.S. 2019. NMR spectroscopy for metabolomics research. *Metabolites*, 9(7):123.

Ewald, S., Nasuhidehnavi, A., Feng, T.Y., Lesani, M. and McCall, L.I. 2024. The intersection of host *in vivo* metabolism and immune responses to infection with kinetoplastid and apicomplexan parasites. *Microbiology and Molecular Biology Reviews*, 1:e00164-22.

Fonseca, P.D.M., Corral, M.A., Cosenza-Contreras, M., Meisel, D.M.C.L., Melo, G.B., Antunes, M.M.S., Santo, M.C.E., Gryschek, R.C.B., Costa-Cruz, J.M., Castro-Borges, W. and Paula, F.M. 2020. Shotgun proteomics of *Strongyloides venezuelensis* infective third stage larvae: Insights into host–parasite interaction and novel targets for diagnostics. *Molecular and Biochemical Parasitology*, 235:111249.

Gao, Y. and Yates, Y.R. 2019. Protein analysis by shotgun proteomics. In: Tao, W.A. and Zhang, Y. (eds.) *Mass spectrometry-based chemical proteomics*. John Wiley & Sons, pp. 1–38.

Gilchrist, C.A., Campo, J.J., Pablo, J.V., Ma, J.Z., Teng, A., Oberai, A., Shandling, A.D., Alam, M., Kabir, M., Faruque, A.S.G. and Haque, R. 2023. Specific *Cryptosporidium* antigens associate with reinfection immunity and protection from cryptosporidiosis. *Journal of Clinical Investigation*, 133(16):e166814.

Gilmore, J.M. and Washburn, M.P. 2010. Advances in shotgun proteomics and the analysis of membrane proteomes. *Journal of Proteomics*, 73(11):2078–91.

Goncalves-Silva, G., Vieira, L.G.M.D.S., Cosenza-Contreras, M., Souza, A.F.P., Costa, D.C. and Castro-Borges, W. 2022. Profiling the serum proteome during *Schistosoma mansoni* infection in the BALB/c mice: a focus on the altered lipid metabolism as a key modulator of host-parasite interactions. *Frontiers in Immunology*, 13:955049.

González-Miguel, J., Becerro-Recio, D., Sotillo, J., Simón, F. and Siles-Lucas, M. 2020. Set up of an *in vitro* model to study early host-parasite interactions between newly excysted juveniles of *Fasciola hepatica* and host intestinal cells using a quantitative proteomics approach. *Veterinary Parasitology*, 278:109028.

Gowda, G.A., Zhang, S., Gu, H., Asiago, V., Shanaiah, N. and Raftery, D. 2008. Metabolomics-based methods for early disease diagnostics. *Expert Review of Molecular Diagnostics*, 8(5):617–633.

Grisi, L., Leite, R.C., Martins, J.R.D.S., Barros, A.T.M.D., Andreotti, R., Cançado, P.H.D., León, A.A.P.D., Pereira, J.B. and Villela, H.S. 2014. Reavaliação do potencial impacto econômico de parasitos de bovinos no Brasil. *Revista Brasileira de Parasitologia Veterinária*, 23:150–156.

Grzelak, S., Stachyra, A. and Bień-Kalinowska, J. 2021. The first analysis of *Trichinella spiralis* and *Trichinella britovi* adult worm excretory-secretory proteins by two-dimensional electrophoresis coupled with LC-MS/MS. *Veterinary Parasitology*, 297:09096.

Guidi, A., Petrella, G., Fustaino, V., Saccoccia, F., Lentini, S., Gimmelli, R., Di Pietro, G., Bresciani, A., Cicero, D.O. and Ruberti, G. 2020. Drug effects on metabolic profiles of *Schistosoma mansoni* adult male parasites detected by 1H-NMR spectroscopy. *PLoS Neglected Tropical Diseases*, 14(10):e0008767.

Han, X., Aslanian, A. and Yates, J.R. 2008. Mass spectrometry for proteomics. *Current Opinion in Chemical Biology*, 12(5):483–490.

Hesterberg, U.W., Bagnall, R., Perrett, K., Horner, R. and Gummow, B. 2007. A questionnaire survey of perceptions and preventive measures related to animal health amongst cattle owners of rural communities in KwaZulu-Natal, South Africa. *Journal of the South African Veterinary Association*, 78(4):205–208.

Holzmuller, P., Geiger, A., Nzoumbou-Boko, R., Pissarra, J., Hamrouni, S., Rodrigues, V., Dauchy, F.A., Lemesre, J.L., Vincendeau, P. and Bras-Gonçalves, R. 2018. Trypanosomatid infections: How do parasites and their excreted-secreted factors modulate the inducible metabolism of l-Arginine in macrophages? *Frontier in Immunology*, 9:778.

Hossain, E.K.R.A.M., Khanam, S., Dean, D.A., Wu, C., Lostracco-Johnson, S., Thomas, D., Kane, S.S., Parab, A.R., Flores, K., Katemauswa, M. and Gosmanov, C. 2020. Mapping of host-parasite-microbiome interactions reveals metabolic determinants of tropism and tolerance in Chagas disease. *Science Advances*, 6(30):eaaz2015.

Iii, E.G.H. and Elenberg, F. 2020. Ethical challenges posed by big data. *Innovations in Clinical Neuroscience*, 17(10–12):24–30.

Isaac, C., Turay, P.N., Inegbenosun, C.U., Ezekiel, S.A., Adamu, H.O. and Ohiolei, J.A. 2019. Prevalence of soil-transmitted helminths in primary school playgrounds in Edo State, southern Nigeria. *Helminthologia*, 56(4):282.

Ivanisevic, T. and Sewduth, R.N. 2023. Multi-omics integration for the design of novel therapies and the identification of novel biomarkers. Proteomes, 11(4):34.

Jendoubi, T. 2021. Approaches to integrating metabolomics and multi-omics data: a primer. *Metabolites*, 11(3):184.

Jia, Z., Hasi, S., Zhan, D., Vogl, C. and Burger, P.A. 2024. Transcriptomic profiling of different developmental stages reveals parasitic strategies of *Wohlfahrtia magnifica*, a myiasis-causing flesh fly. *BMC Genomics*, 25(1):111.

Jiménez, L., Díaz-Zaragoza, M., Hernández, M., Navarro, L., Hernández-Ávila, R., Encarnación-Guevara, S., Ostoa-Saloma, P. and Landa, A. 2023. Differential protein expression of *Taenia crassiceps* ORF strain in the murine cysticercosis model using resistant (C57BL/6) mice. *Pathogens*, 12(5):678.

Jousse, C., Dalle, C., Abila, A., Traïkia, M., Diogon, M., Lyan, B., El Alaoui, H., Vidau, C. and Delbac, F. 2020. A combined LC-MS and NMR approach to reveal metabolic changes in the hemolymph of honeybees infected by the gut parasite Nosema ceranae. *Journal of Invertebrate Pathology*, 176:107478.

Kafsack, B.F. and Llinás, M. 2010. Eating at the table of another: metabolomics of host-parasite interactions. *Cell Host & Microbe*, 7(2):90–99.

Khan, M.N., Sajid, M.S., Rizwan, H.M., Qudoos, A., Abbas, R.Z., Riaz, M. and Khan, M.K. 2017. Comparative efficacy of six anthelmintic treatments against natural infection of fasciola species in sheep. *Pakistan Veterinary Journal*, 37(1):65–68.

Kim, M.R. and Kim, C.W. 2007, Human blood plasma preparation for two-dimensional gel electrophoresis. *Analytical Technologies in the Biomedical and Life Science*, 849(1–2):203–210.

Kloehn, J., Blume, M., Cobbold, S.A., Saunders, E.C., Dagley, M.J. and McConville, M.J. 2016. Using metabolomics to dissect host–parasite interactions. *Current Opinion in Microbiology*, 32:59–65.

Krishnan, A. and Soldati-Favre, D. 2021. Amino acid metabolism in apicomplexan parasites. *Metabolites*, 11(2):61.

Krumsiek, J., Bartel, J. and Theis, F.J. 2016. Computational approaches for systems metabolomics. *Current Opinion in Biotechnology*, 39:198–206.

Le, C., Chu, S., Tan, S., Yin, X., Jiang, Y., Dai, X., Gong, X., Fang, X. and Tian, D. 2021. Towards higher sensitivity of mass spectrometry: A perspective from the mass analyzers. *Frontier in Chemistry*, 9:813359.

Li, T., Liu, H., Jiang, N., Wang, Y., Wang, Y., Zhang, J., Shen, Y. and Cao, J. 2021. Comparative proteomics reveals *Cryptosporidium parvum* manipulation of the host cell molecular expression and immune response. *PLoS Neglected Tropical Diseases*, 15(11):e0009949.

Lin, H.C., Chu, L.J., Huang, P.J., Cheng, W.H., Zheng, Y.H., Huang, C.Y., Hong, S.W., Chen, L.C., Lin, H.A., Wang, J.Y. and Chen, R.M. 2020. Proteomic signatures of metronidazole-resistant *Trichomonas vaginalis* reveal novel proteins associated with drug resistance. *Parasites & Vectors*, 13:1–14.

Lorenzatto, K.R., Kim, K., Ntai, I., Paludo, G.P., Camargo de Lima, J., Thomas, P.M., Kelleher, N.L. and Ferreira, H.B. 2015. Top down proteomics reveals mature proteoforms expressed in subcellular fractions of the *Echinococcus granulosus* preadult stage. *Journal of Proteome Research*, 14(11):4805–4814.

Manzano-Román, R. and Fuentes, M. 2020. Relevance and proteomics challenge of functional posttranslational modifications in Kinetoplastid parasites. *Journal of Proteomics*, 220:103762.

McConville, M.J. and Naderer, T. 2011. Metabolic pathways required for the intracellular survival of Leishmania. *Annual Review of Microbiology*, 6:543–561.

McDonald, W.H. and Yates, J.R. 3rd. 2002. Shotgun proteomics and biomarker discovery. *Disease Markers*, 18(2):99–105.

McWilliam, H.E., Driguez, P., Piedrafita, D., McManus, D.P. and Meeusen, E.N. 2014. Discovery of novel *Schistosoma japonicum* antigens using a targeted protein microarray approach. *Parasites & Vectors*, 7:1–11.

Misra, B.B., Langefeld, C., Olivier, M. and Cox, L.A. 2019. Integrated omics: tools, advances and future approaches. *Journal of Molecular Endocrinology*, 62(1):R21–R45.

Molina-Mora, J.A., Chinchilla-Montero, D., Castro-Peña, C. and García, F. 2020. Two-dimensional gel electrophoresis (2D-GE) image analysis based on CellProfiler: Pseudomonas aeruginosa AG1 as model. *Medicine (Baltimore)*, 99(49):e23373.

Morante, T., Shepherd, C., Constantinoiu, C., Loukas, A. and Sotillo, J. 2017. Revisiting the *Ancylostoma caninum* secretome provides new information on hookworm–host interactions. *Proteomics*, 17(23–24):1700186.

Mukherjee, S., Mukherjee, N., Gayen, P., Roy, P. and Babu, S.P. 2016. Metabolic inhibitors as antiparasitic drugs: Pharmacological, biochemical and molecular perspectives. *Current Drug Metabolism*, 17(10):937–970.

Nagorny, S., Aleshukina, A., Aleshukina, I., Denisenko, V., Ermakova, L. and Pshenichnaya, N. 2022. Application of mathematical models for MALDI-TOF MS on the example of dirofilariasis. *International Journal of Infectious Diseases*, 116:S95.

Nahed-Toral, J., López-Tirado, Q., Mendoza-Martınez, G., Aluja-Schunemann, A. and Trigo-Tavera, F.J. 2003. Epidemiology of parasitosis in the Tzotzil sheep production system. *Small Ruminant Research*, 49(2):199–206.

Negrao, F., Fernandez-Costa, C., Zorgi, N., Giorgio, S., Nogueira Eberlin, M. and Yates III, J.R. 2019. Label-free proteomic analysis reveals parasite-specific protein alterations in macrophages following *Leishmania amazonensis, Leishmania major*, or *Leishmania infantum* Infection. *ACS Infectious Diseases*, 5(6):851–862.

Olson, W.J., Martorelli Di Genova, B., Gallego-Lopez, G., Dawson, A.R., Stevenson, D., Amador-Noguez, D. and Knoll, L.J. 2020. Dual metabolomic profiling uncovers *Toxoplasma* manipulation of the host metabolome and the discovery of a novel parasite metabolic capability. *PLoS Pathogens*, 16(4):e1008432.

Olszewski, K.L. and Llinás, M. 2011. Central carbon metabolism of *Plasmodium* parasites. *Molecular Biochemistry and Parasitology*, 175(2):95–103.

Olszewski, K.L., Morrisey, J.M., Wilinski, D., Burns, J.M., Vaidya, A.B., Rabinowitz, J.D. and Llinás, M. 2009. Host-parasite interactions revealed by *Plasmodium falciparum* metabolomics. *Cell Host & Microbe*, 5(2):191–199.

Ouarti, B., Laroche, M., Righi, S., Meguini, M.N., Benakhla, A., Raoult, D. and Parola, P. 2020. Development of MALDI-TOF mass spectrometry for the identification of lice isolated from farm animals. *Parasite*, 27:28.

Parab, A.R. and McCall, L.I. 2021. Tryp-ing up metabolism: role of metabolic adaptations in kinetoplastid disease pathogenesis. *Infection and Immunity*, 89(4):10–1128.

Park, Y.H., Shi, Y.P., Liang, B., Medriano, C.A.D., Jeon, Y.H., Torres, E., Uppal, K., Slutsker, L. and Jones, D.P. 2015. High-resolution metabolomics to discover potential parasite-specific biomarkers in a *Plasmodium falciparum* erythrocytic stage culture system. *Malaria Journal*, 14:1–9.

Perera, D., Golizeh, M. and Ndao, M. 2020. A procedure for analyzing the proteomic proteomics profile of *Schistosoma mansoni* Cercariae. In: Timson, D.J. (ed.) *Schistosoma mansoni: Methods and protocols*. Springer US, pp. 75–84.

Pergande, M.R. and Cologna, S.M. 2017. Isoelectric point separations of peptides and proteins. *Proteomes*, 5(1):4.

Pinu, F.R., Beale, D.J., Paten, A.M., Kouremenos, K., Swarup, S., Schirra, H.J. and Wishart, D. 2019. Systems biology and multi-omics integration: viewpoints from the metabolomics research community. *Metabolites*, 9(4):76.

Prasopdee, S., Thitapakorn, V., Sathavornmanee, T. and Tesana, S. 2019. A comprehensive review of omics and host-parasite interplays studies, towards control of *Opisthorchis viverrini* infection for prevention of cholangiocarcinoma. *Acta Tropica*, 196:76–82.

Price, D.R., Nisbet, A.J., Frew, D., Bartley, Y., Oliver, E.M., McLean, K., Inglis, N.F., Watson, E., Corripio-Miyar, Y. and McNeilly, T.N. 2019. Characterisation of a niche-specific excretory–secretory peroxiredoxin from the parasitic nematode *Teladorsagia circumcincta*. *Parasites & Vectors*, 12:1–14.

Que, X. and Reed, S.L. 2000. Cysteine proteinases and the pathogenesis of amebiasis. *Clinical Microbiology Review*, 13(2):196–206.

Rex, D.A.B., Patil, A.H., Modi, P.K., Kandiyil, M.K., Kasaragod, S., Pinto, S.M., Tanneru, N., Sijwali, P.S. and Prasad, T.S.K. 2022. Dissecting *Plasmodium yoelii* pathobiology: Proteomic approaches for decoding novel translational and post-translational modifications. *ACS Omega*, 7(10):8246–8257.

Riekenberg, P.M., Briand, M.J., Moléana, T., Sasal, P., van der Meer, M.T.J., Thieltges, D.W., & Letourneur, Y. 2021. Isotopic discrimination in helminths infecting coral reef fishes depends on parasite group, habitat within host, and host stable isotope value. *Scientific Reports*, 11(1):4638.

Robinson, M.W. and Cwiklinski, K. 2021. Proteomics of host-helminth interactions. *Pathogens*, 10(10):1317.

Sánchez-Juanes, F., Calvo Sánchez, N., Belhassen García, M., Vieira Lista, C., Román, R.M., Álamo Sanz, R., Muro Álvarez, A. and Muñoz Bellido, J.L. 2022. Applications of MALDI-TOF mass spectrometry to the identification of parasites and arthropod vectors of human diseases. *Microorganisms*, 10(11):2300.

Sánchez-Ovejero, C., Benito-Lopez, F., Díez, P., Casulli, A., Siles-Lucas, M., Fuentes, M. and Manzano-Román, R. 2016. Sensing parasites: Proteomic and advanced bio-detection alternatives. *Journal of Proteomics*, 136:145–156.

Schmid-Hempel, P. 2009. Immune defence, parasite evasion strategies and their relevance for 'macroscopic phenomena' such as virulence. *Philosophical Transactions of the Royal Society of London. Series B, Biological Sciences*, 364(1513):85–98.

Sen, P. and Orešič, M. 2023. Integrating omics data in genome-scale metabolic modeling: A methodological perspective for precision medicine. *Metabolites*, 13(7):855.

Stryiński, R., Łopieńska-Biernat, E. and Carrera, M. 2020. Proteomic insights into the biology of the most important foodborne parasites in Europe. *Foods*, 9(10):1403.

Subramanian, I., Verma, S., Kumar, S., Jere, A. and Anamika, K. 2020. Multi-omics data integration, interpretation, and its application. *Bioinformatics and Biology Insights*, 14:1177932219899051.

Sumner, L.W., Amberg, A., Barrett, D., Beale, M.H., Beger, R., Daykin, C.A., Fan, T.W., Fiehn, O., Goodacre, R., Griffin, J.L., Hankemeier, T., Hardy, N., Harnly, J., Higashi, R., Kopka, J., Lane, A.N., Lindon, J.C., Marriott, P., Nicholls, A.W., Reily, M.D., Thaden, J.J. and Viant, M.R. 2007. Proposed minimum reporting standards for chemical analysis Chemical Analysis Working Group (CAWG) Metabolomics Standards Initiative (MSI). *Metabolomics*, 3(3):211–221.

Tabrizi, F., Tabaei, S.J.S., Ahmadi, N.A. and Oskouie, A.A. 2021. A nuclear magnetic resonance-based metabolomic study to identify metabolite differences between Iranian isolates of *Leishmania major* and *Leishmania tropica*. *Iranian Journal of Medical Sciences*, 46(1):43.

Templin, M.F., Stoll, D., Schrenk, M., Traub, P.C., Vöhringer, C.F. and Joos, T.O. 2002. Protein microarray technology. *Drug Discovery Today*, 7(15):815–822.

Tolmachev, A.V., Monroe, M.E., Purvine, S.O., Moore, R.J., Jaitly, N., Adkins, J.N., Anderson, G.A. and Smith, R.D. 2008. Characterization of strategies for obtaining confident identifications in bottom-up proteomics measurements using hybrid FTMS instruments. *Annals of Chemistry*, 80:8514–8525.

Tose, L., Ramirez, C.E., Michalkova, V., Nouzova, M., Noriega, F.G. and Fernandez-Lima, F. 2022.Coupling stable isotope labeling and liquid chromatography-trapped ion mobility spectrometry-time-of-flight-tandem mass spectrometry for de novo mosquito ovarian lipid studies. *Analytical Chemistry*, 94(16):6139–6145.

Tounta, V., Liu, Y., Cheyne, A. and Larrouy-Maumus, G. 2021. Metabolomics in infectious diseases and drug discovery. *Molecular Omics*, 17(3):376–393.

Urban, P.L. 2016. Quantitative mass spectrometry: an overview. *Philosophical Transactions: Mathematical, Physical and Engineering Sciences*, 374(2079):20150382.

Vengesai, A., Manuwa, M., Midzi, H., Mandeya, M., Muleya, V., Mujeni, K., Chipako, I., Goldring, D. and Mduluza, T. 2023. Identification of *Schistosoma haematobium* and *Schistosoma mansoni* linear B-cell epitopes with diagnostic potential using in silico immunoinformatic tools and peptide microarray technology. *medRxiv*, 2023-12.

Vincent, I.M. and Barrett, M.P. 2015. Metabolomic-based strategies for anti-parasite drug discovery. *Journal of Biomolecular Screening*, 20(1):44–55.

Wadhawan, M., Ahmad, F., Yadav, S. and Rathaur, S. 2022. Proteomic analysis reveals differential protein expression induced by inhibition of prolyl oligopeptidase in filarial parasites. *The Protein Journal*, 41(6):613–624.

Wandy, J. and Daly, R. 2021. GraphOmics: an interactive platform to explore and integrate multi-omics data. *BMC Bioinformatics*, 22:1–19.

Wang, J., Jiang, N., Sang, X., Yang, N., Feng, Y., Chen, R., Wang, X. and Chen, Q. 2021. Protein modification characteristics of the malaria parasite *Plasmodium falciparum* and the infected erythrocytes. *Molecular Cell Proteomics*, 20:100001.

Wangchuk, P., Yeshi, K. and Loukas, A. 2023. Metabolomics and lipidomics studies of parasitic helminths: molecular diversity and identification levels achieved by using different characterisation tools. *Metabolomics*, 19(7):63.

Wanichthanarak, K., Fahrmann, J.F. and Grapov, D. 2015. Genomic, proteomic, and metabolomic data integration strategies. *Biomarker Insights*, 10:BMI–S29511.

Wendel, T.P., Feucherolles, M., Rehner, J., Poppert, S., Utzinger, J., Becker, S.L. and Sy, I. 2021. Evaluating different storage media for identification of *Taenia saginata* proglottids using maldi-tof mass spectrometry. *Microorganisms*, 9:2006.

Whitman, J.D., Sakanari, J.A. and Mitreva, M. 2021. Areas of metabolomic exploration for helminth infections. *ACS Infectious Diseases*, 7(2):206–214.

Yannell, K.E., Ferreira, C.R., Tichy, S.E. and Cooks, R.G. 2018. Multiple reaction monitoring (MRM)-profiling with biomarker identification by LC-QTOF to characterize coronary artery disease. *Analyst*, 143(20):5014–5022.

Yu, X.T. and Zeng, T. 2018. Integrative analysis of omics big data. *Methods in Molecular Biology*, 1754:109–135.

Zhao, Y., Li, X., Zhou, R., Zhang, L., Chen, L., Tachibana, H., Feng, M. and Cheng, X. 2022. Quantitative proteomics reveals metabolic reprogramming in host cells induced by trophozoites and intermediate subunit of gal/galnac lectins from *Entamoeba histolytica*. *Msystems*, 7(2):e01353-21.

Zhou, D.H., Zhao, F.R., Nisbet, A.J., Xu, M.J., Song, H.Q., Lin, R.Q., Huang, S.Y. and Zhu, X.Q. 2014. Comparative proteomic analysis of different *Toxoplasma gondii* genotypes by two-dimensional fluorescence difference gel electrophoresis combined with mass spectrometry. *Electrophoresis*, 35(4):533–545.

6 Integrative Omics in Parasitology

Raja Adil Sarfraz[1], Hafiz Muhammad Rizwan[2],
Nadia Nazish[3], Muhammad Sulman Ali Taseer[4],
and Syed Soban Hassan[5]

[1]Department of Chemistry, Faculty of Science, University of Agriculture, Faisalabad, Pakistan

[2]Section of Parasitology, Department of Pathobiology, KBCMA College of Veterinary and Animal Sciences, Narowal, Sub-campus University of Veterinary and Animal Sciences, Lahore, Pakistan

[3]Department of Zoology, University of Sialkot, Sialkot, Pakistan

[4]Section of Pathology, Department of Pathobiology, KBCMA College of Veterinary and Animal Science, Narowal, Sub-campus University of Veterinary and Animal Sciences, Lahore, Pakistan

[5]Faculty of Veterinary Sciences, KBCMA College of Veterinary and Animal Sciences, Narowal, Sub-campus University of Veterinary and Animal Sciences, Lahore, Pakistan

6.1 INTRODUCTION

Medical and veterinary research has been transformed by high-throughput technologies. The discipline of "integrative genetics" emerged as a result of the development of genotyping arrays, which made it possible to conduct extensive genome-wide association studies and techniques for analysing global transcript levels (Hasin et al., 2017). The fields of transcriptomics, proteomics, metabolomics, and genomics in livestock species have enhanced our understanding of the complex molecular pathways behind anti-parasitic resistance in many important parasites. These technologies are still in their early stages (Kumar et al., 2021). Improved technologies have made it easier to identify potential biomarkers of resistant parasites, to identify the actual genes causing resistance, and to identify regulatory networks and parasite pathways controlling the development of anti-parasitic resistance, which includes the nature of parasitic infection and host–parasite interaction (Mukherjee et al., 2023). Developments in

DOI: 10.1201/9781032651071-6

mass spectrometry, computational biology, and nucleic acid sequencing have made it easier to identify, mark up, and analyse genes, transcripts, proteins, and metabolic products in model nematodes (*Pristionchus pacificus* and *Caenorhabditis elegans*) and socioeconomically significant parasitic species (Ma et al., 2020).

Integrating multi-omics data with collaborative modelling and analysis is a highly effective and precise way to comprehend the systems biology of animal immune system that is both healthy and sustainable (Suravajhala et al., 2016). Notable advancements have been made in the identification of novel targets in protozoan diseases through the application of genomics and integrative omics-based approaches (Cowell and Winzeler, 2019). Molecular biomarkers are specific molecules or a class of molecules that show promise in the diagnosis or prognosis of diseases (Doroszkiewicz et al., 2022). Transcriptomics and proteomics are two examples of the vast amounts of molecular "omics" data that have been collected over the past few decades due to advancements in high-throughput technology. These omics data make it possible to screen for diseases or abnormalities utilising biomarkers (Shi et al., 2020).

Interestingly, using many "omics" techniques simultaneously (also known as "multi-omics" or "integrated omics") makes it easier to independently and globally integrate the various components of complex biological processes (Zhou et al., 2021a). Successful integration of more than two omics technologies is extremely rare, despite the need and importance of integrating omics research into a variety of fields of study, such as disease biology (Pathak and Dave, 2014), microbiome analysis (Muller et al., 2014), and systems microbiology (Mochida and Shinozaki, 2011). Data analysis is now the main focus instead of data collection due to technological advancements. Large-scale data from transcriptomics, proteomics, and metabolomics research are now available, which raises additional concerns about appropriate integrated analysis techniques (Misra et al., 2019). We can integrate knowledge from several levels and get a more comprehensive understanding of the system under investigation by using integrative analysis approaches. The common results and method-specific results overlap significantly, despite the fact that the underlying mathematical assumptions differ greatly (Tomescu et al., 2014).

Yugi et al. (2016) proposed a trans-omics concept of dynamic networks that integrates more recent datasets, such as allosteric regulation, DNA–protein interactions, phosphoproteomics, and others, which can reveal important components of dynamic biological networks when omics data are successfully integrated. In the ever-expanding omics age, novel computational and statistical approaches are needed for data integration and the discovery of molecular signatures and biomarkers (Thaddi et al., 2024).

6.2 INTEGRATING MULTIPLE OMICS DATA FOR A HOLISTIC PERSPECTIVE

The majority of early omic techniques were devoted to extracting a single "layer" of data from the entire cell. Nonetheless, it is clear that changes in the host's molecular structure occur at several levels as a result of pathogenic invasion and other biological processes (Coiras et al., 2008). These molecular layers, such as the genetic code, mRNA transcripts, proteins, lipids, and metabolites, are also related to one another and influence and enhance one another (Sun and Hu, 2016). By combining proteomics with other omic techniques, several multi-omic approaches have been used in recent years to explore pathogenic infection. These methods have been helpful in figuring out the parasite's coding capacity, identifying important virulence factors, and defining the host's systemic response to a pathogenic infection (Rebollar et al., 2016). The primary focus in gaining practical understanding of cellular processes is now on analysing multi-omics data in combination with clinical information. It appears that integrating multi-omics data that provides details on proteins from several layers may help us comprehend complex biology in a systematic and holistic way (Yan et al., 2018). To comprehend the interactions between molecules, integrated techniques incorporate individual omics data in a chronological or simultaneous fashion (Bersanelli et al., 2016). They aid in evaluating the information transfer between omics levels and, hence, aid in closing the gap between genotype and phenotype (Subramanian et al., 2020).

Integrative techniques can eventually contribute to improved treatment and prevention since they can research biological phenomena holistically, which can enhance prognostics and the accuracy with which disease phenotypes are predicted (Hasin et al., 2017). High-throughput omics techniques, such as transcriptomics, proteomics, metabolomics, and genomics, are being rapidly adopted to evaluate biological materials. As a result, every analysis can produce daily data files that range from tera to petabytes in size (Reska et al., 2021). Different multi-dimensional omics data are difficult to integrate into biologically meaningful contexts because of their file sizes and the nomenclature discrepancies among different data kinds (Misra et al., 2019). Generating multiple datasets from a single sample through the application of "omic" techniques, such as proteomics/meta-proteomics, genome/metagenomics, transcriptomics/meta-transcriptomics, and metabolomics, has made it easier to generate hypotheses that have led to the identification of biological, molecular, and ecological functions and processes, as well as connections and correlations (Santiago-Rodriguez and Hollister, 2021).

All areas of life science are seeing a rise in the application of numerous omics approaches, such as transcriptomics, proteomics, metabolomics, and genomics. When considering biological systems under study, omics techniques offer a more holistic molecular perspective than conventional methods (Pinu et al., 2019). High-throughput omics (HTO) technologies, including transcriptomics, proteomics, metabolomics, genomics, and epigenomics, have advanced dramatically in recent years, affecting every aspect of biology. The systems biology era's advancement, particularly its applications to animal production and health qualities, has been driven by this (Suravajhala et al., 2016). Omics research analysing thousands to millions of markers with comparable biochemical characteristics is made possible by high-throughput methods (e.g. transcriptomics for RNA transcripts). Nevertheless, a single "omics" layer can only offer a limited amount of information about the basic pathways behind a disease (Vailati-Riboni et al., 2017). Thousands of single nucleotide polymorphisms for complex diseases and traits have been found through genome-wide association studies, yet little is known about the functional consequences and underlying processes of the linked loci (Sun and Hu, 2016). Based on the open-source Mergeomics R software, the Mergeomics web server is a dynamic online resource for multi-omics data integration to identify biological pathways, networks, and critical drivers crucial to disease aetiology (Ding et al., 2021).

6.3 APPLICATIONS OF INTEGRATIVE OMICS IN VETERINARY PARASITOLOGY

While *Caenorhabditis (C.) elegans* is a valuable model for supporting molecular investigations of parasitic nematodes, its application to investigating processes unique to parasitism within host animals is restricted. Utilising integrative omics techniques and significantly increased resources is necessary to have a thorough understanding of parasitic nematodes like *Haemoncus (H.) contortus* (Ma et al., 2020). Opportunities for thorough investigations of the transcriptomes (mRNA and miRNA), proteomes (somatic, excretory/secretory, and phosphorylated proteins), and lipidomes (e.g. polar and neutral lipids) of this nematode are made possible by the enhanced genome and well-established *in vitro* larval culture system. These tools ought to make it possible to investigate its developmental biology in depth at a degree that wasn't previously feasible (Ma et al., 2020). In the area of tropical and sub-tropical animal research, however, the integration of omics techniques with animal production affected by the parasites has received less attention. This type of focus is extremely narrow and distinct from those found in industrialised nations' temperate zones (Ribeiro et al., 2020). Recent developments in eukaryotic genome sequencing technologies, proteomics, transcriptomics, and metabolomics have made it possible to use molecular diagnostic tools to identify target molecules for control strategy formulation and to discover parasites early (Debnath et al., 2010).

In the field of veterinary parasitology, it also results in the introduction of many vaccinations that have been purified (Kumar et al., 2021). Countless datasets with ground-breaking applications in drug resistance, molecular epidemiology, diagnostic biomarkers (Figure 6.1), and possible therapeutic targets or vaccine candidates are made available by parasite integrated omics (Deblais et al., 2020). It is an extensive vocabulary covering several disciplinary biological domains, such as sequencing, function, evolution, and editing, together with genomic information, e.g. in case of *Plasmodium* spp. (Diab and Younis, 2022). It will be crucial to integrate findings from omics techniques on *Opisthorchis (O.) viverrini* and host interactions in order to create long-lasting and efficient strategies for the prevention and management of opisthorchiasis and opisthorchiasis-induced cholangiocarcinoma (Prasopdee et al., 2019).

The draft genome, transcriptomes relevant to each stage of development, and proteomic datasets for the somatic proteome, secretome, extracellular vesicles, and glycoproteome of the outer tegumental surface are among the extensive collection of omics datasets now accessible for *Fasciola (F.) hepatica* (Cwiklinski et al., 2021). With the use of these databases, researchers can now examine the complex details of the *Fasciola* life cycle, with a focus on how life history variables affect gene flow among liver fluke populations, which in turn affects the development of virulence, pathogenicity traits, and medication resistance (Cwiklinski and Dalton, 2018). Integrated omics has already yielded new molecular understanding of filarial worms and led to the discovery of novel targets for drugs, potential vaccines, and infection biomarkers (Lustigman et al., 2017). Future use of these diverse novel datasets is expected to advance our knowledge of these uncommon parasites and their

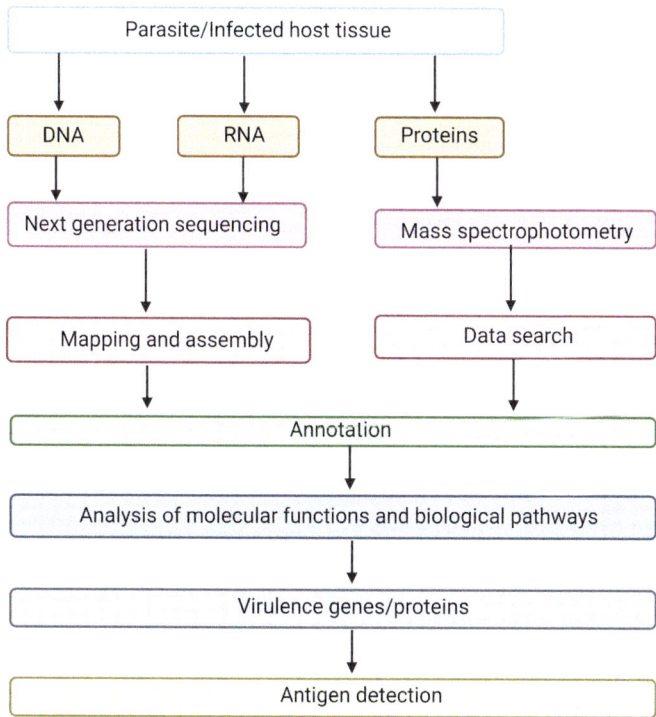

FIGURE 6.1 Integrative omics.: A promising approach for parasite diagnosis.

interactions with their host, ultimately assisting us in achieving the WHO's determination of permanently eradicating filarial infections (Hopkins, 2016).

6.4 APPLYING INTEGRATIVE OMICS APPROACHES IN PARASITE CONTROL

Due to intensive fish farming operations, the increasing need for fish products has resulted in health issues associated with disease. The aquaculture sector may be impacted by high fish mortality rates resulting from parasite-induced fish disease infections (Shinn et al., 2015). To better understand how to increase fish resistance to parasitic infection, a methodical approach to solving fish disease issues using multi-omics technologies has been employed recently. It is anticipated that the integration of several omics will improve our understanding of fish immune processes during disease infection (Su et al., 2024). This is because distinct omics data layers can be utilised to represent an organism's characteristics at various biomolecule levels (Natnan et al., 2021).

The landscape of genes, transcripts, proteins, lipids, and functional information for *H. contortus*, has been revealed by recent developments in genomics, transcriptomics, proteomics, and lipidomics, as well as functional genomics (Ma et al., 2020).

The biological elements of *H. contortus*'s development and reproduction, adaptability, parasitism, and drug resistance have been revealed by analysis of individual genome, transcriptome, proteome, and lipidome datasets (Marks et al., 2019). We are able to gain a comprehensive and global image of the function of several acetyl-CoA sources in *Toxoplasma (T.) gondii* physiology by employing molecular and multiomics techniques (Blume and Seeber, 2018). Acetyl-CoA found in the cytosol is necessary for the production of fatty acids unique to parasites (Mazumdar and Striepen, 2007). In contrast, metabolic adjustments made at the transcriptional, translational, and post-translational levels can cause the loss of mitochondrial acetyl-CoA, resulting in the control of parasites (Kloehn et al., 2020). Novel insights into malaria pathophysiology and immunity may be obtained through systems-scale analysis of various layers of molecular and cellular data (Tang et al., 2019).

The adaptability of *Anaplasmataceae* species is essential for their survival in a variety of microenvironments (Pruneau et al., 2014). They have to get past the immune system when they are extracellular and infectious. To survive and/or proliferate inside the host/vector cells, they must disrupt biological processes and resist the innate immune response (Marcelino et al., 2012). The study of how the expression of genes and proteins is altered based on environmental factors is made easier by functional genomics (Jaenisch and Bird, 2003). An overview of differentially expressed genes and proteins can be obtained through an initial high-throughput screening of gene and protein expression using omics techniques on the parasite, host, or vector. The second step entails applying conventional methodologies to further understand parasite biology and pathogenesis by concentrating on particular processes, gene function, and pathways of interest (Pruneau et al., 2014).

A more comprehensive gene expression study is made possible by the multiomics approach in order to comprehend *Entamoeba histolytica*'s adaptive response to growth stress (Singh et al., 2022). The power of omics approaches lies in their capacity to yield comprehensive gene, transcript, protein, and metabolite profiles, exceeding the limitations of traditional genetic/biochemical studies that focus on single or small numbers of target molecules (Singh et al., 2023). This broadens our understanding of parasite biology and, consequently, enhances parasite control efforts and diagnostic procedures. In the context of microbiota, parasitome, host co-metabolism, and infection response, omics technologies offer exciting possibilities capable of leading to the discovery of novel critical pathways that may improve diagnostic and therapeutic methods for gastrointestinal (GI) diseases connected to parasites (Marzano et al., 2017).

6.5 APPLYING INTEGRATIVE OMICS APPROACHES IN PARASITE DIAGNOSIS

Molecular barcoding and *Plasmodium (P.) falciparum* metabolomics offer distinct approaches for diagnosis, particularly in asymptomatic individuals (Tripathi et al., 2021). Studies on the resistance of *Plasmodium* have led to the identification of molecular genetic markers in resistant strains, which are useful instruments for tracking treatment resistance (Diab and Younis, 2022). In endemic areas, multi-omics data could support diagnostic and treatment approaches for the mass screening of malaria caused by mixed or other parasite species (Abdrabou, 2022). Additionally, establishing a worldwide database for clinical data and creating biosensors for detecting ultra-low parasitemia could help understand the relationship between parasitemia and disease severity for prognostic purposes. This approach may contribute to identifying diverse, globally relevant biomarker candidates through artificial intelligence-driven analysis (Boniolo et al., 2021). This will contribute to the UN goal of eliminating malaria worldwide by facilitating prompt diagnosis and effective treatment (Aggarwal et al., 2021).

In the current proteogenomics investigation, Pawer et al. (2014) mapped 43% of the *Leishmania (L.) major* proteome, demonstrating the importance of high-resolution mass spectrometry data in proteomic profiling and genome annotation of *L. major*. Promastigotes express a wide range of putative proteins. In addition, they found genuine virulence factors that have been linked to *Leishmania* pathogenesis and survival in infected hosts. Despite being the first *Leishmania* genome sequenced with thorough annotation, the *L. major* genome still yielded 26 genome search-specific peptides (GSSPs) during six-frame translated genome searches. These findings led to corrections in 15 gene models (Nirujogi, 2015). In addition, Pawer et al. (2014) found three additional genes in the *L. major* genome using GSSP evidence.

The widespread use of omics techniques in fish disease research has made it easier to comprehend various fish disease mechanisms and identify different biomarkers of disease virulence and host defence mechanisms (Natnan et al., 2021). These high-throughput technologies, when paired with bioinformatics, can create vast amounts of data to accelerate the identification of prospective biomarkers for different diagnostic and therapeutic advancements (Quezada et al., 2017). Numerous fish illness investigations have found potential molecular biomarkers such as genes, mRNAs, proteins, metabolites, and other substances (Natnan et al., 2021). These indicators may identify and distinguish between various elements that drive an organism to react in a specific way to an illness (Liu et al., 2014).

Aside from that, biomarkers are employed to detect the early stage of an infection and to interconnect the numerous systems that relate to other aspects associated with disease (Trzeciak et al., 2020). The metabolic fingerprint of rodents in response to schistosome infection can be summarised as decreased levels of tricarboxylic acid cycle intermediates, stimulated glycolysis, disrupted amino acid metabolism, disruptions in the gut microbiota, and a phenomenon unique to *S. japonicum* infection, i.e. inhibition of short-chain fatty acids (Wu et al., 2010). Despite significant advances in rodent models, clinical diagnosis of schistosomiasis with metabonomics still lags behind other omics approaches because the physiological systems of rodents in laboratories and humans are vastly different (Wang and Hu, 2014).

6.6 APPLYING INTEGRATIVE OMICS APPROACHES IN DRUG DISCOVERY FOR PARASITES

Neglected diseases have long been understudied, resulting in inefficient treatments with dangerous adverse effects. To reverse this scenario, an intense search for prospective therapeutic candidates has just begun under the framework of the non-profit organisation Drugs for Neglected Diseases Initiative (Bacchi et al., 1992). In previous work, scientists sought to create a first visualisation of proteins shared by *Trypanosoma (Tr.) cruzi*, *Tr. brucei*, and *L. major* that have interesting features as possible therapeutic targets, in order to identify particular candidates on which to focus in the future. As a result, they found a prioritised list of 319 common candidates with interesting properties that could be used as pharmacological targets (Ros-Lucas et al., 2022; Rivara-Espasandín et al., 2023). Further research would be required to experimentally verify these candidates (Rivara-Espasandín et al., 2023).

Metal complexes' potential use in medicine is an important subject in bioinorganic chemistry (Sekhon, 2011). High-throughput omics techniques can provide detailed information about the mechanism of action of novel metal-based drugs (Wang et al., 2020). The discovery of novel metallodrugs against *Tr. cruzi* is a rapidly developing field (Ravera et al., 2018). The combination of metallomics, proteomics, and transcriptomics enables the identification of various molecular targets and parasitic metabolic pathways affected by possible anti-parasitic medications such as vanadium (V), platinum (Pt), and palladium (Pd). In particular, metallomics investigations using Pd and Pt comparable compounds reveal that Pt is more readily absorbed by parasites than Pd, and both accumulate similarly in the parasite DNA fraction. Unexpectedly, vanadium did not interact with DNA (Gambino and Otero, 2019). The articles reviewed demonstrate the application of omics methods to identify molecular targets for possible therapeutic drugs (Scalese et al., 2022).

The integration of genomes, transcriptomics, and proteomics resulted in a widely applicable method for identifying putative target proteins in parasites that is both cost-effective and time-saving (Trapp et al., 2014). The predicted binding ligands can now be further investigated for their efficacy in acanthocephalan control (Schmidt et al., 2022). Existing helminth-targeting medications (anthelmintics) typically belong to only a few families of chemicals and target a limited number of proteins and biological reactions in these parasites, leading to widespread multidrug resistance and the need for new anthelmintics (Fontaine, 2017). Until recently, there was a lack of molecular and genomic data related to most helminths due to the difficulties associated with working with parasitic worms (Wit and Gilleard, 2017). Clinical applications of drug discovery by integrative omics are given in Figure 6.2.

The emergence of Next-Generation Sequencing has led to vast amounts of omics data. Coupled with chemogenomic screening and advancements in high-throughput screening techniques for specific helminth species and *C. elegans*, it's now feasible to perform data-driven, large-scale searches for new targets. This allows for experimental testing of drugs and drug-like compounds associated with these targets (Tyagi et al., 2019). A few years ago, a considerable number of genes/proteins from omic-based research were exclusively reported for *Schistosoma* spp., mainly *S. mansoni*, in the field of trematodology (Wang and Hu, 2014). The omic-based technique has resulted in the discovery of compounds that are presently thought to be promising for schistosomiasis immunotherapy (de Sousa et al., 2013). Integrated techniques, particularly with bioinformatic tools, will be useful in strategically identifying individual proteins of interest from a whole trematode proteome, which may be utilised as a protective commercialised product (Haçarız and Sayers, 2016).

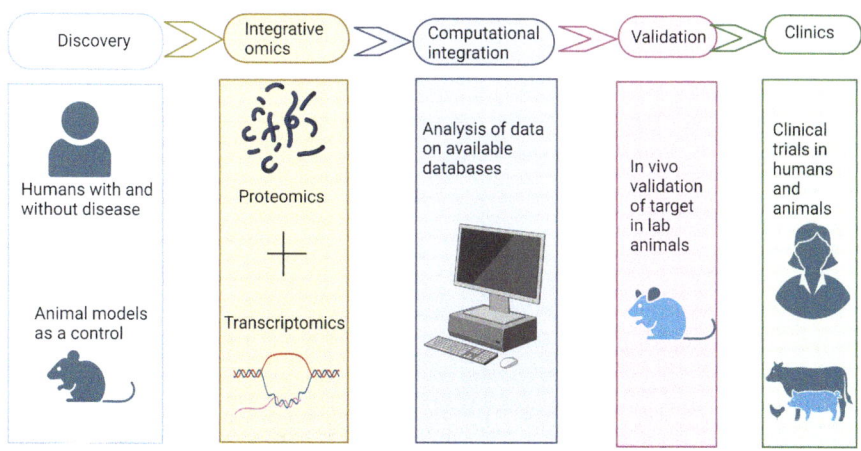

FIGURE 6.2   Clinical applications of drug discovery by integrative omics.

6.7   CHALLENGES AND FUTURE DIRECTIONS IN INTEGRATIVE OMICS FOR PARASITE RESEARCH

The integrated omics approaches present several broad experimental challenges, such as (i) comprehending the statistical behaviour of read-outs from each omics regime independently, (ii) identifying relationships between omics regimes that are not immediately apparent within their original biological context, and (iii) utilising time resolution in omics data to inform directionality (Buescher and Driggers, 2016). Distinct types of individual datasets have distinct requirements for quality assurance, control, data normalisation, and reduction strategies, making heterogeneous datasets difficult to manage. For example, RNA-Seq data is normalised and scaled differently from small RNA-Seq data; the former generally contains tens of thousands of transcripts, whilst the latter typically has fewer than 2000 short RNAs (Zhou et al., 2021b). As single-cell sequencing technologies, longer-read sequencing technologies, and applications for genomic and transcriptome investigations advance rapidly, new issues emerge, such as proper sequence coverage and statistical analysis of single-cell data (Menon, 2018).

The major problem of omics application in practical fields is that it is not yet feasible since these omics technologies have not yet passed the regulatory bodies' standards, and there is a continual need to conduct regulatory omics studies (Sauer et al., 2017). Major issues include a lack of standards for data formats and analytic pipelines, chemical variability of tiny molecules, the platform used, heterogeneity in sample processing, and varied quantification approaches (Spicer et al., 2017). The omics approaches produce massive volumes of data. Analysing, synthesising, and saving these data sets is an important undertaking because they greatly exceed everything that has previously been preserved (Prat and Degli-Esposti, 2019). The identification of biomarkers in the early stages of the onset of disease is still challenging (Banerjee et al., 2021). A significant disadvantage of dynamic omics is the time-consuming nature of 2D separation. It is expected that in the future, some great flash analysis techniques will be devised, potentially eliminating the need for the arduous liquid chromatography separation process entirely (Yan et al., 2015). "Multi-omics" data can help develop personalised treatments and vaccines for parasite infections, potentially addressing drug resistance issues (Zhou et al., 2021a).

6.8 CONCLUSION

In summary, omics methodologies are expected to play a crucial role in understanding the biological traits of parasites. Additionally, they can aid in creating innovative strategies to repel parasites and potentially develop helminth-based therapies for autoimmune diseases. The development of efficient, effective, and precise methodologies for researchers to identify proteins of interest from the parasite's proteome pool will be critical to maximising the benefits of this omics era. Based on the historical success of omic-based studies in various domains, we anticipate that the results of the relevant studies will translate into useful products to combat parasitic infections in the near future. We expect that further developments in integrative omics will lead to a decrease in the ratio of anti-parasitic drug resistance.

REFERENCES

Abdrabou, W.S. 2022. *Multi-omics analysis of host-parasite interactions in Plasmodium falciparum Malaria* (Doctoral dissertation, New York University).
Aggarwal, S., Peng, W.K. and Srivastava, S. 2021. Multi-omics advancements towards *Plasmodium vivax* malaria diagnosis. *Diagnostics*, 11(12):2222.
Bacchi, C.J., Nathan, H.C., Yarlett, N., Goldberg, B., McCann, P.P., Bitonti, A.J. and Sjoerdsma, A. 1992. Cure of murine *Trypanosoma brucei* rhodesiense infections with an S-adenosylmethionine decarboxylase inhibitor. *Antimicrobial Agents and Chemotherapy*, 36(12):2736–2740.
Banerjee, S., Prabhu Basrur, N. and Rai, P.S. 2021. Omics technologies in personalized combination therapy for cardiovascular diseases: Challenges and opportunities. *Personalized Medicine*, 18(6):595–611.
Bersanelli, M., Mosca, E., Remondini, D., Giampieri, E., Sala, C., Castellani, G. and Milanesi, L. 2016. Methods for the integration of multi-omics data: mathematical aspects. *BMC Bioinformatics*, 17:167–177.
Blume, M. and Seeber, F. 2018. *Metabolic interactions between Toxoplasma gondii and its host*. F1000Res, 7:F1000 Faculty Rev-1719.
Boniolo, F., Dorigatti, E., Ohnmacht, A.J., Saur, D., Schubert, B. and Menden, M.P. 2021. Artificial intelligence in early drug discovery enabling precision medicine. *Expert Opinion on Drug Discovery*, 16(9):991–1007.
Buescher, J.M. and Driggers, E.M. 2016. Integration of omics: more than the sum of its parts. *Cancer & Metabolism*, 4:1–8.
Coiras, M., Camafeita, E., López-Huertas, M.R., Calvo, E., López, J.A. and Alcamí, J. 2008. Application of proteomics technology for analyzing the interactions between host cells and intracellular infectious agents. *Proteomics*, 8(4):852–873.
Cowell, A.N. and Winzeler, E.A. 2019. Advances in omics-based methods to identify novel targets for malaria and other parasitic protozoan infections. *Genome Medicine*, 11:1–17.

Cwiklinski, K. and Dalton, J.P. 2018. Advances in *Fasciola hepatica* research using 'omics' technologies. *International Journal for Parasitology*, 48(5):321–331.

Cwiklinski, K., Verissimo, C.D.M., McVeigh, P., Donnelly, S. and Dalton, J.P. 2021. Applying'omics' technologies to understand Fasciola spp. biology. In: J.P. Dalton (ed.) *Fasciolosis*, CABI, pp. 338–378.

de Sousa, T.N., de Menezes Neto, A. and de Brito, C.F.A. 2013. "Omics" in the study of the major parasitic diseases malaria and schistosomiasis. *Infection, Genetics and Evolution*, 19:258–273.

Deblais, L., Kathayat, D., Helmy, Y.A., Closs, G. and Rajashekara, G. 2020. Translating 'big data': better understanding of host-pathogen interactions to control bacterial foodborne pathogens in poultry. *Animal Health Research Reviews*, 21(1):15–35.

Debnath, M., Prasad, G.B. and Bisen, P.S. 2010. *Molecular diagnostics: Promises and possibilities*. Springer Science & Business Media.

Diab, R. and Younis, S. 2022. Omics: Approaches and applications related to diagnosis, treatment, and control of parasitic diseases. Part I: *Plasmodium spp. Parasitologists United Journal*, 15(2):144–153.

Ding, J., Blencowe, M., Nghiem, T., Ha, S.M., Chen, Y.W., Li, G. and Yang, X. 2021. Mergeomics 2.0: a web server for multi-omics data integration to elucidate disease networks and predict therapeutics. *Nucleic Acids Research*, 49(W1):W375–W387.

Doroszkiewicz, J., Groblewska, M. and Mroczko, B. 2022. Molecular biomarkers and their implications for the early diagnosis of selected neurodegenerative diseases. *International Journal of Molecular Sciences*, 23(9):4610.

Fontaine, P. 2017. *The transcription factor Skn-1 confers resistance to benzimidazole drugs in caenorhabditis elegans via the Phase II drug detoxification gene Ugt-22* (Doctoral dissertation, University of Florida).

Gambino, D. and Otero, L. 2019. Metal compounds in the development of antiparasitic agents: rational design from basic chemistry to the clinic. *Metal Ions in Life Sciences*, 19:331–358.

Haçarız, O. and Sayers, G.P. 2016. The omic approach to parasitic trematode research—a review of techniques and developments within the past 5 years. *Parasitology Research*, 115(7):2523–2543.

Hasin, Y., Seldin, M. and Lusis, A. 2017. Multi-omics approaches to disease. *Genome Biology*, 18(1):1–15.

Hopkins, A.D. 2016. Neglected tropical diseases in Africa: a new paradigm. *International Health*, 8:i28–i33.

Jaenisch, R. and Bird, A. 2003. Epigenetic regulation of gene expression: how the genome integrates intrinsic and environmental signals. *Nature Genetics*, 33(3):245–254.

Kloehn, J., Oppenheim, R.D., Siddiqui, G., De Bock, P.J., Kumar Dogga, S., Coute, Y., Hakimi, M.A., Creek, D.J. and Soldati-Favre, D. 2020. Multi-omics analysis delineates the distinct functions of sub-cellular acetyl-CoA pools in *Toxoplasma gondii*. BMC biology, 18:1–26.

Kumar, S., Gupta, S., Mohmad, A., Fular, A., Parthasarathi, B.C. and Chaubey, A.K. 2021. Molecular tools-advances, opportunities and prospects for the control of parasites of veterinary importance. *International Journal of Tropical Insect Science*, 41:33–42.

Liu, R., Wang, X., Aihara, K. and Chen, L. 2014. Early diagnosis of complex diseases by molecular biomarkers, network biomarkers, and dynamical network biomarkers. *Medicinal Research Reviews*, 34(3):455–478.

Lustigman, S., Grote, A. and Ghedin, E. 2017. The role of'omics' in the quest to eliminate human filariasis. *PLoS Neglected Tropical Diseases*, 11(4):e0005464.

Ma, G., Gasser, R.B., Wang, T., Korhonen, P.K. and Young, N.D. 2020. Toward integrative 'omics of the barber's pole worm and related parasitic nematodes. *Infection, Genetics and Evolution*, 85:104500.

Marcelino, I., De Almeida, A.M., Ventosa, M., Pruneau, L., Meyer, D.F., Martinez, D., Lefrançois, T., Vachiéry, N. and Coelho, A.V. 2012. Tick-borne diseases in cattle: applications of proteomics to develop new generation vaccines. *Journal of Proteomics*, 75(14):4232–4250.

Marks, N.D., Winter, A.D., Gu, H.Y., Maitland, K., Gillan, V., Ambroz, M., Martinelli, A., Laing, R., MacLellan, R., Towne, J. and Roberts, B. 2019. Profiling microRNAs through development of the parasitic nematode *Haemonchus* identifies nematode-specific miRNAs that suppress larval development. *Scientific Reports*, 9(1):17594.

Marzano, V., Mancinelli, L., Bracaglia, G., Del Chierico, F., Vernocchi, P., Di Girolamo, F., Garrone, S., Tchidjou Kuekou, H., D'Argenio, P., Dallapiccola, B. and Urbani, A. 2017. Omic" investigations of protozoa and worms for a deeper understanding of the human gut parasitome. *PLoS Neglected Tropical Diseases*, 11(11):e0005916.

Mazumdar, J. and Striepen, B. 2007. Make it or take it: fatty acid metabolism of apicomplexan parasites. *Eukaryotic Cell*, 6(10):1727–1735.

Menon, V. 2018. Clustering single cells: a review of approaches on high-and low-depth single-cell RNA-seq data. *Briefings in Functional Genomics*, 17(4):240–245.

Misra, B.B., Langefeld, C., Olivier, M. and Cox, L.A. 2019. Integrated omics: tools, advances and future approaches. *Journal of Molecular Endocrinology*, 62(1):R21–R45.

Mochida, K. and Shinozaki, K. 2011. Advances in omics and bioinformatics tools for systems analyses of plant functions. *Plant and Cell Physiology*, 52(12):2017–2038.

Mukherjee, A., Kar, I. and Patra, A.K. 2023. Understanding anthelmintic resistance in livestock using "omics" approaches. *Environmental Science and Pollution Research,* 30(60):125439-125463.

Muller, E.E., Pinel, N., Laczny, C.C., Hoopmann, M.R., Narayanasamy, S., Lebrun, L.A., Roume, H., Lin, J., May, P., Hicks, N.D. and Heintz-Buschart, A. 2014. Community-integrated omics links dominance of a microbial generalist to fine-tuned resource usage. *Nature Communications*, 5(1):5603.

Natnan, M.E., Low, C.F., Chong, C.M., Bunawan, H. and Baharum, S.N. 2021. Integration of omics tools for understanding the fish immune response due to microbial challenge. *Frontiers in Marine Science*, 8:668771.

Nirujogi, R.S. 2015. *Proteomic and proteogenomic analysis of kinetoplastid protozoan parasite Leishmania Donovani* (Doctoral dissertation). Institute of Bioinformatics, Pondicherry University, India.

Pathak, R.R. and Dave, V. 2014. Integrating omics technologies to study pulmonary physiology and pathology at the systems level. *Cellular Physiology and Biochemistry*, 33(5):1239–1260.

Pawar, H., Renuse, S., Khobragade, S.N., Chavan, S., Sathe, G., Kumar, P., Mahale, K.N., Gore, K., Kulkarni, A., Dixit, T. and Raju, R. 2014. Neglected tropical diseases and omics science: proteogenomics analysis of the promastigote stage of *Leishmania major* parasite. *Omics: A Journal of Integrative Biology*, 18(8):499–512.

Pinu, F.R., Beale, D.J., Paten, A.M., Kouremenos, K., Swarup, S., Schirra, H.J. and Wishart, D. 2019. Systems biology and multi-omics integration: viewpoints from the metabolomics research community. *Metabolites*, 9(4):76.

Prasopdee, S., Thitapakorn, V., Sathavornmanee, T. and Tesana, S. 2019. A comprehensive review of omics and host-parasite interplays studies, towards control of *Opisthorchis viverrini* infection for prevention of cholangiocarcinoma. *Acta Tropica*, 196:76–82.

Prat, O. and Degli-Esposti, D. 2019. New challenges: omics technologies in ecotoxicology. In: Gross, E. and Garric, J. (eds.) *Ecotoxicology*. ISTE Press - Elsevier, pp. 181–208.

Pruneau, L., Moumène, A., Meyer, D.F., Marcelino, I., Lefrançois, T. and Vachiéry, N. 2014. Understanding Anaplasmataceae pathogenesis using "Omics" approaches. *Frontiers in Cellular and Infection Microbiology*, 4:86.

Quezada, H., Guzmán-Ortiz, A.L., Díaz-Sánchez, H., Valle-Rios, R. and Aguirre-Hernández, J. 2017. Omics-based biomarkers: current status and potential use in the clinic. *Boletín Médico Del Hospital Infantil de México (English Edition)*, 74(3): 219–226.

Ravera, M., Moreno-Viguri, E., Paucar, R., Pérez-Silanes, S. and Gabano, E. 2018. Organometallic compounds in the discovery of new agents against kinetoplastid-caused diseases. *European Journal of Medicinal Chemistry*, 155:459–482.

Rebollar, E.A., Antwis, R.E., Becker, M.H., Belden, L.K., Bletz, M.C., Brucker, R.M., Harrison, X.A., Hughey, M.C., Kueneman, J.G., Loudon, A.H. and McKenzie, V. 2016. Using "omics" and integrated multi-omics approaches to guide probiotic selection to mitigate chytridiomycosis and other emerging infectious diseases. *Frontiers in Microbiology*, 7:68.

Reska, D., Czajkowski, M., Jurczuk, K., Boldak, C., Kwedlo, W., Baucr, W., Koszclcw, J. and Kretowski, M. 2021. Integration of solutions and services for multi-omics data analysis towards personalized medicine. *Biocybernetics and Biomedical Engineering*, 41(4):1646–1663.

Ribeiro, D.M., Salama, A.A., Vitor, A.C., Argüello, A., Moncau, C.T., Santos, E.M., Caja, G., de Oliveira, J.S., Balieiro, J.C., Hernández-Castellano, L.E. and Zachut, M. 2020. The application of omics in ruminant production: A review in the tropical and sub-tropical animal production context. *Journal of Proteomics*, 227:103905.

Rivara-Espasandín, M., Palumbo, M.C., Sosa, E.J., Radío, S., Turjanski, A.G., Sotelo-Silveira, J., Fernandez Do Porto, D. and Smircich, P., 2023. Omics data integration facilitates target selection for new antiparasitic drugs against TriTryp infections. *Frontiers in Pharmacology*, 14:1136321.

Ros-Lucas, A., Martinez-Peinado, N., Bastida, J., Gascón, J. and Alonso-Padilla, J. 2022. The use of AlphaFold for in silico exploration of drug targets in the parasite trypanosoma cruzi. *Frontiers in Cellular and Infection Microbiology*, July 14, 12:944748.

Santiago-Rodriguez, T.M. and Hollister, E.B. 2021. Multi 'omic data integration: A review of concepts, considerations, and approaches. *Seminars in Perinatology*, 45(6):151456.

Sauer, U.G., Deferme, L., Gribaldo, L., Hackermüller, J., Tralau, T., van Ravenzwaay, B., Yauk, C., Poole, A., Tong, W. and Gant, T.W. 2017. The challenge of the application of'omics technologies in chemicals risk assessment: Background and outlook. *Regulatory Toxicology and Pharmacology*, 91:S14–S26.

Scalese, G., Kostenkova, K., Crans, D.C. and Gambino, D. 2022. Metallomics and other omics approaches in antiparasitic metal-based drug research. *Current Opinion in Chemical Biology*, 67:102127.

Schmidt, H., Mauer, K., Glaser, M., Dezfuli, B.S., Hellmann, S.L., Silva Gomes, A.L., Butter, F., Wade, R.C., Hankeln, T. and Herlyn, H. 2022. Identification of antiparasitic drug targets using a multi-omics workflow in the acanthocephalan model. *BMC Genomics*, 23(1):1–16.

Sekhon, B.S. 2011. Inorganics/bioinorganics: biological, medicinal and pharmaceutical uses. *Journal of Pharmaceutical Education and Research*, 2(1):1.

Shi, K., Lin, W. and Zhao, X.M. 2020. Identifying molecular biomarkers for diseases with machine learning based on integrative omics. *IEEE/ACM Transactions on Computational Biology and Bioinformatics*, 18(6):2514–2525.

Shinn, A., Pratoomyot, J., Bron, J., Paladini, G., Brooker, E. and Brooker, A. 2015. Economic impacts of aquatic parasites on global finfish production. *Global Aquaculture Advocate*, 2015:58–61.

Singh, S.S., Mansuri, M.S., Naiyer, S., Kaur, D., Agrahari, M., Srinivasan, S., Jhingan, G.D., Bhattacharya, A. and Bhattacharya, S. 2022. Multi-omics analysis to characterize molecular adaptation of *Entamoeba histolytica* during serum stress. *Proteomics*, 22(22):2200148.

Singh, S.S., Sarma, D.K., Verma, V., Nagpal, R. and Kumar, M. 2023. Unveiling the future of metabolic medicine: omics technologies driving personalized solutions for precision treatment of metabolic disorders. *Biochemical and Biophysical Research Communications*, 682:1–20.

Spicer, R.A., Salek, R. and Steinbeck, C. 2017. A decade after the metabolomics standards initiative it's time for a revision. *Scientific Data*, 4(1):1–3.

Su, G., Yu, C., Liang, S., Wang, W. and Wang, H. 2024. Multi-omics in food safety and authenticity in terms of food components. *Food Chemistry*, 437:137943.

Subramanian, I., Verma, S., Kumar, S., Jere, A. and Anamika, K. 2020. Multi-omics data integration, interpretation, and its application. *Bioinformatics and Biology Insights*, 14:1177932219899051.

Sun, Y.V. and Hu, Y.J. 2016. Integrative analysis of multi-omics data for discovery and functional studies of complex human diseases. *Advances in Genetics*, 93:147–190.

Suravajhala, P., Kogelman, L.J. and Kadarmideen, H.N. 2016. Multi-omic data integration and analysis using systems genomics approaches: methods and applications in animal production, health and welfare. *Genetics Selection Evolution*, 48(1):1–14.

Tang, Y., Joyner, C.J., Cordy, R.J., Galinski, M.R., Lamb, T.J. and Styczynski, M.P. 2019. Multi-omics integrative analysis of acute and relapsing Malaria in a non-human primate model of *P. Vivax* Infection. BioRxiv:564195. https://doi.org/10.1101/564195

Thaddi, B.N., Dabbada, V.B., Ambati, B. and Kilari, E.K. 2024. Decoding cancer insights: recent progress and strategies in proteomics for biomarker discovery. *Journal of Proteins and Proteomics,* 15:67–87.

Tomescu, O.A., Mattanovich, D. and Thallinger, G.G. 2014. Integrative omics analysis. A study based on *Plasmodium falciparum* mRNA and protein data. *BMC Systems Biology*, 8(2):1–16.

Trapp, J., Armengaud, J., Salvador, A., Chaumot, A. and Geffard, O. 2014. Next-generation proteomics: toward customized biomarkers for environmental biomonitoring. *Environmental Science & Technology*, 48(23):13560–13572.

Tripathi, M., Khatri, A., Lakra, V., Kaushik, J. and Rathore, S. 2021. Malaria in the era of omics: challenges and way forward. In: Hameed, S. and Fatima, Z. (eds.) *Integrated Omics Approaches to Infectious Diseases*. Springer, Singapore. pp. 483–506.

Trzeciak, A., Pietropaoli, A.P. and Kim, M. 2020. Biomarkers and associated immune mechanisms for early detection and therapeutic management of sepsis. *Immune Network*, 20(3):e23.

Tyagi, R., Rosa, B.A. and Mitreva, M. 2019. Omics-driven knowledge-based discovery of anthelmintic targets and drugs. *In:* Roy, K. (ed.) *Silico Drug Design*. Academic Press, pp. 329–358.

Vailati-Riboni, M., Palombo, V. and Loor, J.J. 2017. What are omics sciences?. In: Ametaj, B.N. (eds.) *Periparturient Diseases of* Dairy Cows: *A* Systems Biology *Approach*. Springer Cham. pp. 1–7.

Wang, H., Zhou, Y., Xu, X., Li, H. and Sun, H. 2020. Metalloproteomics in conjunction with other omics for uncovering the mechanism of action of metallodrugs: mechanism-driven new therapy development. *Current Opinion in Chemical Biology*, 55:171–179.

Wang, S. and Hu, W. 2014. Development of "-omics" research in *Schistosoma spp.* and-omics-based new diagnostic tools for schistosomiasis. *Frontiers in Microbiology*, 5:313.

Wit, J. and Gilleard, J.S. 2017. Resequencing helminth genomes for population and genetic studies. *Trends in Parasitology*, 33(5):388–399.

Wu, J., Xu, W., Ming, Z., Dong, H., Tang, H. and Wang, Y. 2010. Metabolic changes reveal the development of schistosomiasis in mice. *PLoS Neglected Tropical Diseases*, 4(8):807.

Yan, J., Risacher, S.L., Shen, L. and Saykin, A.J. 2018. Network approaches to systems biology analysis of complex disease: integrative methods for multi-omics data. *Briefings in Bioinformatics*, 19(6):1370–1381.

Yan, S.K., Liu, R.H., Jin, H.Z., Liu, X.R., Ye, J., Shan, L. and Zhang, W.D. 2015. "Omics" in pharmaceutical research: overview, applications, challenges, and future perspectives. *Chinese Journal of Natural Medicines*, 13(1):3–21.

Yugi, K., Kubota, H., Hatano, A. and Kuroda, S. 2016. Trans-omics: how to reconstruct biochemical networks across multiple 'omic' layers. *Trends in Biotechnology*, 34(4):276–290.

Zhou, M., Varol, A. and Efferth, T. 2021a. Multi-omics approaches to improve malaria therapy. *Pharmacological Research*, 167:105570.

Zhou, Y., Yang, B., Wang, J., Zhu, J. and Tian, G. 2021b. A scaling-free minimum enclosing ball method to detect differentially expressed genes for RNA-seq data. *BMC Genomics,* June 26, 22(1):479.

7 Omics-Based Biomarkers for Parasitic Infections

Hafiz Muhammad Rizwan[1],
Muhammad Sohail Sajid[2], Muhammad Younus[1],
Haroon Ahmad[2], Hizqeel Ahmed Muzaffar[3],
Muhammad Nadeem Saleem[4], and
Muhammad Zeeshan[2]

[1]Section of Parasitology, Department of Pathobiology, KBCMA College of Veterinary and Animal Sciences, Narowal, Sub-campus University of Veterinary and Animal Sciences, Lahore, Pakistan

[2]Department of Parasitology, Faculty of Veterinary Sciences, University of Agriculture, Faisalabad, Pakistan

[3]Faculty of Veterinary Sciences, KBCMA College of Veterinary and Animal Sciences, Narowal, Sub-campus University of Veterinary and Animal Sciences, Lahore, Pakistan

[4]Section of Animal Breeding and Genetics Section, Department of Animal Sciences, KBCMA College of Veterinary and Animal Sciences, Narowal, Sub-campus University of Veterinary and Animal Sciences, Lahore, Pakistan

7.1 INTRODUCTION

Omics research, which highly depends upon experimental technologies, develops informative data in enormous amounts and has successfully led to the development of various diagnostic techniques for the detection of parasitic infections (Wang and Hu, 2014). Advancements in DNA sequencing, RNA sequencing, operation of mass spectrometers, and bioinformatics have led us to the identification, interpretation, and analysis of various proteins, genes, and transcripts in parasites of different classes (Ma et al., 2020a). The latest advancements in omics technologies have led to the detection of biomolecules essential for parasites in their transmission between different hosts and the identification of new drug and vaccine targets (Prasopdee et al., 2019) and biomarkers of infection. By utilising these techniques, it is expected that host–parasite interaction can be well understood (Lustigman et al., 2017). In the

DOI: 10.1201/9781032651071-7

past 20 years, omics research has significantly advanced medical parasitology data-sets for phylogenetic analysis, host–parasite interactions, and parasite system biology. Examples of these datasets include transcriptomes, proteomics, metabolomics, and genomes (Swann et al., 2015). Genome-wide association studies, in conjunction with bioinformatics, have allowed researchers to discover interesting therapeutic targets, diagnostic biomarkers, and possible vaccine candidates for use in the detection, management, and prevention of several neglected tropical diseases (Bah et al., 2018).

There are two types of omics approaches: structural (genomics) and functional (post-genomics) (Diab and Younis, 2022). Nuclear staining dye is used to stain iRBCs on a microarray chip containing whole blood cells, and the results are correlated with microscopy findings to further develop phenome-based diagnoses. The technique is quick, simple to apply, and has shown consistent results (Yatsushiro et al., 2016). Small subunit ribosomal RNA (ssrRNA) is used in the nucleic acid-based diagnostic method to amplify the genus and species-specific stretch, which is used to identify parasite species (Aggarwal et al., 2021). Serum proteomics is one proteome-based test that has steadily grown in the field of diagnostic applications for the highly sensitive identification of diseases (Anderson and Anderson, 2002). By examining the changes in the host proteome, it can also help to clarify the relationship between the host and parasite (Aggarwal et al., 2021). Protein-based biomarkers are based on antigen and antibody interaction assays like point of care (POC) diagnostic tests (Das et al., 2018). Moreover, the ability of parasite proteins to develop constantly expressed proteins is demonstrated by parasite proteomics. Sorting these proteins will yield a list of proteins that could be used as possible biomarker candidates (Venkatesh et al., 2020).

With the right information and technologies at hand, the integrated omics approach facilitates the understanding of pathobiology's complexities (Tomescu et al., 2014). When exposed to a disease that arises from alterations in the biochemical, physiological, or a mix of both, the infected individual displays symptoms. The first step in understanding the disease is to examine physiological changes, such as a change in the shape of red blood cells like when *Plasmodium* is present. These changes can be verified by the use of microscopy (Payne, 1988). The changed form can be investigated further by utilising cutting-edge technologies like proteomics, genomics, and metabolomics methods to determine the molecular causes of the altered morphology (Olivier et al., 2019). Omics-based biomarkers also help in the understanding of the pathogenesis of parasites within their hosts (Aggarwal et al., 2021). In this chapter, biomarkers like genomics-based, transcriptomics-based, proteomics approaches in biomarker discovery, metabolomics approaches in biomarker discovery, epigenomics RNAs as potential biomarkers, non-coding RNAs as potential biomarkers, integrative omics approaches for biomarker identification, challenges in omics-based biomarker research, and future perspectives in omics-based biomarker research for parasitic infections are discussed.

7.2 GENOMICS AS BIOMARKERS

Among the omics sciences, genomics is the most advanced field of research. Genomic research in the veterinary and medical fields looks for genetic polymorphisms linked to illness, therapy response, or future prognosis of the patient (Klopfleisch, 2015). Genome-wide association studies (GWAS) are an effective method that has been utilised in numerous instances to find thousands of genetic variations linked to complex disorders. Thousands of parasites are genotyped for over a million genetic markers in these kinds of investigations, and statistically significant changes in minor allele frequencies between case and control groups are taken as indications of association (Perera et al., 2022). The GWAS research has been a tremendous asset to our comprehension of complex traits (Tam et al., 2019). Genotype arrays, exome sequencing, and Next-Generation Sequencing (NGS) for whole-genome sequencing are related technologies (Hasin et al., 2017).

If we study the gastrointestinal (GI) nematodes of sheep, then the application of genomics tells us that in the case of *Haemonchus contortus*, various interaction genes, e.g. CAT, are enhanced with the Wnt receptor signalling pathway and up-regulation of NFκ β transcription factor function. Another gene known as FCER1A, which encodes a high-affinity receptor for the fragment crystallisable (Fc) region of the antibody E (IgE), is directly responsible for innate immunity to GI parasites in sheep. These biomarkers are also associated with T-cell regulation and B-cell regulation (Kadarmideen et al., 2011). To improve the genetic response to selection for GI parasite resistance, molecular markers may be employed. Still, it has been difficult to identify potential GI parasite resistance genes (Álvarez et al., 2019). In the case of protozoal infections like malaria caused by *Plasmodium* species, not only can symptomatic infections be detected, asymptomatic infections can also be detected because Pfg17 is an excellent biomarker in this condition (Essuman et al., 2017).

The scientific community has made significant contributions to the enormous advancements in cancer research over the past few years, including the discovery of biomarkers linked to helminths (Van-Tong et al., 2017). In this context, improved knowledge of the pathogenetic evolution of cancer may have a beneficial effect on clinical practices, particularly in the areas of diagnosis and treatment. Changes in the molecular makeup of cancer cells (mRNA, DNA, lipids, and sugars) can serve as "sentinels" for monitoring the course of the disease, risk assessment, differential diagnosis, therapy response prediction, and prognosis determination (Scholte et al., 2018). The knowledge of genomics as biomarkers can also help us to understand susceptible and resistant genes in parasitic infections. The effectiveness of breeding programmes for farm animals can be improved by the identification of genetic markers of resistance and susceptibility (Wakchaure et al., 2015).

A study of relationships between gene variants related to the host immune response and phenotypic resistant features was the initial strategy employed to look for genetic markers linked to host resistance (Aboshady et al., 2020). The majority of the time, parasitic resistance has been linked to genetic markers from the major histocompatibility complex (MHC) region (Valilou et al., 2015). To provide guidance on treatment options and possible interactions between drugs and vaccines, genomic data collected from animal models and pathogens can be coupled with host genetics and patient health records. Africa, however, produces the least amount of research on infectious disease genetics, despite bearing the greatest burden of infectious diseases (Bah et al., 2018). Unprecedented insights into the biology and successful establishment of apicomplexans as a parasitic phylum are made possible by the availability and analysis of apicomplexan genomes and associated metadata (Swapna and Parkinson, 2017).

7.3 TRANSCRIPTOMICS AS BIOMARKERS

Transcriptomics is a popular method used to examine the processes of both the parasite and the host in infectious disorders. Progress in technology and bioinformatics has enabled more comprehensive examinations of the relationship between RNA expression and basic biology, immunity, pathophysiology, diagnostics, and prognosis (Menyhárt and Győrffy, 2021). Now, a previously unachievable objective—the simultaneous investigation of RNA expression in host and parasite to enhance understanding of their interactions—can be realised through the application of transcriptomic techniques (Lee et al., 2018a). Transcriptomics is basically the quantitative or qualitative study of RNAs on a genome-wide scale (Hasin et al., 2017). Studies of gene expression have gained popularity as a means of examining how the host reacts to parasitic infections and immunological disruption (Barton et al., 2017). Another benefit of transcriptomics biomarkers is that they make measurements faster and less annoying than traditional clinical or parasitological assessments. Additionally, they might make it easier to plan smaller, yet effective clinical trials, which could hasten the regulatory review and approval of treatments (Veras et al., 2018).

DNA microarrays have been developed within the past two years in order to improve gene expression analysis and the identification of new genes involving the genome sequencing of vertebrates and parasites (Geiger et al., 2011). The study of coordinated expression of functionally related gene sets using microarrays started to shed light on the biology of protozoan parasites and the diseases they cause (Duncan, 2004). River blindness, caused by *Onchocerca volvulus*, is a significant concern. Transcriptome data from various parasite stages are obtained through RNA sequencing. This data helps in verifying the parasite's genome and understanding stage-specific mRNA expression (Bennuru et al., 2016). In protozoal infections like malaria, genes that are more expressed in hosts include MMP8, OLFM4, DEFA3, and ELANE (Lee et al., 2018b). In the case of *Fasciola hepatica*, secretory proteins responsible for host–parasite interaction are released by the expression of sequence tags (Robinson et al., 2009). In leishmaniasis, macrophages are impacted. Affected macrophages lack the up-regulation of genes related to the retinoid X receptor pathway, associated with lipid metabolism (Bichiou et al., 2021).

Transcriptomics from infected tissue samples showed significant up-regulation of genes in pathways linked to immune cell activation, including antigen-presenting cells, natural killer cells, granulocytes, and lymphocytes (Cantacessi et al., 2015). It is obvious that the advent of high-throughput transcriptomic technology has led to a rapid growth in the already large amount of knowledge regarding the molecular connections that parasites and their hosts have. Additionally, these technologies have made it possible to go forward with the investigation of the molecular connections between parasites and their vectors (Kima, 2014).

7.4 PROTEOMICS AS BIOMARKERS

Proteomics is a valuable tool for detecting parasites and host alterations within micro-detection platforms. It is expected that these techniques will provide a novel solution to combat parasitic diseases (Sánchez-Ovejero et al., 2016). A potential field of study is the identification of biomarkers of parasitic infections using differential protein profiling of certain hosts or parasitic compounds. This method mostly relies on changes in protein variations, peptide degradations, or post-translational modifications caused by parasites (De-Bock et al., 2010). Given that proximal biofluids and human and animal tissues serve as the route and destination points for parasites and/or their secretions, these fluids may hold molecular information about the physiological and pathological states of the organism. Proximal biofluid proteomic characterisation may yield complete and valuable data for prognostic, predictive, and diagnostic biomarkers. Finding extremely low-abundance protein circulating biomarkers, which offer more downstream information than nucleic acids and may be crucial for early diagnosis, is the challenging part of the research (Qoronfleh and Lindpaintner, 2010).

Mass spectrometry is a technique that allows us to examine body components to find variations in the expression of proteins that are then identified as biomarkers of different diseases. In the case of urinary schistosomiasis, Actin 1, heat shock protein, phosphopyruvate hydrase, histone-4, elongation factor 1-alpha, and a few other proteins derived from the *Schistosome* species can be used as biomarkers for the diagnosis of disease (Onile et al., 2017). In the case of blood parasites, if we want an early diagnosis, mass spectrometry of serum protein profile of blood proteome can be a promising approach (Pérez-Montoto et al., 2009). For example, malaria, a disease caused by the blood parasite *Plasmodium*, is diagnosed by identifying different proteins like histidine-rich proteins, lactate dehydrogenase, and *Plasmodium*-associated aldolase as biomarkers (Mathema and Na-Bangchang, 2015). Similarly, when the technique of proteomics is carried out in malaria-infected patients, inflammatory proteins, erythrocyte-derived proteins, PFI0875w, PFL0480w, and PF080054 can be used as biomarkers to detect malaria (Huang et al., 2012). In the case of cystic echinococcosis, proteins like the Src Kinases and the Lyn Kinases are potential biomarkers (Fratini et al., 2020). In the case of Onchocerciasis, major antigen/OVOC11613, OVOC1523/ATP synthase, OVOC11626/PLK5, OVOC11613, and OVOC247/laminin are the proteins that can be detected as biomarkers (Rosa et al., 2023).

Comprehensive mapping of protein expression, proteoforms, and protein–protein interactions in several biological systems, including *Leishmania*, has been made possible by the development of mass spectrometry-based proteomics (Capelli-Peixoto et al., 2019). The Tandem Mass Tag proteomic technique made it possible to identify novel serum proteins whose concentrations alter following treatment for canine leishmaniosis. These proteins play a role in a variety of pathological processes, including inflammatory, coagulation, and defensive systems. Some of these proteins have not previously been identified in canine leishmaniosis. As such, they may be useful biomarkers for tracking the course of this disease's treatment (Martinez-Subiela et al., 2017). Because of our increased engagement with the wild, the globe is currently facing an increasing number of zoonotic illnesses. Developing novel intervention options requires a detailed comprehension of this parasite-new host interaction. Proteomics techniques based on mass spectrometry have been useful in providing a more profound understanding of the host–pathogen relationship and the evolution of its products (Lodhiya et al., 2022).

7.5   METABOLOMICS AS BIOMARKERS

Metabolomics, which involves measuring every molecule in an organism, and metabolite profiling, which measures a selection of metabolites, have gained recognition as valuable technologies for measuring organismal metabolism in "real time." Metabolomic analysis's potential for identifying biomarkers for the precise diagnosis of parasitic infections has been established through the application of machine learning algorithms and multivariate statistical techniques (Denery et al., 2010). Together with transcriptomics, proteomics, and genomics, metabolomics has proven to be a very useful technique for understanding host–pathogen interactions at the small-molecule level. Numerous infectious diseases and applications have been studied through the use of metabolomics. Metabolomics is most commonly used for prognostic and diagnostic purposes, i.e. Nuclear Magnetic Resonance (NMR) or mass spectrometry-based metabolomics for the screening of disease-specific biomarkers (Tounta et al., 2021). Infections caused by helminths are among the very first experimental structures that are employed in metabolomics. The results are positive, and they have led us to great expectations for the future (Tyagi et al., 2019).

Irregularities of the microbiota, significant alteration in the metabolism of lipids, and remodelling of the metabolism of amino acids are the major metabolic traits that have been revealed by metabolomics after experimental studies on helminth infections. For example, rabbits infected with *Schistosoma japonicum* show changes in their serum lipid profile (Kokova and Mayboroda, 2019). Similarly, the concentration of essential amino acids like valine is lower in cases of infection caused by *Echinostoma caproni* (Li et al., 2011) and is higher in cases of infection caused by *Schistosoma* and *Fasciola* (Wu et al., 2010). In the case of *Brugia malayi*, metabolomics has revealed that the parasite's ability to switch between anaerobic and aerobic pathways and the ability to catabolise glutamate to aspartate produces energy essential for the parasite's survival (Whitman et al., 2021). Similarly, when individuals infected with *Echinostoma caproni* were examined, it was found that there is an increase in urinary mannitol. The reason behind this increase might be that there is increased intestinal permeability compared to healthy individuals (Saric et al., 2008). Areas of metabolomics exploration for helminth infections. are given in Figure 7.1.

In the case of *Schistosoma haematobium* infections, metabolomics has explained that the levels of sex steroids in hosts have declined, while there is an increase in lipids like ganglioside, catechols, and benzenoids (Adebayo et al., 2018). In the case of malarial patients, metabolites such as N-acetyl putrescine, N-acetylspermidine, 1,3-diacetylpropane, alanine, taurine, succinic acid, and pipecolic are the major metabolites that are detected through metabolomics (Abdelrazig et al., 2017). The results of the biochemical indices showed that infection with *Clonorchis sinensis* would impact the biochemical indices of liver function, particularly those related to cholinesterase, total bile acid, glutamyl transpeptidase (GGT), aspartate transaminase

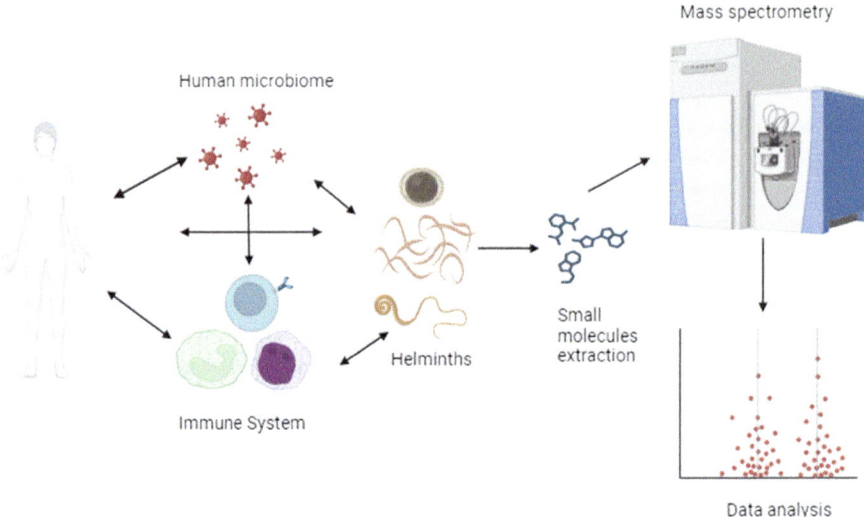

FIGURE 7.1   Areas of metabolomics exploration for helminth infections.

(AST), and high-density lipoprotein (Qiu et al., 2022). Glycerophospholipid metabolism constitutes one of the primary pathways impacted by *Trichinella* infection, and glycerophospholipids are the primary metabolite class found (Chienwichai et al., 2023). The identification of distinct biomarkers for infectious diseases by worldwide evaluation of metabolites and metabolite pathway dysregulation is made possible by metabolic-based methodologies. This consequently makes it possible to provide treatments and build diagnostic tools (Midzi et al., 2023). An effective method for comprehending the biology of protozoan parasites and host–parasite interactions is global metabolite analysis (Kafsack and Llinás, 2010).

7.6   EPIGENOMICS AS POTENTIAL BIOMARKERS

The study of chemical changes to DNA and histones that control gene expression or cellular phenotype is known as epigenomics. However, in the past ten years, this phrase has changed in response to the discovery of several mechanisms (such as microRNAs and the nuclear arrangement of chromosomes) that control the expression of certain genes (García-Giménez et al., 2012). The interplay between host–parasite interactions is regulated by epigenetic processes (Afrin et al., 2019). It is now possible to forecast for the first time how epigenetic mechanisms and regulatory small RNAs may affect the regulation and evolution of animal and microbial genomes because of recent developments in molecular biology and genome sequencing technologies (Kim et al., 2016). Transcriptional programming in the host following pathogen infection eventually results in cellular responses, including the dysregulation of the cell cycle, apoptosis, and immune-related gene regulation. Such interactions result in a modification of the host's epigenetic profile. Thus, it can be concluded that epigenetic changes like histone modifications, non-coding RNAs, and DNA methylation are brought about by host–parasite interactions (Fol et al., 2020).

Understanding the interactions between diverse epigenetic factors is crucial. These factors drive transcriptional changes in parasites and hosts during infection. Recognising the parasite's mode of action and reciprocal communication with the host is essential throughout this process (Kanyal et al., 2019). Pathogen-associated molecular patterns (PAMPs) from viruses, bacteria, and parasites cause an alteration in the epigenetic landscape of the host's immune cells directly involved in pathogen recognition (Kulkarni et al., 2022). *Leishmania donovani* causes DNA methylation of macrophages. *Leishmania major* uses microRNA epigenetic mechanisms affecting human peripheral blood mononuclear cells (Afrin et al., 2019). *Plasmodium chabaudi* causes DNA methylation of hepatic cells. *Toxoplasma gondii* causes histone modification of macrophages (Gendlina et al., 2017). *Schistosoma japonicum* uses epigenetic mechanisms affecting hepatic cells (Syn et al., 2016). The RNAs unique to *Echinococcus* species exhibit considerable promise as early echinococcosis diagnostic biomarkers and may also shed light on the aetiology of the illness (Habibi et al., 2023).

When combined with novel technology, genomic sequences associated with the primary *Schistosoma* species provide a route for the discovery of biomarkers and strategies for the diagnosis, management, and control of schistosomiasis. Histone methylation epigenetic marks can serve as useful indicators and targets for treatment. When an individual becomes infected with *Schistosoma mansoni*, the protein known as HMGB1 becomes elevated, leading to fibrosis of hepatic cells (Assenço et al., 2021). Together with genomic research, epigenomics examines global studies of epigenetic modifications throughout the entire genome, illuminating how the genome is folded within the nucleus of cells, bound by proteins, and altered by enzymes that control gene expression without modifying DNA (Mu et al., 2022). Data from these studies have the potential to enhance our understanding of the functional interpretation of genetic variants found in those regions. It also provides insight into epigenetic markers linked to disease independent of genetic variation. Additionally, it offers information on epigenetic modifications correlating with diseases (Roadmap et al., 2015).

7.7 NON-CODING RNAS AS POTENTIAL BIOMARKERS

Non-coding RNAs, originally regarded as genomic garbage, are now considered to be essential regulators of cellular function (Wei et al., 2017). Other classes of RNAs, including mRNA, rRNA, and tRNA, are regulated and processed by non-coding RNAs (Collins et al., 2011). Non-coding RNAs (ncRNAs) are among the many diverse molecules involved in the interactions between parasites and hosts. It is currently understood that ncRNAs are i) transferred by the vector to potentially influence vertebrate host responses and promote vector survival, and ii) regulated in the host by parasites to promote parasite survival. The ncRNAs interfere with vertebrate host responses to vectors and host responses to parasites at every level of the parasite-vector-host interaction. Due to their diversity, small non-coding RNAs (18–200 nt)—which include piwi-interacting RNAs (piRNAs), microRNAs (miRNAs), and small interfering RNAs (siRNAs)—are gaining more attention (Bensaoud et al., 2019).

An important non-invasive biomarker for the pathological diagnosis and prognosis of several illnesses, particularly infectious diseases, may be abnormal expression of miRNAs (Correia et al., 2017). The ability of a parasite to respond through miRNA-mediated gene expressions to developmental and external stimuli may be necessary for the parasite's life cycle. Thousands of miRNAs have been found in helminthic and protozoan parasites during the past few years, and an abundance of data has shown how important miRNAs are to the life cycle of the parasites (Liu et al., 2010). As predictive and diagnostic biomarkers for infectious diseases, the detection of these miRNAs in the biofluids of infected hosts is expanding quickly (Ghalehnoei et al., 2020). Furthermore, parasites rely on the cellular machinery of their hosts for infection and completing their biological cycles. Parasite miRNAs have the potential to influence the host's reaction, underscoring the significance of miRNA machinery in the search for novel therapeutic approaches against parasites (Manzano-Román and Siles-Lucas, 2012).

Different ncRNAs have been identified as biomarkers in different parasitic infections. For example, miR-451 and miR-16 in malaria, and miR-671, miR-361-3p, and miR-193b with leishmaniasis (Tamgue et al., 2021). The sRNA derived from the non-coding 7SL RNA can be detected in the serum of animals infected with trypanosomiasis. This ncRNA has high sensitivity and can be detected even before the onset of parasitemia. It can also differentiate between the different species of *Trypnasoma*, thus leading to accurate diagnosis (Chiweshe et al., 2019). Similarly, serum miRNA levels increase in the case of *Schistosoma mansoni* infection, which can be employed as a biomarker for diagnosis (Hoy et al., 2014). The phenomenon of host miRNA levels altering after parasite infection and the specific miRNA sequences that are specific to parasites are well-established. However, comprehensive details regarding the direct involvement of parasites in host miRNA level alteration and how parasites regulate this at the molecular level are still lacking (Lemaire et al., 2013). Circulating miRNAs have good potential as non-invasive biomarkers because they can be found in bodily fluids such as serum, saliva, and others. miRNAs are appealing targets for disorder treatment due to their role as master regulators of gene expression. The miRNA machinery and related events can be manipulated with ease. Additionally, miRNA-based treatments appear to lack side effects when administered (Manzano-Román and Siles-Lucas, 2012). The fact that the variable abundance of endogenous miRNAs in serum can come from a variety of cell types and be linked to unrelated illnesses presents a potential barrier to their use as biomarkers (Hoy and Buck, 2012).

7.8   INTEGRATIVE OMICS APPROACHES FOR BIOMARKER IDENTIFICATION

Certain molecules, or a group of molecules, are known as molecular biomarkers, and they can aid in the diagnosis or prognosis of illnesses. With the development of high-throughput technologies during the past few decades, an enormous amount of molecular "omics" data, such as transcriptomics and proteomics, has been gathered. Screening for diseases or disorders using biomarkers is made possible by the availability of these omics data (Shi et al., 2020). Large-scale omics datasets (transcriptomics, proteomics, metabolomics, metagenomics, phenomics, etc.) are now widely available, revolutionising biology and promoting the development of systems techniques to improve our comprehension of biological processes (Figure 7.2). Biostatisticians, biomathematicians, computational biologists, and biologists face enormous hurdles as well as fascinating prospects due to the reduced time and cost required to generate these datasets through omics data integration (Misra et al., 2019).

Although it is important to integrate omics researchers into various fields of study, including systems microbiology (Mochida and Shinozaki, 2011), microbiome analysis (Muller et al., 2014), and disease biology (Pathak and Dave, 2014). The successful implementation of more than two omics technologies is very rare. These integrated omics approaches present several broad experimental challenges, such as (i) comprehending the statistical behaviour of read-outs from each omics regime independently, (ii) identifying relationships between omics regimes that are not immediately apparent within their original biological context, and (iii) utilising time resolution in omics data to inform directionality (Buescher and Driggers, 2016). In addition to the three layers of omics datasets that are most frequently used—transcriptomics, proteomics, and metabolomics—Yugi et al. (2016) proposed a trans-omics concept of dynamic networks that incorporates more recent datasets like phosphoproteomics, DNA–protein interactions, protein–protein interactions, and allosteric regulation.

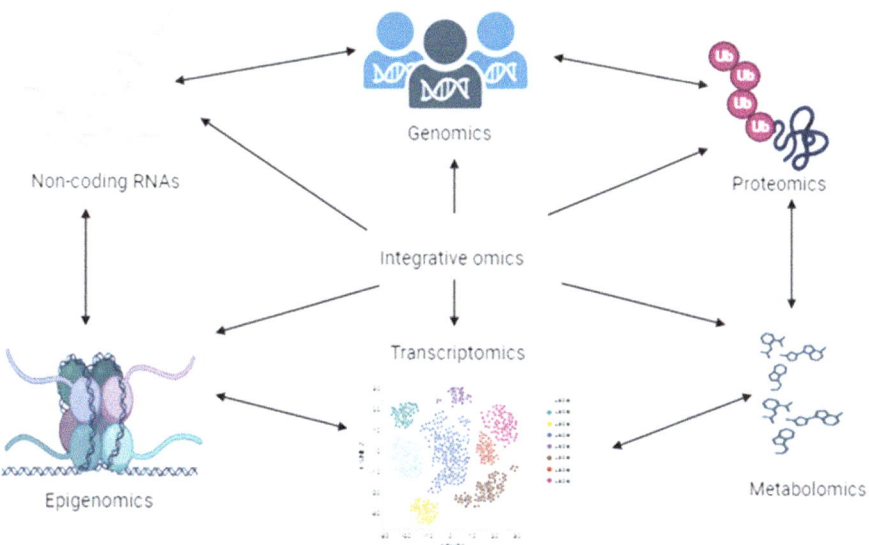

FIGURE 7.2 Integrative omics approaches.

These datasets can reveal crucial elements of dynamic biological networks when omics data are successfully integrated.

Novel computational and statistical approaches are required for data integration and the discovery of biomarkers and molecular signatures in the ever-expanding omics age (Hendrickx et al., 2020). Data Integration Analysis for Biomarker discovery using Latent cOmponents (DIABLO) is a multi-omics integrative technique that selects a subset of molecular features to discriminate between distinct phenotypic groups and looks for common information across different data types (Singh et al., 2019). *Haemonchus (H.) contortus* landscape of genes, transcripts, proteins, lipids, and functional information has been uncovered by recent developments in genomics, transcriptomics, proteomics, and lipidomics, as well as functional genomics. Specifically, investigations of individual genome, transcriptome, proteome, and lipidome data sets have uncovered some fascinating biological features of *H. contortus* development and reproduction, adaptability, parasitism, and medication resistance (Ma et al., 2020a). Advanced omics technologies can define the components of extracellular vesicles secreted by *H. contortus*, including proteins, lipids, miRNAs, and mRNAs. These insights can illuminate host–parasite interactions and disease processes. Integrative genomics has provided some understanding of *H. contortus*'s developmental biology, but significant obstacles remain in fully grasping its "systems biology" (Ma et al., 2020b).

7.9 CHALLENGES IN OMICS-BASED BIOMARKER RESEARCH

Even if any individual omics dataset might not contain all four Vs—velocity, variety, volume, and veracity—that are linked with the integration of "big data." They however present comparable difficulties, particularly in research with sizeable sample sizes. Variations among samples become enormous and sparse for high-dimensional datasets exceeding 1000 variables, known as the "curse of dimensionality." This makes cluster analysis uninformative and presents additional hurdles for analysing integrated omic datasets (Ronan et al., 2016). Since different types of individual datasets have different requirements for quality assurance, control, normalisation of data, and reduction techniques, heterogeneous datasets present challenges. For instance, the normalisation and scale of RNA-seq data differ from small RNA-seq data. The former typically contains tens of thousands of transcripts, while the latter typically contains fewer than 2000 small RNAs. As single-cell sequencing technologies, longer-read sequencing technologies, and applications for genomic and transcriptomic analyses develop quickly, new challenges are also arising, such as appropriate sequence coverage and statistical analysis of single-cell data (Menon, 2018).

Despite continuous efforts through the proteomics standards initiative, the community has not yet reached an agreement on data formats, cleaning, and normalisation. For example, the usage of ion intensity versus peptide-to-spectrum matches (Deutsch et al., 2017). One significant restriction relates to the interpretation of transcriptome and genome data concerning biological function, specifically the impact of particular variants on phenotypic variation (Lappalainen et al., 2013). Due to the absence of protein amplification techniques, proteomics procedures still require large sample sizes and encounter challenges with membrane protein isolation, low abundance protein detection, and insoluble protein identification. Even untargeted proteomic techniques will not include data for every protein in a given biological sample, as the representation of nuclear proteins in a proteomic dataset, for instance, usually needs enrichment of nuclei (Freeman and Hemby, 2004; Novikova et al., 2022). Top-down and bottom-up proteomics variability in protein quantification is increased by the use of chromatography to separate complicated chemistries, such as various charged states and post-translational modifications (Dupree et al., 2020).

Peptide identification is also subject to variance because of differences in peptide structure, charge, and hydrophobicity. These biochemical characteristics influence peptide and protein detection and identification using NMR or mass spectrometry (Háda et al., 2018). Analysis pipelines for proteomic data need to handle normalisation, absolute versus relative quantification, and absent data, i.e. is the peptide not identified because it is not ionised efficiently, or is it not there in the sample (Bantscheff et al., 2012). However, just like proteins, metabolites cannot be amplified, and only 15–30% of the total mass spectra are recognisable and measurable, which reduces the amount of information that may be usefully extracted. Furthermore, a problem with score-based spectral identification of molecules is false positives. Major problems include a lack of standards for data formats for data and analysis pipelines, chemical variability of small molecules, the platform employed, variability in sample processing, and diverse quantification methodologies (Spicer et al., 2017).

The major challenge of omics application in practical fields is that it is not yet possible because these omics technologies have not yet met the regulatory authorities' requirements, and there is a consistent need to perform regulatory omics studies (Sauer et al., 2017). The omics techniques generate enormous amounts of data. Analysing, synthesising, and storing these data sets is a significant task because they significantly outweigh all that has previously been saved (Prat and Degli-Esposti, 2019). The identification of biomarkers in the early stages of the onset of disease is still challenging (Banerjee et al., 2021). When analysing omics data on a daily basis, integrating heterogeneous and large-scale data presents both a conceptual and a practical difficulty. There is general agreement over the availability of appropriate tools for the analysis of individual data types in omics research (Mougin et al., 2018). Most software is thought to be primarily accessible to researchers with programming experience. While opinions on the availability of user-friendly tools are divided, it is evident that new analysis tools must be created in the field. Other factors with comparable status include the necessity for new analysis tools, the availability of user-friendly software, and the exclusivity of tools for programmers (Gomez-Cabrero et al., 2014).

7.10   FUTURE PERSPECTIVES IN OMICS-BASED BIOMARKER RESEARCH

A major drawback of dynamic omics is the time-consuming nature of 2D separation. It is anticipated that in the future, some excellent flash analysis techniques will be created, potentially removing the need for the laborious liquid chromatography separation process altogether (Yan et al., 2015). To advance our understanding of health and disease complexities, we need to integrate data from sequenced genomes, functional genomics, protein profiling, metabolomics, and bioinformatics. Effective use of potent new technologies already available is crucial for conducting thorough systems-based analyses (Matthews et al., 2016).

There is near-universal agreement that new tools for knowledge bases, causal discovery, explorative data analysis, public data availability, and organisation are needed. The creation of tools as both OpenSource and user-friendly software is a crucial prerequisite (Gomez-Cabrero et al., 2014). These omics technologies have increased our knowledge towards the understanding of potential drug targets, developing new drugs, and various methods of treatment for different parasitic diseases (Rabaan et al., 2022). "Multi-omics" data revealing individual differences can facilitate the development of new medications and vaccines. These data may open up new avenues for customised clinical management of parasite infections. They can address the issue of drug resistance that currently exists (Zhou et al., 2021).

REFERENCES

Abdelrazig, S., Ortori, C.A., Davey, G., Deressa, W., Mulleta, D., Barrett, D.A., Amberbir, A. and Fogarty, A.W. 2017. A metabolomic analytical approach permits identification of urinary biomarkers for *Plasmodium falciparum* infection: a case–control study. *Malaria Journal*, 16(1):1–8.

Aboshady, H.M., Stear, M.J., Johansson, A., Jonas, E. and Bambou, J.C. 2020. Immunoglobulins as biomarkers for gastrointestinal nematodes resistance in small ruminants: A systematic review. *Scientific Reports*, 10(1):7765.

Adebayo, A.S., Mundhe, S.D., Awobode, H.O., Onile, O.S., Agunloye, A.M., Isokpehi, R.D., Shouche, Y.S., Santhakumari, B. and Anumudu, C.I. 2018. Metabolite profiling for biomarkers in *Schistosoma haematobium* infection and associated bladder pathologies. *PLoS Neglected Tropical Diseases*, 12(4):0006452.

Afrin, F., Khan, I. and Hemeg, H.A. 2019. *Leishmania*-host interactions—an epigenetic paradigm. *Frontiers in Immunology*, 10:492.

Aggarwal, S., Peng, W.K. and Srivastava, S. 2021. Multi-omics advancements towards *Plasmodium vivax* malaria diagnosis. *Diagnostics*, 11(12):2222.

Álvarez, I., Fernández, I., Soudré, A., Traoré, A., Pérez-Pardal, L., Sanou, M., Tapsoba, S.A., Menéndez-Arias, N.A. and Goyache, F. 2019. Identification of genomic regions and candidate genes of functional importance for gastrointestinal parasite resistance traits in Djallonké sheep of Burkina Faso. *Archives Animal Breeding*, 62(1):313–323.

Anderson, N.L. and Anderson, N.G. 2002. The human plasma proteome: history, character, and diagnostic prospects. *Molecular & Cellular Proteomics*, 1(11):845–867.

Assenço, R.G., Mota, E.A., De Oliveira, V.F., Borges, W.D.C. and Guerra-Sá, R. 2021. Epigenetic markers associated with schistosomiasis. *Helminthologia*, 58(1):28–40.

Bah, S.Y., Morang'a, C.M., Kengne-Ouafo, J.A., Amenga–Etego, L. and Awandare, G.A. 2018. Highlights on the application of genomics and bioinformatics in the fight against infectious diseases: challenges and opportunities in Africa. *Frontiers in Genetics*, 9:575.

Banerjee, S., Prabhu Basrur, N. and Rai, P.S. 2021. Omics technologies in personalized combination therapy for cardiovascular diseases: Challenges and opportunities. *Personalized Medicine*, 18(6):595–611.

Bantscheff, M., Lemeer, S., Savitski, M.M. and Kuster, B. 2012. Quantitative mass spectrometry in proteomics: critical review update from 2007 to the present. *Analytical and Bioanalytical Chemistry*, 404:939–965.

Barton, A.J., Hill, J., Pollard, A.J. and Blohmke, C.J. 2017. Transcriptomics in human challenge models. *Frontiers in Immunology*, 8:1839.

Bennuru, S., Cotton, J.A., Ribeiro, J.M., Grote, A., Harsha, B., Holroyd, N., Mhashilkar, A., Molina, D.M., Randall, A.Z., Shandling, A.D. and Unnasch, T.R. 2016. Stage-specific transcriptome and proteome analyses of the filarial parasite *Onchocerca volvulus* and its Wolbachia endosymbiont. *MBio*, 7(6):10–1128.

Bensaoud, C., Hackenberg, M. and Kotsyfakis, M. 2019. Noncoding RNAs in parasite–vector–host interactions. *Trends in Parasitology*, 35(9):715–724.

Bichiou, H., Bouabid, C., Rabhi, I. and Guizani-Tabbane, L. 2021. Transcription factors interplay orchestrates the immune-metabolic response of *Leishmania* infected macrophages. *Frontiers in Cellular and Infection Microbiology*, 11:660415.

Buescher, J.M. and Driggers, E.M. 2016. Integration of omics: more than the sum of its parts. *Cancer & Metabolism*, 4:1–8.

Cantacessi, C., Dantas-Torres, F., Nolan, M.J. and Otranto, D. 2015. The past, present, and future of Leishmania genomics and transcriptomics. *Trends in Parasitology*, 31(3):100–108.

Capelli-Peixoto, J., Mule, S.N., Tano, F.T., Palmisano, G. and Stolf, B.S. 2019. Proteomics and leishmaniasis: potential clinical applications. *PROTEOMICS–Clinical Applications*, 13(6):1800136.

Chienwichai, P., Thiangtrongjit, T., Tipthara, P., Tarning, J., Adisakwattana, P. and Reamtong, O. 2023. Untargeted serum metabolomics analysis of *Trichinella spiralis*-infected mouse. *PLOS Neglected Tropical Diseases*, 17(2):0011119.

Chiweshe, S.M., Steketee, P.C., Jayaraman, S., Paxton, E., Neophytou, K., Erasmus, H., Labuschagne, M., Cooper, A., MacLeod, A., Grey, F.E. and Morrison, L.J. 2019. Parasite specific 7SL-derived small RNA is an effective target for diagnosis of active trypanosomiasis infection. *PLoS Neglected Tropical Diseases*, 13(2):0007189.

Collins, L.J., Schönfeld, B. and Chen, X.S. 2011. The epigenetics of non-coding RNA. In: Tollefsbol, T. (ed.) *Handbook of epigenetics*. Academic Press. pp. 49–61.

Correia, C.N., Nalpas, N.C., McLoughlin, K.E., Browne, J.A., Gordon, S.V., MacHugh, D.E. and Shaughnessy, R.G. 2017. Circulating microRNAs as potential biomarkers of infectious disease. *Frontiers in Immunology*, 8:118.

Das, S., Peck, R.B., Barney, R., Jang, I.K., Kahn, M., Zhu, M. and Domingo, G.J. 2018. Performance of an ultra-sensitive *Plasmodium falciparum* HRP2-based rapid diagnostic test with recombinant HRP2, culture parasites, and archived whole blood samples. *Malaria Journal*, 17(1):1–7.

De-Bock, M., De Seny, D., Meuwis, M.A., Chapelle, J.P., Louis, E., Malaise, M., Merville, M.P. and Fillet, M. 2010. Challenges for biomarker discovery in body fluids using SELDI-TOF-MS. *Journal of Biomedicine and Biotechnology*, 2010:906082.

Denery, J.R., Nunes, A.A., Hixon, M.S., Dickerson, T.J. and Janda, K.D. 2010. Metabolomics-based discovery of diagnostic biomarkers for onchocerciasis. *PLoS Neglected Tropical Diseases*, 4(10):834.

Deutsch, E.W., Orchard, S., Binz, P.A., Bittremieux, W., Eisenacher, M., Hermjakob, H., Kawano, S., Lam, H., Mayer, G., Menschaert, G. and Perez-Riverol, Y. 2017. Proteomics standards initiative: Fifteen years of progress and future work. *Journal of Proteome Research*, 16(12):4288–4298.

Diab, R. and Younis, S. 2022. Omics: Approaches and applications related to diagnosis, treatment, and control of parasitic diseases. Part I: *Plasmodium spp. Parasitologists United Journal*, 15(2):144–153.

Duncan, R. 2004. DNA microarray analysis of protozoan parasite gene expression: outcomes correlate with mechanisms of regulation. *Trends in Parasitology*, 20(5):211–215.

Dupree, E.J., Jayathirtha, M., Yorkey, H., Mihasan, M., Petre, B.A. and Darie, C.C. 2020. A critical review of bottom-up proteomics: the good, the bad, and the future of this field. *Proteomes*, 8(3):14.

Essuman, E., Grabias, B., Verma, N., Chorazeczewski, J.K., Tripathi, A.K., Mlambo, G., Addison, E.A., Amoah, A.G., Quakyi, I., Oakley, M.S. and Kumar, S. 2017. A novel gametocyte biomarker for superior molecular detection of the *Plasmodium falciparum* infectious reservoirs. *The Journal of Infectious Diseases*, 216(10):1264–1272.

Fol, M., Włodarczyk, M. and Druszczyńska, M. 2020. Host epigenetics in intracellular pathogen infections. *International Journal of Molecular Sciences*, 21(13):4573.

Fratini, F., Tamarozzi, F., Macchia, G., Bertuccini, L., Mariconti, M., Birago, C., Iriarte, A., Brunetti, E., Cretu, C.M., Akhan, O. and Siles-Lucas, M. 2020. Proteomic analysis of plasma exosomes from Cystic Echinococcosis patients provides *in vivo* support for distinct immune response profiles in active vs inactive infection and suggests potential biomarkers. *PLoS Neglected Tropical Diseases*, 14(10):0008586.

Freeman, W.M. and Hemby, S.E. 2004. Proteomics for protein expression profiling in neuroscience. *Neurochemical Research*, 29(6):1065–1081.

García-Giménez, J.L., Sanchis-Gomar, F., Lippi, G., Mena, S., Ivars, D., Gomez-Cabrera, M.C., Viña, J. and Pallardó, F.V. 2012. Epigenetic biomarkers: A new perspective in laboratory diagnostics. *Clinica Chimica Acta*, 413(19–20):1576–1582.

Geiger, A., Simo, G., Grébaut, P., Peltier, J.B., Cuny, G. and Holzmuller, P. 2011. Transcriptomics and proteomics in human African trypanosomiasis: Current status and perspectives. *Journal of Proteomics*, 74(9):1625–1643.

Gendlina, I., Silmon de Monerri, N. and Kim, K. 2017. Modification of the host epigenome by parasitic protists. In: Doerfler, W. and Casadesús, J. (eds.) *Epigenetics of infectious diseases. Epigenetics and human health*. Springer, pp. 189–220.

Ghalehnoei, H., Bagheri, A., Fakhar, M. and Mishan, M.A. 2020. Circulatory microRNAs: promising non-invasive prognostic and diagnostic biomarkers for parasitic infections. *European Journal of Clinical Microbiology & Infectious Diseases*, 39:395–402

Gomez-Cabrero, D., Abugessaisa, I., Maier, D., Teschendorff, A., Merkenschlager, M., Gisel, A., Ballestar, E., Bongcam-Rudloff, E., Conesa, A. and Tegnér, J. 2014. Data integration in the era of omics: current and future challenges. *BMC Systems Biology*, 8(2):1–10.

Habibi, B., Gholami, S., Bagheri, A., Fakhar, M., Moradi, A. and Khazeei Tabari, M.A. 2023. Cystic echinococcosis microRNAs as potential noninvasive biomarkers: current insights and upcoming perspective. *Expert Review of Molecular Diagnostics*, 23(10):885–894.

Háda, V., Bagdi, A., Bihari, Z., Timári, S.B., Fizil, Á. and Szántay Jr, C. 2018. Recent advancements, challenges, and practical considerations in the mass spectrometry-based analytics of protein biotherapeutics: A viewpoint from the biosimilar industry. *Journal of Pharmaceutical and Biomedical Analysis*, 161:214–238.

Hasin, Y., Seldin, M. and Lusis, A. 2017. Multi-omics approaches to disease. *Genome Biology*, 18(1):1–15.

Hendrickx, J.O., van Gastel, J., Leysen, H., Martin, B. and Maudsley, S. 2020. High-dimensionality data analysis of pharmacological systems associated with complex diseases. *Pharmacological Reviews*, 72(1):191–217.

Hoy, A.M. and Buck, A.H. 2012. Extracellular small RNAs: what, where, why? *Biochemical Society Transactions*, 40(4):886–890.

Hoy, A.M., Lundie, R.J., Ivens, A., Quintana, J.F., Nausch, N., Forster, T., Jones, F., Kabatereine, N.B., Dunne, D.W., Mutapi, F. and MacDonald, A.S. 2014. Parasite-derived microRNAs in host serum as novel biomarkers of helminth infection. *PLoS Neglected Tropical Diseases*, 8(2):2701.

Huang, H., Mackeen, M.M., Cook, M., Oriero, E., Locke, E., Thézénas, M.L., Kessler, B.M., Nwakanma, D. and Casals-Pascual, C. 2012. Proteomic identification of host and para-site biomarkers in saliva from patients with uncomplicated *Plasmodium falciparum* malaria. *Malaria Journal*, 11(1):1–9.

Kadarmideen, H.N., Watson-Haigh, N.S. and Andronicos, N.M. 2011. Systems biology of ovine intestinal parasite resistance: disease gene modules and biomarkers. *Molecular Biosystems*, 7(1):235–246.

Kafsack, B.F. and Llinás, M. 2010. Eating at the table of another: metabolomics of host-parasite interactions. *Cell, Host & Microbe*, 7(2):90–99.

Kanyal, A., Nahata, S. and Karmodiya, K. 2019. Epigenetics in infectious disease. In: Sharma, S. (ed.) *Prognostic Epigenetics*. Academic Press, pp. 171–201.

Kim, D., Thairu, M.W. and Hansen, A.K. 2016. Novel insights into insect-microbe interac-tions—role of epigenomics and small RNAs. *Frontiers in Plant Science*, 7:1164.

Kima, P.E. 2014. *Leishmania* molecules that mediate intracellular pathogenesis. *Microbes and Infection*, 16(9):721–726.

Klopfleisch, R. 2015. Personalised medicine in veterinary oncology: one to cure just one. *The Veterinary Journal*, 205(2):128–135.

Kokova, D. and Mayboroda, O.A. 2019. Twenty years on: metabolomics in helminth research. *Trends in Parasitology*, 35(4):282–288.

Kulkarni, S., Arumugam, T., Chuturgoon, A., An, P. and Ramsuran, V. 2022. Epigenetics of infectious diseases. *Frontiers in Immunology*, 13:1054151

Lappalainen, T., Sammeth, M., Friedländer, M.R., 't Hoen, P.A., Monlong, J., Rivas, M.A., Gonzalez-Porta, M., Kurbatova, N., Griebel, T., Ferreira, P.G. and Barann, M. 2013. Transcriptome and genome sequencing uncovers functional variation in humans. *Nature*, 501(7468):506–511.

Lee, H.J., Georgiadou, A., Otto, T.D., Levin, M., Coin, L.J., Conway, D.J. and Cunnington, A.J. 2018b. Transcriptomic studies of malaria: A paradigm for investigation of sys-temic host-pathogen interactions. *Microbiology and Molecular Biology Reviews*, 82(2):10–1128.

Lee, H.J., Georgiadou, A., Walther, M., Nwakanma, D., Stewart, L.B., Levin, M., Otto, T.D., Conway, D.J., Coin, L.J. and Cunnington, A.J. 2018a. Integrated pathogen load and dual transcriptome analysis of systemic host-pathogen interactions in severe malaria. *Science Translational Medicine*, 10(447):3619.

Lemaire, J., Mkannez, G., Guerfali, F.Z., Gustin, C., Attia, H., Sghaier, R.M., Sysco-Consortium, Dellagi, K., Laouini, D. and Renard, P. 2013. MicroRNA expression pro-file in human macrophages in response to *Leishmania major* infection. *PLoS Neglected Tropical Diseases*, 7(10):2478.

Li, J.V., Saric, J., Wang, Y., Keiser, J., Utzinger, J. and Holmes, E. 2011. Chemometric analysis of biofluids from mice experimentally infected with *Schistosoma mansoni*. *Parasites & Vectors*, 4(1):1–16.

Liu, Q., Tuo, W., Gao, H. and Zhu, X.Q. 2010. MicroRNAs of parasites: Current status and future perspectives. *Parasitology Research*, 107:501–507.

Lodhiya, T., Devassy, D. and Mukherjee, R. 2022. Parasite proteomics. In: Parija, S.C. and Chaudhury, A. (eds.) *Textbook of Parasitic Zoonoses*. Springer, pp. 39–49.

Lustigman, S., Grote, A. and Ghedin, E. 2017. The role of 'omics' in the quest to eliminate human filariasis. *PLoS Neglected Tropical Diseases*, 11(4):0005464.

Ma, G., Gasser, R.B., Wang, T., Korhonen, P.K. and Young, N.D. 2020a. Toward integrative 'omics of the barber's pole worm and related parasitic nematodes. *Infection, Genetics and Evolution*, 85:104500.

Ma, G., Wang, T., Korhonen, P.K., Hofmann, A., Sternberg, P.W., Young, N.D. and Gasser, R.B. 2020. Elucidating the molecular and developmental biology of parasitic nematodes: Moving to a multiomics paradigm. *Advances in Parasitology*, 108:175–229.

Manzano-Román, R. and Siles-Lucas, M. 2012. MicroRNAs in parasitic diseases: Potential for diagnosis and targeting. *Molecular and Biochemical Parasitology*, 186(2):81–86.

Martinez-Subiela, S., Horvatic, A., Escribano, D., Pardo-Marin, L., Kocaturk, M., Mrljak, V., Burchmore, R., Ceron, J.J. and Yilmaz, Z. 2017. Identification of novel biomarkers for treatment monitoring in canine leishmaniosis by high-resolution quantitative proteomic analysis. *Veterinary Immunology and Immunopathology*, 191:60–67.

Mathema, V.B. and Na-Bangchang, K. 2015. A brief review on biomarkers and proteomic approach for malaria research. *Asian Pacific Journal of Tropical Medicine*, 8(4):253–262.

Matthews, H., Hanison, J. and Nirmalan, N. 2016. "Omics"-informed drug and biomarker discovery: Opportunities, challenges and future perspectives. *Proteomes*, 4(3):28.

Menon, V., 2018. Clustering single cells: A review of approaches on high-and low-depth single-cell RNA-seq data. *Briefings in Functional Genomics*, 17(4):240–245.

Menyhárt, O. and Győrffy, B. 2021. Multi-omics approaches in cancer research with applications in tumor subtyping, prognosis, and diagnosis. *Computational and Structural Biotechnology Journal*, 19:949–960.

Midzi, H., Vengesai, A., Muleya, V., Kasambala, M., Mduluza-Jokonya, T.L., Chipako, I., Siamayuwa, C.E., Mutapi, F., Naicker, T. and Mduluza, T. 2023. Metabolomics for biomarker discovery in schistosomiasis: A systematic scoping review. *Frontiers in Tropical Diseases*, 4:1108317.

Misra, B.B., Langefeld, C., Olivier, M. and Cox, L.A. 2019. Integrated omics: tools, advances and future approaches. *Journal of Molecular Endocrinology*, 62(1):R21–R45.

Mochida, K. and Shinozaki, K. 2011. Advances in omics and bioinformatics tools for systems analyses of plant functions. *Plant and Cell Physiology*, 52(12):2017–2038.

Mougin, F., Auber, D., Bourqui, R., Diallo, G., Dutour, I., Jouhet, V., Thiessard, F., Thiebaut, R. and Thebault, P. 2018. Visualizing omics and clinical data: Which challenges for dealing with their variety? *Methods*, 132:3–18.

Mu, J., Cao, J., Feng, G. and Zhang, Q. 2022. Cellular and molecular basis in parasitic diseases control: Research trends. *Frontiers in Cell and Developmental Biology*, 10:897858.

Muller, E.E., Pinel, N., Laczny, C.C., Hoopmann, M.R., Narayanasamy, S., Lebrun, L.A., Roume, H., Lin, J., May, P., Hicks, N.D. and Heintz-Buschart, A. 2014. Community-integrated omics links dominance of a microbial generalist to fine-tuned resource usage. *Nature Communications*, 5(1):5603.

Novikova, S., Tolstova, T., Kurbatov, L., Farafonova, T., Tikhonova, O., Soloveva, N., Rusanov, A., Archakov, A. and Zgoda, V. 2022. Nuclear proteomics of induced leukemia cell differentiation. *Cells*, 11(20):3221.

Olivier, M., Asmis, R., Hawkins, G.A., Howard, T.D. and Cox, L.A. 2019. The need for multi-omics biomarker signatures in precision medicine. *International Journal of Molecular Sciences*, 20(19):4781.

Onile, O.S., Calder, B., Soares, N.C., Anumudu, C.I. and Blackburn, J.M. 2017. Quantitative label-free proteomic analysis of human urine to identify novel candidate protein biomarkers for schistosomiasis. *PLOS Neglected Tropical Diseases*, 11(11):0006045.

Pathak, R.R. and Dave, V. 2014. Integrating omics technologies to study pulmonary physiology and pathology at the systems level. *Cellular Physiology and Biochemistry*, 33(5):1239–1260.

Payne, D. 1988. Use and limitations of light microscopy for diagnosing malaria at the primary health care level. *Bulletin of the World Health Organization*, 66(5):621.

Perera, T.R., Skerrett-Byrne, D.A., Gibb, Z., Nixon, B. and Swegen, A. 2022. The future of biomarkers in veterinary medicine: Emerging approaches and associated challenges. *Animals*, 12(17):2194.

Pérez-Montoto, L.G., Prado-Prado, F., Ubeira, F.M. and González-Díaz, H. 2009. Study of parasitic infections, cancer, and other diseases with mass-spectrometry and quantitative proteome-disease relationships. *Current Proteomics*, 6(4):246–261.

Prasopdee, S., Thitapakorn, V., Sathavornmanee, T. and Tesana, S. 2019. A comprehensive review of omics and host-parasite interplays studies, towards control of *Opisthorchis viverrini* infection for prevention of cholangiocarcinoma. *Acta Tropica*, 196:76–82.

Prat, O. and Degli-Esposti, D. 2019. New challenges: Omics technologies in ecotoxicology. In: Gross, E. and Garric, J (eds.) *Ecotoxicology*. ISTE Press – Elsevier, pp. 181–208.

Qiu, Y.Y., Chang, Q.C., Gao, J.F., Bao, M.J., Luo, H.T., Song, J.H., Hong, S.J., Mao, R.F., Sun, Y.Y., Chen, Y.Y. and Liu, M.Y. 2022. Multiple biochemical indices and metabolomics of *Clonorchis sinensis* provide a novel interpretation of biomarkers. *Parasites & Vectors*, 15(1):172.

Qoronfleh, M.W. and Lindpaintner, K. 2010. Protein biomarker immunoassays opportunities and challenges. *Drug Discovery World*, 11(1):19–28.

Rabaan, A.A., Bakhrebah, M.A., Mohapatra, R.K., Farahat, R.A., Dhawan, M., Alwarthan, S., Aljeldah, M., Al Shammari, B.R., Al-Najjar, A.H., Alhusayyen, M.A. and Al-Absi, G.H. 2022. Omics approaches in drug development against leishmaniasis: Current scenario and future prospects. *Pathogens*, 12(1):39.

Roadmap, E.C., Kundaje, A., Meuleman, W., Ernst, J., Bilenky, M., Yen, A., Heravi-Moussavi, A., Kheradpour, P., Zhang, Z., Wang, J. and Ziller, M.J. 2015. Integrative analysis of 111 reference human epigenomes. *Nature*, 518(7539):317–330.

Robinson, M.W., Menon, R., Donnelly, S.M., Dalton, J.P. and Ranganathan, S. 2009. An integrated transcriptomics and proteomics analysis of the secretome of the helminth pathogen *Fasciola hepatica*: Proteins associated with invasion and infection of the mammalian host. *Molecular & Cellular Proteomics*, 8(8):1891–1907.

Ronan, T., Qi, Z. and Naegle, K.M. 2016. Avoiding common pitfalls when clustering biological data. *Science Signaling*, 9(432):re6.

Rosa, B.A., Curtis, K., Gilmore, P.E., Martin, J., Zhang, Q., Sprung, R., Weil, G.J., Townsend, R.R., Fischer, P.U. and Mitreva, M. 2023. Direct proteomic detection and prioritization of 19 onchocerciasis biomarker candidates in humans. *Molecular & Cellular Proteomics*, 22(1):100454.

Sánchez-Ovejero, C., Benito-Lopez, F., Díez, P., Casulli, A., Siles-Lucas, M., Fuentes, M. and Manzano-Román, R. 2016. Sensing parasites: Proteomic and advanced bio-detection alternatives. *Journal of Proteomics*, 136:145–156.

Saric, J., Li, J.V., Wang, Y., Keiser, J., Bundy, J.G., Holmes, E. and Utzinger, J. 2008. Metabolic profiling of an *Echinostoma caproni* infection in the mouse for biomarker discovery. *PLoS Neglected Tropical Diseases*, 2(7):254.

Sauer, U.G., Deferme, L., Gribaldo, L., Hackermüller, J., Tralau, T., van Ravenzwaay, B., Yauk, C., Poole, A., Tong, W. and Gant, T.W. 2017. The challenge of the application of'omics technologies in chemicals risk assessment: Background and outlook. *Regulatory Toxicology and Pharmacology*, 91:14–26.

Scholte, L.L., Pascoal-Xavier, M.A. and Nahum, L.A. 2018. Helminths and cancers from the evolutionary perspective. *Frontiers in Medicine*, 5:90.

Shi, K., Lin, W. and Zhao, X.M. 2020. Identifying molecular biomarkers for diseases with machine learning based on integrative omics. *IEEE/ACM Transactions on Computational Biology and Bioinformatics*, 18(6):2514–2525.

Singh, A., Shannon, C.P., Gautier, B., Rohart, F., Vacher, M., Tebbutt, S.J. and Lê Cao, K.A. 2019. DIABLO: An integrative approach for identifying key molecular drivers from multi-omics assays. *Bioinformatics*, 35(17):3055–3062.

Spicer, R.A., Salek, R. and Steinbeck, C. 2017. A decade after the metabolomics standards initiative it's time for a revision. *Scientific Data*, 4(1):1–3.

Swann, J., Jamshidi, N., Lewis, N.E. and Winzeler, E.A. 2015. Systems analysis of host–parasite interactions. Wiley interdisciplinary reviews. *Systems Biology and Medicine*, 7(6):381–400.

Swapna, L.S. and Parkinson, J. 2017. Genomics of apicomplexan parasites. *Critical Reviews in Biochemistry and Molecular Biology*, 52(3):254–273.

Syn, G., Blackwell, J.M. and Jamieson, S.E. 2016. Epigenetics in infectious diseases. In: García-Giménez, J.L. (ed.) *Epigenetic biomarkers and diagnostics*. Academic Press, pp. 377–400.

Tam, V., Patel, N., Turcotte, M., Bossé, Y., Paré, G. and Meyre, D. 2019. Benefits and limitations of genome-wide association studies. *Nature Reviews Genetics*, 20(8):467–484.

Tamgue, O., Mezajou, C.F., Ngongang, N.N., Kameni, C., Ngum, J.A., Simo, U.S.F., Tatang, F.J., Akami, M. and Ngono, A.N. 2021. Non-coding RNAs in the etiology and control of major and neglected human tropical diseases. *Frontiers in Immunology*, 12:703936.

Tomescu, O.A., Mattanovich, D. and Thallinger, G.G. 2014. Integrative omics analysis. A study based on *Plasmodium falciparum* mRNA and protein data. *BMC Systems Biology*, 8(2):1–16.

Tounta, V., Liu, Y., Cheyne, A. and Larrouy-Maumus, G. 2021. Metabolomics in infectious diseases and drug discovery. *Molecular Omics*, 17(3):376–393.

Tyagi, R., Rosa, B.A. and Mitreva, M. 2019. Omics-driven knowledge-based discovery of anthelmintic targets and drugs. In: Roy, K. (ed.) *In silico drug design*. Academic Press, pp. 329–358.

Valilou, R.H., Rafat, S.A., Notter, D.R., Shojda, D., Moghaddam, G. and Nematollahi, A. 2015. Fecal egg counts for gastrointestinal nematodes are associated with a polymorphism in the MHC-DRB1 gene in the Iranian Ghezel sheep breed. *Frontiers in Genetics*, 6:105.

Van-Tong, H., Brindley, P.J., Meyer, C.G. and Velavan, T.P. 2017. Parasite infection, carcinogenesis and human malignancy. *EBioMedicine*, 15:12–23.

Venkatesh, A., Aggarwal, S., Kumar, S., Rajyaguru, S., Kumar, V., Bankar, S., Shastri, J., Patankar, S. and Srivastava, S. 2020. Comprehensive proteomics investigation of *P. vivax*-infected human plasma and parasite isolates. *BMC Infectious Diseases*, 20(1):1–11.

Veras, P.S.T., Ramos, P.I.P. and De Menezes, J.P.B. 2018. In search of biomarkers for pathogenesis and control of leishmaniasis by global analyses of *Leishmania*-infected macrophages. *Frontiers in Cellular and Infection Microbiology*, 8:326.

Wakchaure, R., Ganguly, S., Praveen, P.K., Kumar, A., Sharma, S. and Mahajan, T. 2015. Marker assisted selection (MAS) in animal breeding: A review. *Journal of Drug Metabolism and Toxicology*, 6(5):127.

Wang, S. and Hu, W. 2014. Development of "-omics" research in *Schistosoma spp.* and-omics-based new diagnostic tools for schistosomiasis. *Frontiers in Microbiology*, 5:313.

Wei, J.W., Huang, K., Yang, C. and Kang, C.S. 2017. Non-coding RNAs as regulators in epigenetics. *Oncology Reports*, 37(1):3–9.

Whitman, J.D., Sakanari, J.A. and Mitreva, M. 2021. Areas of metabolomic exploration for helminth infections. *ACS Infectious Diseases*, 7(2):206–214.

Wu, J., Li, J., Zhu, Z., Li, J., Huang, G., Tang, Y. and Gao, X. 2010. Protective effects of echinocystic acid isolated from *Gleditsia sinensis* Lam. against acute myocardial ischemia. *Fitoterapia*, 81(1):8–10.

Yan, S.K., Liu, R.H., Jin, H.Z., Liu, X.R., Ye, J., Shan, L. and Zhang, W.D. 2015. " Omics" in pharmaceutical research: overview, applications, challenges, and future perspectives. *Chinese Journal of Natural Medicines*, 13(1):3–21.

Yatsushiro, S., Yamamoto, T., Yamamura, S., Abe, K., Obana, E., Nogami, T., Hayashi, T., Sesei, T., Oka, H., Okello-Onen, J. and Odongo-Aginya, E.I. 2016. Application of a cell microarray chip system for accurate, highly sensitive and rapid diagnosis for malaria in Uganda. *Scientific Reports*, 6(1):30136.

Yugi, K., Kubota, H., Hatano, A. and Kuroda, S. 2016. Trans-omics: how to reconstruct biochemical networks across multiple 'omic'layers. *Trends in Biotechnology*, 34(4):276–290.

Zhou, M., Varol, A. and Efferth, T. 2021. Multi-omics approaches to improve malaria therapy. *Pharmacological Research*, 167:105570.

8 Omics and Discoveries of Anti-Parasitic Drugs

Amina Basheer[1], Syed Babar Jamal[1],
Sumra Wajid Abbasi[1],
Muhammad Waqar Arshad[2], and Shumaila Naz[1]

[1]Department of Biological Sciences, National University of Medical Sciences, Rawalpindi, Pakistan

[2]Departments of Urology and Biochemistry and Molecular Genetics, Northwestern University, Feinberg School of Medicine, Chicago, Illinois, USA

8.1 INTRODUCTION

Advancements in technology have revolutionised our ability to gather a wide range of molecular data from tissues and cells. Progress began with the mapping and sequencing of the human genome (Satam et al., 2023). Thanks to these technologies, we can now capture a detailed snapshot of the biological processes at work within a biological system at a level of detail never before imaginable. In general, the term "omics" encompasses the scientific disciplines involved in high-throughput measurements of biological molecules (Arivaradarajan and Misra, 2018). Over time, omics research has made significant strides, greatly enriching our understanding of biology, genetics, and the intricate workings of living systems. Omics technologies have unlocked the ability to scrutinise biological samples at the level of their genes, transcripts, proteins, metabolites, and interaction networks in the pursuit of novel target molecules (Mohammadi-Shemirani et al., 2023).

Historically, the selection of molecular targets for drug discovery has relied on accumulating experimental data that support the hypothesis that altering the function of a particular molecule will have a meaningful impact on a disease (Stewart et al., 2002). This process depends on the utilisation of bioinformatics tools and databases that enable the collection and integration of diverse sources of evidence connecting potential therapeutic targets with specific diseases (Varshney et al., 2022). Bioinformatics, an interdisciplinary field within the life sciences, aims to provide the methodologies and computational techniques necessary to organise, interpret, and analyse vast amounts of biological data, encompassing various "omics" data types, such as genomics and proteomics (Bayat, 2002). The significance of computational tools in illuminating and comprehending the intricate mechanisms underlying diseases, especially complex ones, cannot be overstated. These tools have become

DOI: 10.1201/9781032651071-8

indispensable for the progress of research pertaining to drug target discovery (DTD). Contemporary bioinformatics methodologies for DTD draw from a diverse array of data sources, including experimental data, mechanistic insights, pharmacological information, and, in recent times, omics-based molecular profiles (Paananen & Fortino, 2020a).

Recent advancements in sequencing, microarray, and mass spectrometry (MS) technologies have empowered scientists to generate genomes, transcriptomics, proteomics, and other -omic datasets with unprecedented precision (Ahmed, 2022). These technologies have been widely employed in research to elucidate the molecular underpinnings of complex diseases and provide insights into pharmacological treatments (Karna et al., 2020).

Research employing omics technologies also presents a potential avenue for personalised medicine, in which treatments can be tailored to individual patients. For instance, there is evidence showing that genetic variations can assist healthcare providers in anticipating how effective a particular targeted medication might be or whether it could potentially lead to adverse effects for patients with specific molecular profiles (Singh et al., 2023). The routine integration of disease-related omics-driven molecular profiles with data on pharmacological treatments and exposures has the potential to greatly accelerate the processes of drug discovery and development (Paananen & Fortino, 2020b). Conventional drug development has typically adhered to the "one drug, one target" paradigm, with the primary goal of identifying a solitary molecular target, usually a specific protein, and ensuring high selectivity to minimise unintended effects on other biological targets, commonly referred to as "off-targets" (Konc, 2019). However, numerous diseases are characterised by intricate interactions among genetic and environmental factors. In such complex scenarios, the traditional approach of developing single-target drugs may prove inadequate in achieving a meaningful therapeutic effect.

Bioinformatics and omics are being developed together to become new resources for finding therapeutic drug targets and drug screenings. If enough data are available, bioinformatics helps identify therapeutic targets for any disease, which is the biggest impact on drug development. The following analytical features shown in Figure 8.1 can be used to organise computational frameworks for omics-based approaches that allow for systematic target selection, rational target prioritisation, and clinical relevance.

8.2 GENOMICS AND DRUG DISCOVERY IN PARASITIC INFECTIONS

The study of genomics now includes a wider range of research fields, such as functional genomics, comparative genomics, and structural genomics, in addition to genome sequencing (Giani et al., 2020). The goal of functional genomics is to comprehend how genes interact with other genes and gene products during biological activities. This field is heavily reliant on methods like transcriptomics, which evaluate gene expression (Moreno et al., 2022), and proteomics, which examine the

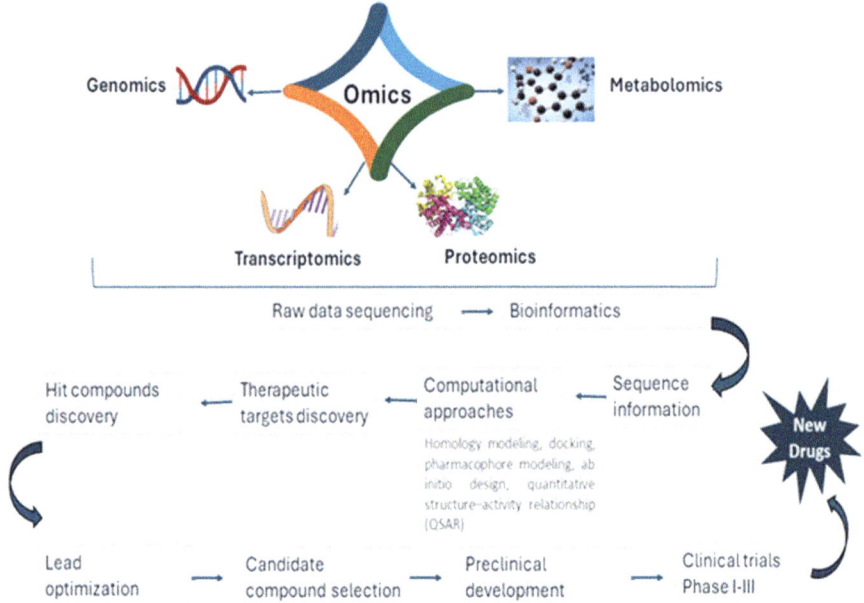

FIGURE 8.1 The flow chart of omics-based drug discovery.

full protein complement (Caudai et al., 2021). Comparative genomics compares the genomes of various species to find patterns and differences. This strategy aids in the identification of conserved genes and functional components as well as evolutionary links (Yanai et al., 2002). The study of the three-dimensional structures of proteins and other macromolecules encoded by the genome is known as structural genomics, and this knowledge is essential for comprehending protein function and medication discovery (Michalska & Joachimiak, 2021). The artificial intelligence (AI) driven AlphaFold and RoseTTAFold were introduced. The utilisation of AlphaFold's models clearly provides suitable beginning points for molecular dynamics simulations pertaining to both types of drugs, hence delivering models that are advanced and accurate (Nussinov et al., 2023).

Genomics and drug discovery in parasitic infections is a multidisciplinary effort that incorporates the study of genetics, bioinformatics, molecular biology, and pharmacology to discover novel treatments for parasitic diseases (Aulner et al., 2019). Parasitic diseases pose a considerable worldwide threat, particularly in developing nations. These infections are caused by a variety of parasites, including protozoa and helminths (Pisarski, 2019). The identification of potential drug targets and the study of parasite biology are both greatly facilitated by genomic research (Cowell & Winzeler, 2019).

Numerous factors and research studies show how the remarkable development of genomics has paved the way for a more profound and in-depth study of parasitic diseases. The genomes of many parasitic organisms have been sequenced, yielding vital insights into their biology and evolution. For example, *Plasmodium (P.) falciparum's* genome sequencing has revealed new therapeutic targets in the malaria parasite (Coghlan et al., 2018; Garrido-Cardenaset al., 2018). Similarly, the genome of the agent that causes African trypanosomiasis, *Trypanosoma (T.) brucei*, has been sequenced. Researchers can also use genomic data to pinpoint the genes and proteins vital for the survival and propagation of parasites. Potential therapeutic targets can be derived from these genes and proteins. An example is the intensive examination of genes involved in the development of surface proteins, metabolic pathways, and drug resistance in trypanosomes that have been identified as possible targets (Maslov et al., 2019).

Functional genomics techniques, such as RNA interference (RNAi), have been used to knock down individual genes in parasites, allowing researchers to better understand their function and assess their potential as therapeutic targets. *Leishmania* spp. and other parasites have been studied using this method. High-throughput screening of chemical libraries can be guided by genomic data to find prospective therapeutic candidates (Hentzschelet al.,2020). The search for antimalarial drugs has employed this strategy. Monitoring drug resistance in parasitic diseases is another function of genomics. Researchers can track the development of drug-resistant strains and modify treatment approaches by sequencing parasite populations over time. By locating antigens that trigger protective immune reactions, genomics aids in the creation of vaccines to prevent parasite diseases. For instance, research on schistosomiasis vaccines has benefited from genomics. By enabling customised therapeutics based on a person's susceptibility to parasite infections and their drug response, genomic information can support the development of personalised treatment approaches (Okombo et al., 2021; Verjee, 2020).

8.2.1 Understanding Host–Parasite Interactions Using Genomics

Genetic information about the host, such as susceptibility factors and immunological responses, can be determined through genomic studies of the host organism (such as people, animals, or plants). The susceptibility of host populations to parasitic diseases can vary genetically. The biology of parasites, particularly virulence factors, surface antigens, and treatment resistance mechanisms, can be better understood by studying their genomes (Ebert & Fields, 2020). Genome data on *P. falciparum* have shed light on malaria parasite biology and drug resistance. The host immune responses to parasite infections are studied using omics methods including transcriptomics and proteomics, which make it possible to identify the genes and pathways involved in the immune response (Sexton et al., 2019)

Pattern recognition receptors (PRRs) have evolved in hosts and identify PAMPs, or pathogen-associated molecular patterns. The PRRs and their ligands have been found through genomic investigations, shedding light on host defence mechanisms. Parasites use several strategies to sidestep host immune reactions. The molecular mechanisms of immune evasion, such as antigenic variation or host immune pathway inhibition, can be uncovered by genomic analysis (van-Hensbergen & Hu, 2024). Some parasites can adjust to various host species or strains. Genomic analyses can identify alterations relevant to host adaptability and host switching events (Mourier et al., 2021).

Co-evolution is a phenomenon in which changes in one partner's genome induce changes in the other's; it occurs frequently in host–parasite interactions and genomics can shed light on the co-evolutionary dynamics between hosts and parasites (Buckingham & Ashby, 2022). Genomes of both hosts and parasites can be analysed to identify prospective therapeutic targets. Targeted medicines can be created by better understanding host–parasite interactions. The selection of parasite antigens that vaccines can target is guided by genomic information. For the creation of vaccines that work, this information is crucial. The development of more targeted therapies is made possible by genomic investigations, which offer a thorough understanding of the molecular mechanisms of host–parasite interactions (Cuesta-Astroz et al., 2019). Personalised medicine strategies to treat parasitic diseases can be informed by knowledge of genetic factors impacting host vulnerability. Strategies to stop parasite transmission and lessen the danger of new infectious diseases emerging can be influenced by knowledge of co-evolutionary dynamics. The discovery of immunomodulatory treatments for parasite infections benefits from our growing understanding of immune responses and immune evasion mechanisms (Alvarez et al., 2022).

8.2.2 Vaccine Development Using Genomics for Parasitic Diseases

The first stage in developing a vaccine is sequencing the genome of the parasite that causes the sickness. This provides a thorough list of the genes, proteins, and possible antigens present in the parasite, and the process involves sequencing of the genome, identification of desired genes and proteins, prediction of antigens, and selection of vaccine candidates, which leads to vaccine development (Oli et al., 2020). The details are given in Figure 8.2. Genomic information is analysed to find antigens, which are proteins or glycoproteins found on the parasite surface or in its cells and are necessary for the parasite's survival or engaged in interactions with the host. Potential vaccination candidates include these antigens. Epitopes are specific areas of antigens that are likely to elicit an immune response, and their prediction is made possible by bioinformatics algorithms in immunoinformatics (De Groot et al., 2020).

To create recombinant proteins or subunit vaccines, mRNAs encoding selected antigens are cloned and expressed. The safe manufacture and development of vaccine components is ensured by the following process:

- **Human clinical trials**: Vaccine candidates proceed to human clinical trials if they exhibit success in animal investigations. In these studies, healthy volunteers are used to examine vaccine efficacy, immunogenicity, and safety (Van Tilbeurgh et al., 2021).
- **Genomic monitoring of vaccine efficacy**: Genomic analysis can be utilised to track the genetic diversity of the parasite population during clinical trials. These data aid in assessing how well vaccination protects against various parasite strains (Moser et al., 2020).

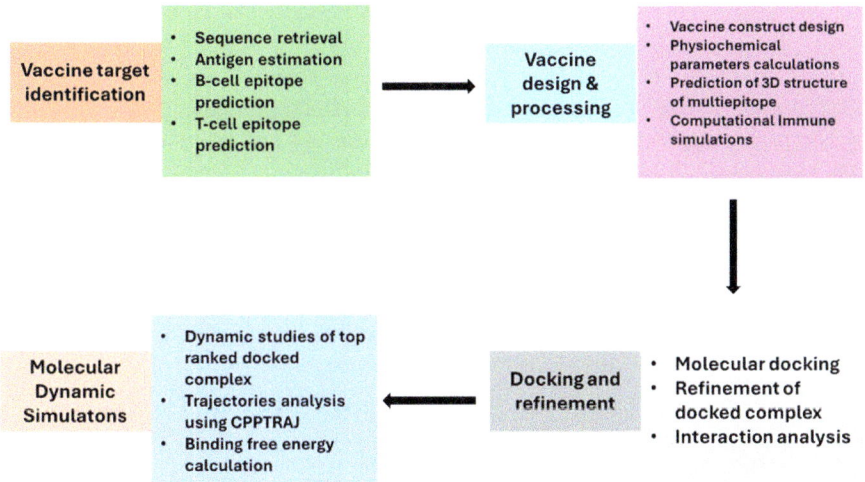

FIGURE 8.2   Flow chart of *in-silico* vaccine design and construct.

- **Vaccine formulation**: Vaccine formulation and delivery strategy optimisation can be guided by genomic data to increase the efficacy of vaccines by identifying antigenic variants and improving vaccine delivery systems (Cotugno et al., 2019).
- **Immunogenicity testing**: Recombinant antigens are evaluated in animal models to determine their immunogenicity and capacity to elicit defence-related immune reactions. This process aids in the selection of vaccine candidates with high potential (Rainard et al., 2022).

8.2.3   DRUG RESISTANCE SURVEILLANCE IN PARASITIC INFECTIONS USING GENOMICS

Anti-parasitic resistance must be detected and monitored early to guide treatment regimens, provide effective patient care, and limit the spread of resistant strains. The discovery of novel drug resistance signs and processes is aided by genomic surveillance, which promotes the creation of alternative treatments (Wijnant et al., 2022). Public health organisations can carry out focused interventions, such as altering medication regimens or deploying combination medicines, by monitoring the frequency of drug-resistant parasites. A deeper understanding of the evolutionary mechanisms of drug resistance in parasites is made possible by genomic monitoring data (Ippolitoet al., 2021).

The initial stage in drug resistance surveillance is collecting clinical samples from infected persons, such as blood, tissue, or faeces. Genomic DNA is isolated from the collected samples. Depending on the parasite and the characteristics of the sample, different techniques can be employed to extract DNA (Mutombo et al., 2019). Using NGS technology, the collected DNA is submitted for genomic sequencing.

Massive volumes of DNA sequence data are produced using NGS, which completely covers the parasite genome. Sequencing reads are then mapped or matched to a parasite strain that is drug-sensitive or a reference genome, and single nucleotide polymorphisms (SNPs), insertions, deletions, and structural variations are identified by comparing the sequencing data from drug-resistant and drug-sensitive samples (Mthethwa et al., 2021).

The study focuses on genes or loci known to be related to resistance for the specific parasite and medication under investigation. Through laboratory tests like drug susceptibility assays, detected mutations are connected to drug resistance phenotypes. This supports the finding that resistance is related to chromosomal changes (Rocamora & Winzeler, 2020).

8.3 TRANSCRIPTOMICS AND DRUG TARGET DISCOVERY

The study of an organism's transcriptome, which includes all RNA molecules in a particular cell or tissue at a certain moment, including mRNA, non-coding RNA, and small RNA, is an essential aspect of omics (Zhang et al., 2019). Transcriptomics is essential to understand the parasite gene expression dynamics and regulatory mechanisms, providing insights into their biology and potential therapeutic targets (Sexton et al., 2019). Many techniques that have been implemented to analyse transcriptomics data are discussed below.

8.3.1 RNA SEQUENCING

RNA-seq is a high-throughput sequencing approach that offers detailed information about the transcriptome, including gene expression levels, alternative splicing, and the discovery of new transcripts (Moreno et al., 2022). RNA fragments from the parasite are represented by millions of short reads produced by high-throughput sequencing systems like Illumina. Following sequencing, computational analysis is carried out to build de novo transcripts or align the reads to a reference genome, allowing for the discovery of gene expression levels, differential expression, and novel genes (Han et al., 2015).

8.3.2 MICROARRAYS

In earlier years, microarrays were commonly utilised for transcriptome profiling. The two main features required to set up a microarray are probe design and sample hybridisation. DNA microarrays are made up of immobilised DNA probes, each of which represents a different parasite gene or gene portion. Labelled cDNA created from parasite RNA is hybridised to the microarray, and the strength of the signal reflects the levels of gene expression (Negi et al., 2022).

8.3.3 COMPARATIVE AND FUNCTIONAL GENOMICS

Comparative transcriptomics compares the transcriptomes of different parasite strains or species to identify potential drug targets (Guleria & Jaiswal, 2020). For a transcriptomics analysis, parasite samples from various strains or life stages are collected and prepared. These samples are subjected to high-throughput sequencing (such as RNA-seq), and computational analysis of the transcriptome comparisons is used to discover differentially expressed genes (Suhre et al., 2020). To assess the identified potential of genes as therapeutic targets, functional annotation is frequently combined with predictions of protein structure and function (Yang et al., 2020).

Biological functions of parasite genes can be addressed by functional genomics approaches. By using gene knockdown/knockout technology involving CRISPR/ Cas9 or RNAi technology, researchers may selectively silence or delete particular genes in parasites, allowing them to study the effects on parasite survival and virulence (Pal & Dam, 2022). Phenomena like overexpression of a gene can be easily understood using a controlled overexpression strategy, and researchers can study parasite genes to learn more about their roles and potential as therapeutic targets (Maslov et al., 2019).

8.4 PROTEOMICS IN ANTI-PARASITIC DRUG DEVELOPMENT

Proteomics has the capability to profile every protein in a cell. The primary focus of parasite proteomics has been to discover novel proteins that could serve as effective therapeutic targets or potential candidates for vaccinations (Bennett & Robinson, 2021). This emphasis on proteomics is due to the accessibility of advanced technologies in this field. Proteins play a fundamental role in defining an individual phenotype, making them crucial targets for therapeutic interventions. The limited number of drugs available for infectious diseases is often linked to the scarcity of viable pharmacological targets. This shortage of drug targets is particularly notable in the case of protozoan parasites (Suhre et al., 2020). To address this challenge, there is a need to accelerate proteomic research. This involves identifying essential proteins from the vast pool of proteins in parasites. These proteins could potentially be leveraged for therapeutic purposes (Kumar et al., 2024). Proteomics enables the discovery and comparison of proteins under various conditions. These proteins can be categorised based on location and function. Comparative analysis can also be performed to identify transcripts and proteins that are either over-expressed or under-expressed (Graves & Haystead, 2002).

In contemporary research, proteomics plays a pivotal role in scrutinising the proteome of parasites. This approach enables comprehensive analysis of all changes within the proteome and holds the potential to provide valuable insights into host–parasite interactions (Cwiklinski et al., 2021). Such insights are crucial for the development of medications or vaccines aimed at combating infections caused by parasites (Kumar et al., 2024). Proteomics facilitates the identification of proteins that are essential for parasite growth, development, and reproduction (Bennett & Robinson, 2021). By targeting these crucial proteins, researchers can develop drugs that disrupt the biology of the parasite without harming the host. For example, proteins involved in interactions between parasites and hosts, or enzymes vital to key metabolic pathways, represent promising targets for therapeutic interventions (Cuesta-Astroz et al., 2019).

Protein-drug interaction models based on proteome-wide methodologies have become very effective tools for the identification of anti-parasitic medicines. Li et al. (2021) published a study in which they used chemo-proteomics for proteome-wide *Plasmodium* drug discovery. This method facilitates the target deconvolution of novel antimalarial compounds discovered by phenotypic screening but with unknown mechanisms of action. The proteome of *Leishmania* patients has been exploited in a variety of studies to identify therapeutic targets, as well as biomarkers for disease categorisation and prophylaxis (Bharadava et al., 2024; Chávez-Fumagalli et al., 2019).

Drug resistance mechanisms in *Trypanosoma* spp. have been studied using proteomics. Researchers have discovered variations in protein expression and alterations linked to resistance by comparing the proteomes of drug-resistant and susceptible parasites (Van den Kerkhof et al., 2020). Despite decades of research, there is now just one effective medicine, praziquantel, to treat the serious health issue of schistosomiasis. Numerous innovative proteomic studies on various aspects of the structure and evolution of the parasite in the host have been made possible by the recent increase of sequencing databases on *Schistosoma (S.) mansoni* and *S. japonicum* (Carson et al., 2020).

Unprecedented molecular data accumulation is enabling a more rational approach to suggest vaccine and therapeutic targets, such as proteins found on the parasite surface. Successful early trials of two vaccine candidates identified by proteomics at the parasite surface provide reason to believe that such a strategy could give the field a new start (Aulner et al., 2019). These studies highlight the essential role proteomics has played in increasing our knowledge of parasite biology and driving the discovery of anti-parasitic drugs and vaccines. Researchers can discover pharmacological targets, investigate causes of resistance, and create new therapies for these difficult diseases by studying the parasite proteomes (Kumar et al., 2023).

8.5 METABOLOMICS FOR UNDERSTANDING PARASITE METABOLISM AND DRUG RESISTANCE

A complete analysis of metabolic pathways in parasites is made possible by metabolomics, which entails the comprehensive assessment of small molecule metabolites in a biological system. The discovery of novel aspects of parasite metabolism that make appealing pharmacological targets and the clarification of the metabolic targets of anti-parasitic drugs have both been made possible by metabolomics investigations (Wijnant et al., 2022). Studies based on metabolomics are very helpful in analysing drug resistance mechanisms and modes of action in parasitic infections. They have aided in figuring out the mechanism of action of the drug eflornithine, which makes up half of the gold-standard combination therapy used to treat human African trypanosomiasis (Hahnel et al., 2020). Metabolic pathways can be identified by comparing the metabolite profiles of treated and untreated parasites. Researchers can pinpoint alterations in key metabolic pathways crucial for the survival and proliferation of the parasite. This information is vital for developing strategies to overcome drug resistance and improve treatment efficacy. This information enhances our understanding of how eflornithine disrupts essential biological processes in trypanosomes, ultimately leading to parasite death. Metabolomics studies can inform the optimisation of combination therapies for African trypanosomiasis.

Metabolomics has also shed light on the mode of action of the alkyl phospholipid miltefosine in *Leishmania*. The metabolic profile of resistant lines has been examined in antimony resistance in this parasite, providing information about the mode of action of this class of medications (Bharadava et al., 2024). The discovery of metabolic perturbations offers information on the exact metabolic pathways affected by the drug, offering data on its mode of action. Miltefosine's antileishmanial activity is mediated in part by its action on the parasite's lipid metabolism. Metabolomics investigations have indicated changes in lipid profiles after miltefosine administration, including changes in phospholipid composition and fatty acid metabolism. These findings emphasise the importance of lipid metabolism as a target for miltefosine and shed light on its mechanism of action. Metabolomics can reveal metabolic indicators linked to miltefosine sensitivity or resistance in *Leishmania* parasites. These biomarkers can be used to predict treatment outcomes, assess drug efficacy, and guide therapeutic decision-making in clinical environments (Bharadava et al., 2024).

To gain knowledge about the function of the *P. falciparum* chloroquine resistance transporter (PfCRT) protein, a study of chloroquine resistance in *P. falciparum* integrated metabolomics methods with other genetic and proteomic methods (Sanchez et al., 2022). Recent research has also shed light on the mode of action and mechanism of *T. brucei* resistance to a class of halogenated pyrimidines (Hahnel et al., 2020).

The detection of drug-induced changes in parasite metabolism and the identification of the specific metabolites and pathways that were directly affected were achieved using the metabolomic profiling of parasites treated with anti-parasitic drugs. This offered a novel and quick way to identify potential therapeutic targets. Metabolomic profiling can provide a comprehensive picture of metabolic changes, including both anticipated and unexpected changes. By using such a holistic view, researchers can find new metabolic pathways that anti-parasitic drugs might target, which could lead to the discovery of new therapeutic targets. Metabolomic profiling is useful for discovering possible treatment targets in a timely way because it can be performed relatively quickly compared to other omics approaches. Because of the short processing time, researchers can focus on the most promising candidates for further drug discovery efforts (Jacob et al., 2017).

Several antimicrobial drugs were rapidly and objectively categorised according to mechanisms of action thanks to the untargeted nature of metabolomics. Affected metabolic pathways can be quantified and made clearer by metabolomics, both untargeted and targeted (Chernov et al., 2019). The characterisation and classification of metabolites are more difficult than that of genes since they are not specific to a single metabolic pathway.

There has been interest in the use of metabolic markers to help with non-invasive disease diagnosis and disease severity prognosis. The use of metabolic markers to detect *P. falciparum* infection in plasma led to the discovery of significant variations in metabolic profiles based on substances like amino acids and lipids (Uppal et al., 2017). Eflornithine has been shown to be effective against hereditary alpha-tryptasemia caused by *T. brucei* (Amilon et al., 2022). Untargeted metabolomic analysis of protozoan cell cultures was recently utilised to confirm the mechanism of action of eflornithine. This method is thought to be efficient for assessing the mode of action of antiprotozoal drugs unbiasedly (Hahnel et al., 2020).

8.6 APPLICATION OF METAGENOMICS IN IDENTIFYING NEW ANTI-PARASITIC AGENTS

Metagenomics is an effective method for investigating the genetic material of entire microbial communities in their natural habitats, particularly parasites (Garrido-Cardenas et al., 2018). When other, more widely used tests like the polymerase chain reaction (PCR) fail, this method is typically used for surveillance and diagnosis. The failure of these assays could be attributed to the introduction of a new disease, the genetic evolution of an already-known pathogen, or a subpar assay design (Wylezich et al., 2019). The most common samples for metagenomic sequencing in pathogen identification are urine, cerebrospinal fluid (CSF), faeces, blood, or nasopharyngeal swabs, in which researchers have tried to identify the causative agent for an illness or other clinical symptom (Li et al., 2021). For instance, metagenome analysis has facilitated the discovery of the vast genetic diversity of microbes in the environment, and novel antibiotics and antimicrobial compounds. Researchers can find genes that code for antimicrobial compounds by screening metagenomic libraries; these genes could lead to the development of novel treatments (Yadav & Kapley, 2021).

Metagenomics represents a powerful approach that allows simultaneous identification and genomic characterisation of multiple species, all without the need for species-specific procedures (Pérez-Cobas et al., 2020). Recent advances in shotgun metagenomic data collection from faecal samples have provided an unprecedented opportunity to acquire detailed taxonomic and genetic information for a wide array of gut parasitic species (Piombo et al., 2021). Importantly, metagenomics technology offers comprehensive insight into the entire genome, derived from a mixed population of microorganisms, without requiring the isolation of pure cultures. It also grants swift access to the bioactive potential inherent in microbial consortia (Renwick et al., 2021).

When it comes to seeking novel bioactive compounds and other chemicals with potential relevance to the pharmaceutical industry, metagenomic techniques involve extensive data analysis. This analytical approach expedites the process of elucidating the cellular and metabolic pathways within these microbial strains, which are responsible for the production of specific valuable secondary metabolites (Pink et al., 2005). In addition, pathogen characterisation and identification are being done more frequently with shotgun metagenomics and high-throughput sequencing methods (Piombo et al., 2021). Wylezich et al. (2019) used untargeted metagenomics to identify protists and helminths in pre-diagnosed faeces and tissue samples. They also found additional intestinal eukaryotic parasites of unknown pathogenicity, which are frequently missed by standard diagnostic procedures (genera *Hymenolepis*, *Dientamoeba*, *Endolimax*, and *Entamoeba*). In a similar manner, metagenomic samples have yielded bioactive metabolites with enormous medicinal potential, such as erdacin, malacidin, and minimide (Pérez-Cobaset al., 2020). These examples high-light the varied applications of metagenomics in the search for new anti-parasitic drugs, from the discovery of novel chemicals to an understanding of the interactions between microbiota and parasites in various situations. With new opportunities for drug discovery and treatment methods, metagenomics is an important tool in the fight against parasitic infections (Sharpton et al., 2020).

8.7 INTEGRATED OMICS APPROACHES FOR ACCELERATING DRUG DISCOVERY

The interdisciplinary fields of omics and bioinformatics have significantly accel-erated drug discovery and development (Behl et al., 2021). Our understanding of animal and human disorders has greatly improved due to veterinary and medical research in the post-genomic era. Omics technologies have allowed the investigation of various biological samples at gene, protein, and metabolite levels, with interac-tion networks, contributing to the finding of novel therapeutic targets in the process of drug discovery (Kraljevic et al., 2004). Omics approaches have been extensively used in the drug discovery process to obtain a more comprehensive understanding of molecular mechanisms of diseases, locate possible drug targets, enhance the effec-tiveness of drug candidates, and accelerate the whole drug development procedure (Paananen & Fortino, 2020a).

In a similar vein, transcriptomics, which leverages high-throughput sequencing (HTS) technology, delves into the intricacies of a cell's transcriptome. The HTS tech-niques have greatly advanced transcriptomic research, starting with gene expression microarray technology (Guleria & Jaiswal, 2020) and progressing through meth-ods such as serial analysis of gene expression (SAGE), massively parallel signature sequencing (MPSS), and RNA-seq (Yang et al., 2020). By conducting transcriptional profiling across the entire genome, researchers gain profound insights into cellular health and how it responds to various stimuli, whether they be treatments or the contrasting environments of health and disease. This comprehensive understanding is instrumental in advancing drug discovery and development processes (Behl et al., 2021).

Drug discovery is a laborious and expensive undertaking, with costs estimated at around $1.8 billion USD to bring a new drug candidate to the market (Shaker et al., 2021). Proteomics aids in the identification and validation of therapeutic tar-gets. It informs the development of assays for screening potential leads and enables the generation of *in vitro* and *in vivo* biomarkers that serve as surrogate endpoints for assessing efficacy, toxicology, and disease stratification. Much of the research in drug discovery is categorised under functional proteomics, phosphoproteomics, and protein expression profiling, employing MS-based techniques. These methods involve the measurement of protein expression levels, the analysis of protein–pro-tein interactions, and the assessment of signal transduction in comparison to control treatments (Shi-Kai et al., 2015).

However, a crucial aspect of drug development involves identifying protein targets based on phenotypic analyses and understanding the interactions, both intended and unintended, that can occur with potential therapeutic molecules. This challenge is met through chemoproteomics, an emerging technology that combines chemical approaches with MS-based proteomics (Meissner et al., 2022). Chemoproteomics allows for the binding of small compounds with protein targets, facilitating the determination of the required drug quantity to engage a target and induce therapeutic effects. It also helps evaluate interactions with off-target proteins (Uppal et al., 2017).

Proteins constitute major therapeutic targets in various disease states, and proteomics technology plays a pivotal role in identifying these targets. Moreover, for effective molecule design to either inhibit or enhance specific biochemical pathways, a comprehensive understanding of disease-associated pathways is imperative (Gianazza et al., 2020). In this context, proteomics provides essential insights for designing drugs that can modulate these pathways effectively (Meissner et al., 2022). Emerging clinical applications and testing based on metabolomics provide new perspectives into disease causes. Metabolomics has helped researchers identify metabolic origins and biomarkers for chronic diseases such as diabetes, Alzheimer's disease, atherosclerosis, and cancer (Gonzalez-Covarrubias et al., 2022). Effective precision medicine strategies, such as individual drug-response monitoring and personalised phenotyping, can be implemented by metabolomics. For instance, physicians can forecast the pharmacological efficacy of treatment for a specific patient by analysing pre-dose metabolite biofluid profiles (Balashova et al., 2018). Furthermore, data mining algorithms can be employed to assess the efficacy of drug target-disorder interactions. In addition, genomic, transcriptomic, and proteomic data can be employed in innovative ways that are more effective in correlating drug targets to diseases and validating these targets for drug discovery (Paananen & Fortino, 2020b).

8.8 BIOINFORMATIC AND COMPUTATIONAL TOOLS FOR OMICS-BASED DRUG DESIGN

The molecular features of diseases produced from omics data, if systematically integrated, can considerably accelerate the drug discovery and development process. The various omics tools in bioinformatics and computational biology implemented in the drug discovery process are listed and briefly described in Table 8.1.

8.9 CHALLENGES AND OPPORTUNITIES IN OMICS-BASED DRUG DISCOVERY FOR PARASITIC INFECTIONS

Parasitic infections continue to have a devastating impact on animal and human health, especially in tropical areas. Some commonly used drugs are associated with drug resistance and genetic variability. Many drugs used to treat such diseases are outdated and only marginally effective (Kapinder et al., 2023). The advancements in omics and NGS technologies are the most effective in pinpointing not only

TABLE 8.1
Bioinformatics and Computational Tools for Omics-Based Drug Design

Genomics Databases/Tools in Omics-Based Drug Discovery

Databases/Tools	Description	References
GenBank and DNA Data Bank of Japan (DDBJ)	The combined gene entries in GenBank and the DNA Data Bank of Japan (DDBJ) total around 31 million. To accelerate the drug discovery process, these databases serve as the basis for comprehensive pharmacogenomics analysis.	(Clark et al., 2016)
Drug Bank	The Drug Bank stores extensive molecular data on drugs, including details on their mechanisms, interactions, and targets. The most recent versions of Drug Bank include data on the impact different drugs have on metabolite levels, gene expression, and protein expression (pharmacometabolomics, pharmacotranscriptomics, and pharmacoprotoemics, respectively).	(Wishart et al., 2006)
Ensembl	Ensembl is a bioinformatics project to organise biological information based on the sequencing of big genomes. It can provide information about correlations between genetic variations, such as SNPs, structural variants, and diseases.	(Birney et al., 2004)
UCSC Genome Browser	The UCSC Genome Browser is a resource for general bioinformatics, graphical viewer, and a consolidator of omics data. This is helpful in the identification of potential therapeutic targets and the comprehension of the genetic locations of targets.	(Nassar et al., 2023)
PharmGKB	The Pharmacogenomics Knowledgebase (PharmGKB), a comprehensive online database, is used to understand how different hosts respond to drugs based on their genes. It not only provides information about pharmacogenomic data (such as drug dosing guidelines and annotated drug labels) but also information that can accelerate drug discovery and disease processes.	(Gong et al., 2021)
Transcriptomics Databases/Tools in Omics-Based Drug Design		
GEO repository	The Gene Expression Omnibus (GEO) is a database that stores high-throughput gene expression data as well as hybridisation arrays, chips, and microarrays.	(Clough & Barrett, 2016)
Expression Atlas	Expression Atlas can be used for the identification and evaluation of potential drug targets in drug discovery.	(Moreno et al., 2022)
Metabolomics and Pathways Databases/Tools in Omics-Based Drug Design		
MetaboAnalyst and human metabolome database	Integrative omics pathway analysis has been facilitated by the human metabolome database and MetaboAnalyst, which can help in metabolomics and biomarkers discovery.	(Wishart et al., 2018)

(Continued)

TABLE 8.1 (CONTINUED)

Bioinformatics and Computational Tools for Omics-Based Drug Design

Databases/Tools	Description	References
KEGG and Reactome	KEGG and Reactome resources provide annotated pathways and networks that are significant to various disease processes and therapeutic targets.	(Kanehisa et al., 2021)
Madison Metabolomics	Evaluation of the effectiveness and safety of drug targets at the metabolomic level	(Cui et al., 2008)
Cytoscape and STRING	Cystoscape and STRING can be used to visualise biological networks such as protein–protein interaction (PPI) networks, metabolic pathways, and regulatory networks. In the context of drug discovery, this helps construct disease-specific networks.	(Basar et al., 2023)
ToxCast and OpenTox analyse	ToxCast is a high-throughput, *in vitro* assay-based screening platform that assesses the safety of thousands of chemicals and compounds. OpenTox provides the means to construct prediction models of drug toxicity from integrated toxicology data using machine learning and modeling methods.	(Tcheremenskaia et al., 2012)

drug targets but also their mechanisms of action and resistance (Zhou et al., 2021). Chemoproteomics approaches have proven to be valuable not only for determining potential therapeutic targets but also for comprehending the toxicity of off-target effects (Pink et al., 2005).

Despite advancements in improving parasite genomes, the fact that many parasite genomes are still in draft form poses significant challenges in analysing and interpreting the data. This is particularly problematic because many post-genomic applications require comparative genomics at both the gene and single nucleotide levels (Muggia et al., 2020). The limitations of draft genomes, including fragmented genes, erroneous gene models resulting from incorrect allelic sequence assembly, the merging of recently duplicated and divergent sequences into a single locus, and the presence of unorganised contigs within scaffolds, make them insufficient for these types of analyses. As a consequence, various crucial analyses are impeded by the absence of complete or accurate gene models for parasite species. These include parasite drug target discovery, homology modelling, and identification and classification of parasite–host interaction proteins (Chávez-Fumagalli et al., 2019).

To address these limitations, it is imperative not only to refine and upgrade existing parasite genomes but also to expand genomic resources for a broader range of parasitic species (Hahnel et al., 2020). This is especially important because some parasites hold significant socioeconomic, veterinary, and agricultural importance, yet their genomes remain unsequenced (Hupalo et al., 2015). Furthermore, the omics study objects, such as genome, proteome, metabolome, and lipidome, are dynamic and ever-changing, even for the same sample under the same analytical conditions.

The problem is that most omics data being produced currently are static, meaning that they fail to allow for change with time (Jain & Tailor, 2020). In addition to sampling and experimental considerations, the dynamic nature of biological processes may explain why many laboratory results fail to be clinically useful, making it difficult to assure enough repeatability in the development of omics biomarkers. To overcome this obstacle, researchers will need to consider time and conduct their samples at varying stages of time (Shi-Kaiet al., 2015).

8.10 FUTURE PERSPECTIVES AND POTENTIAL IMPACT OF OMICS TECHNIQUES IN PARASITIC DRUG DISCOVERY

Omics approaches facilitate the systematic characterisation of crucial genes, proteins, and metabolic pathways in parasites. The application of genomics and omics-based methods has led to significant advancements in identifying novel targets within parasites. High-throughput omics technologies enable the rapid screening of extensive compound libraries for potential drug candidates, greatly expediting the drug discovery process (Cowell & Winzeler, 2019). Recent progress in genomics, transcriptomics, and proteomics has made it feasible to pinpoint parasite components that play pivotal roles in their function. Omics techniques have been employed in various studies to uncover new drug targets for viruses and parasites. Furthermore, numerous potential antigens have been identified for a diverse range of nematode and platyhelminth parasites affecting both humans and livestock. The increasing effectiveness of omics-guided antigen and target discovery, with genomes as the cornerstone for transcriptomics and proteomics, has been notable (Arivaradarajan & Misra, 2018). Omics research proves invaluable in the development of new vaccines by identifying promising vaccine candidates. The study of an organism's entire gene set marked the onset of the omics era. Genomic studies allow for in-depth exploration of genes, chromosomes, disease variations, and evolutionary relationships with other phyla (Chernov et al., 2019).

REFERENCES

Ahmed, Z. (2022). Multi-omics strategies for personalized and predictive medicine: past, current, and future translational opportunities. *Emerging Topics in Life Sciences*, *6*(2), 215–225. https://doi.org/10.1042/ETLS20210244

Alvarez, M. J. R., Hasanzad, M., Sarhangi, N., & Meybodi, H. R. A. (2022). Precision medicine in infectious disease. *Precision Medicine in Clinical Practice*, 221–257. https://doi.org/10.1007/978-981-19-5082-7_13/COVER

Amilon, C., Boberg, M., Tarning, J., Äbelö, A., Ashton, M., & Jansson-Löfmark, R. (2022). Population pharmacodynamic modeling of eflornithine-based treatments against late-stage gambiense human African trypanosomiasis and efficacy predictions of L-eflornithine-based therapy. *AAPS Journal*, *24*(3), 1–9. https://doi.org/10.1208/S12248-022-00693-2/FIGURES/3

Arivaradarajan, P., & Misra, G. (2018). *Omics approaches, technologies and applications.* Springer, Singapore. https://doi.org/10.1007/978-981-13-2925-8_1

Aulner, N., Danckaert, A., Ihm, J. E., Shum, D., & Shorte, S. L. (2019). Next-generation pheno-typic screening in early drug discovery for infectious diseases. *Trends in Parasitology*, *35*(7), 559–570. https://doi.org/10.1016/j.pt.2019.05.004

Balashova, E., Maslov, D., & Lokhov, P. G. A. (2018). A metabolomics approach to phar-macotherapy personalization. *Mdpi.ComEE Journal of Personalized Medicine, 8*, 28. https://doi.org/10.3390/jpm8030028

Basar, M. A., Hosen, M. F., Kumar Paul, B., Hasan, M. R., Shamim, S. M., & Bhuyian, T. (2023). Identification of drug and protein-protein interaction network among stress and depression: A bioinformatics approach. *Informatics in Medicine Unlocked*, *37*, 101174. https://doi.org/10.1016/J.IMU.2023.101174

Bayat, A. (2002). Science, medicine, and the future: Bioinformatics. *BMJ: British Medical Journal*, *324*(7344), 1018. https://doi.org/10.1136/bmj.324.7344.1018

Behl, T., Kaur, I., Sehgal, A., Singh, S., Bhatia, S., Al-Harrasi, A., Zengin, G., Babes, E. E., Brisc, C., Stoicescu, M., Toma, M. M., Sava, C., & Bungau, S. G. (2021). Bioinformatics accelerates the major tetrad: A real boost for the pharmaceutical industry. *International Journal of Molecular Sciences*, *22*(12), 6184. https://doi.org/10.3390/IJMS22126184

Bennett, A. P. S., & Robinson, M. W. (2021). Trematode proteomics: Recent advances and future directions. *Pathogens 2021*, *10*(3), 348. https://doi.org/10.3390/PATHOGENS10030348

Bharadava, K., Upadhyay, T. K., Kaushal, R. S., Ahmad, I., Alraey, Y., Siddiqui, S., & Saeed, M. (2024). Genomic insight of leishmania parasite: In-depth review of drug resistance mechanisms and genetic mutations. *ACS Omega*. https://doi.org/10.1021/ACSOMEGA .3C09400

Birney, E., Andrews, T. D., Bevan, P., Caccamo, M., Chen, Y., Clarke, L., Coates, G., Cuff, J., Curwen, V., Cutts, T., Down, T., Eyras, E., Fernandez-Suarez, X. M., Gane, P., Gibbins, B., Gilbert, J., Hammond, M., Hotz, H. R., Iyer, V., … Clamp, M. (2004). An overview of ensembl. *Genome Research*, *14*(5), 925. https://doi.org/10.1101/GR.1860604

Buckingham, L. J., & Ashby, B. (2022). Coevolutionary theory of hosts and parasites. *Journal of Evolutionary Biology*, *35*(2), 205–224. https://doi.org/10.1111/JEB.13981

Carson, J. P., Robinson, M. W., Hsieh, M. H., Cody, J., Le, L., You, H., McManus, D. P., & Gobert, G. N. (2020). A comparative proteomics analysis of the egg secretions of three major schistosome species. *Molecular and Biochemical Parasitology*, *240*, 111322. https://doi.org/10.1016/J.MOLBIOPARA.2020.111322

Caudai, C., Galizia, A., Geraci, F., Le Pera, L., Morea, V., Salerno, E., Via, A., & Colombo, T. (2021). AI applications in functional genomics. *Computational and Structural Biotechnology Journal*, *19*, 5762–5790. https://doi.org/10.1016/J.CSBJ.2021.10.009

Chávez-Fumagalli, M. A., Lage, D. P., Tavares, G. S. V., Mendonça, D. V. C., Dias, D. S., Ribeiro, P. A. F., Ludolf, F., Costa, L. E., Coelho, V. T. S., & Coelho, E. A. F. (2019). In silico Leishmania proteome mining applied to identify drug target potential to be used to treat against visceral and tegumentary leishmaniasis. *Journal of Molecular Graphics and Modelling*, *87*, 89–97. https://doi.org/10.1016/J.JMGM.2018.11.014

Chernov, V. M., Chernova, O. A., Mouzykantov, A. A., Lopukhov, L. L., & Aminov, R. I. (2019). Omics of antimicrobials and antimicrobial resistance. *Expert Opinion on Drug Discovery*, *14*(5), 455–468. https://doi.org/10.1080/17460441.2019.1588880

Clark, K., Karsch-Mizrachi, I., Lipman, D. J., Ostell, J., & Sayers, E. W. (2016). GenBank. *Nucleic Acids Research*, *44*(D1), D67–D72. https://doi.org/10.1093/NAR/GKV1276

Clough, E., & Barrett, T. (2016). The gene expression omnibus database. *Methods in Molecular Biology*, *1418*, 93–110. https://doi.org/10.1007/978-1-4939-3578-9_5/COVER

Coghlan, A., Tyagi, R., Cotton, J. A., Holroyd, N., Rosa, B. A., Tsai, I. J., Laetsch, D. R., Beech, R. N., Day, T. A., Hallsworth-Pepin, K., Ke, H. M., Kuo, T. H., Lee, T. J., Martin, J., Maizels, R. M., Mutowo, P., Ozersky, P., Parkinson, J., Reid, A. J., … Berriman, M. (2018). Comparative genomics of the major parasitic worms. *Nature Genetics*, *51*(1), 163–174. https://doi.org/10.1038/s41588-018-0262-1

Cotugno, N., Ruggiero, A., Santilli, V., Manno, E. C., Rocca, S., Zicari, S., Amodio, D., Colucci, M., Rossi, P., Levy, O., Martinon-Torres, F., Pollard, A. J., & Palma, P. (2019). OMIC Technologies and vaccine development: From the identification of vulnerable individuals to the formulation of invulnerable vaccines. *Journal of Immunology Research.* https://doi.org/10.1155/2019/8732191

Cowell, A. N., & Winzeler, E. A. (2019). Advances in omics-based methods to identify novel targets for malaria and other parasitic protozoan infections. *Genome Medicine, 11*(1). https://doi.org/10.1186/S13073-019-0673-3

Cuesta-Astroz, Y., Santos, A., Oliveira, G., & Jensen, L. J. (2019). Analysis of predicted host–parasite interactomes reveals commonalities and specificities related to parasitic lifestyle and tissues tropism. *Frontiers in Immunology, 10*(FEB), 425732. https://doi.org/10.3389/FIMMU.2019.00212/BIBTEX

Cui, Q., Lewis, I. A., Hegeman, A. D., Anderson, M. E., Li, J., Schulte, C. F., Westler, W. M., Eghbalnia, H. R., Sussman, M. R., & Markley, J. L. (2008). Metabolite identification via the madison metabolomics consortium database. *Nature Biotechnology, 26*(2), 162–164. https://doi.org/10.1038/NBT0208-162

Cwiklinski, K., Robinson, M. W., Donnelly, S., & Dalton, J. P. (2021). Complementary transcriptomic and proteomic analyses reveal the cellular and molecular processes that drive growth and development of Fasciola hepatica in the host liver. *BMC Genomics, 22*(1), 1–16. https://doi.org/10.1186/S12864-020-07326-Y/FIGURES/6

De Groot, A. S., Moise, L., Terry, F., Gutierrez, A. H., Hindocha, P., Richard, G., Hoft, D. F., Ross, T. M., Noe, A. R., Takahashi, Y., Kotraiah, V., Silk, S. E., Nielsen, C. M., Minassian, A. M., Ashfield, R., Ardito, M., Draper, S. J., & Martin, W. D. (2020). Better epitope discovery, precision immune engineering, and accelerated vaccine design using Immunoinformatics tools. *Frontiers in Immunology, 11*, 527882. https://doi.org/10.3389/FIMMU.2020.00442/BIBTEX

Ebert, D., & Fields, P. D. (2020). Host–parasite co-evolution and its genomic signature. *Nature Reviews Genetics, 21*(12), 754–768. https://doi.org/10.1038/s41576-020-0269-1

Garrido-Cardenas, J. A., González-Cerón, L., Manzano-Agugliaro, F., & Mesa-Valle, C. (2018). Plasmodium genomics: an approach for learning about and ending human malaria. *Parasitology Research, 118*(1), 1–27. https://doi.org/10.1007/S00436-018-6127-9

Gianazza, E., Brioschi, M., Baetta, R., Mallia, A., Banfi, C., & Tremoli, E. (2020). Platelets in Healthy and Disease States: From Biomarkers Discovery to Drug Targets Identification by Proteomics. *International Journal of Molecular Sciences, 21*(12), 4541. https://doi.org/10.3390/IJMS21124541

Giani, A. M., Gallo, G. R., Gianfranceschi, L., & Formenti, G. (2020). Long walk to genomics: history and current approaches to genome sequencing and assembly. *Computational and Structural Biotechnology Journal, 18*, 9–19. https://doi.org/10.1016/J.CSBJ.2019.11.002

Gong, L., Whirl-Carrillo, M., & Klein, T. E. (2021). PharmGKB, an integrated resource of pharmacogenomic knowledge. *Current Protocols, 1*(8), e226. https://doi.org/10.1002/CPZ1.226

Gonzalez-Covarrubias, V., Martínez-Martínez, E., & Bosque-Plata, L. Del. (2022). The potential of metabolomics in biomedical applications. *Metabolites, 12*(2), 194. https://doi.org/10.3390/METABO12020194

Graves, P. R., & Haystead, T. A. (2002). Molecular biologist's guide to proteomics. *Microbiology and Molecular Biology Reviews, 66*(1), 39–63. https://doi.org/10.1128/MMBR.66.1.39-63.2002

Guleria, V., & Jaiswal, V. (2020). Comparative transcriptome analysis of different stages of Plasmodium falciparum to explore vaccine and drug candidates. *Genomics, 112*(1), 796–804. https://doi.org/10.1016/J.YGENO.2019.05.018

Hahnel, S. R., Dilks, C. M., Heisler, I., Andersen, E. C., & Kulke, D. (2020). Caenorhabditis elegans in anthelmintic research – Old model, new perspectives. *International Journal for Parasitology: Drugs and Drug Resistance*, *14*, 237–248. https://doi.org/10.1016/J .IJPDDR.2020.09.005

Han, Y., Gao, S., Muegge, K., Zhang, W., & Zhou, B. (2015). Advanced applications of RNA sequencing and challenges. *Bioinformatics and Biology Insights*, *9*, BBI–S28991. https://doi.org/10.4137/BBI.S28991

Hentzschel, F., Mitesser, V., Fraschka, S. A. K., Krzikalla, D., Carrillo, E. H., Berkhout, B., Bártfai, R., Mueller, A. K., & Grimm, D. (2020). Gene knockdown in malaria parasites via non-canonical RNAi. *Nucleic Acids Research*, *48*(1), e2–e2. https://doi.org/10.1093 /NAR/GKZ927

Hupalo, D. N., Bradic, M., & Carlton, J. M. (2015). The impact of genomics on population genetics of parasitic diseases. *Current Opinion in Microbiology*, *23*, 49-54. https://doi .org/10.1016/j.mib.2014.11.001

Ippolito, M. M., Moser, K. A., Jean-Bertin, &, Kabuya, B., Cunningham, C., & Juliano, J. J. (2021). Antimalarial Drug Resistance and Implications for the WHO Global Technical Strategy. *Current Epidemiology Reports*, *8*(2), 46–62. https://doi.org/10.1007/S40471 -021-00266-5

Jacob, M., Lopata, A. L., Dasouki, | Majed, Anas, |, Rahman, M. A., & Rahman, A. A. (2017). Metabolomics toward personalized medicine. *Wiley Online Library*, *38*(3), 221–238. https://doi.org/10.1002/mas.21548

Jain, A., & Tailor, V. (2020). Emerging trends of biotechnology in marine bioprospecting: A new vision. *Marine Niche: Applications in Pharmaceutical Sciences: Translational Research*, 1–36. https://doi.org/10.1007/978-981-15-5017-1_1/COVER

Kanehisa, M., Sato, Y., & Kawashima, M. (2021). KEGG mapping tools for uncovering hidden features in biological data. *Protein Science*. https://doi.org/10.1002/PRO.4172

Kapinder, Daram, N., & Verma, A. K. (2023). Drug resistance in helminth parasites: Role of plant-based natural therapeutics. *Natural Product Based Drug Discovery Against Human Parasites*, 553–579. https://doi.org/10.1007/978-981-19-9605-4_25

Karna, E., Szoka, L., Huynh, T. Y. L., & Palka, J. A. (2020). Proline-dependent regulation of collagen metabolism. *Cellular and Molecular Life Sciences*, *77*(10), 1911–1918. https:// doi.org/10.1007/S00018-019-03363-3/FIGURES/2

Konc, J. (2019). Binding site comparisons for target-centered drug discovery. *Expert Opinion on Drug Discovery*, *14*(5), 445–454. https://doi.org/10.1080/17460441.2019.1588883

Kraljevic, S., Stambrook, P. J., & Pavelic, K. (2004). Accelerating drug discovery. *EMBO Reports*, *5*(9), 837–842. https://doi.org/10.1038/SJ.EMBOR.7400236

Kumar, A., Deepika, Sharda, S., & Avasthi, A. (2023). Recent advances in the treatment of parasitic diseases: Current status and future. *Natural Product Based Drug Discovery Against Human Parasites*, 249–286. https://doi.org/10.1007/978-981-19-9605-4_13

Kumar, V., Barwal, A., Sharma, N., Mir, D.S., Kumar, P., Kumar, V. (2024). Therapeutic proteins: Developments, progress, challenges, and future perspectives. *3 Biotech*, *14*(4), 112.

Li, N., Cai, Q., Miao, Q., Song, Z., Fang, Y., & Hu, B. (2021). High-throughput metagenomics for identification of pathogens in the clinical settings. *Small Methods*, *5*(1), 2000792. https://doi.org/10.1002/SMTD.202000792

Maslov, D. A., Opperdoes, F. R., Kostygov, A. Y., Hashimi, H., Lukeš, J., & Yurchenko, V. (2019). Recent advances in trypanosomatid research: genome organization, expression, metabolism, taxonomy and evolution. *Parasitology*, *146*(1), 1–27. https://doi.org /10.1017/S0031182018000951

Meissner, F., Geddes-McAlister, J., Mann, M., & Bantscheff, M. (2022). The emerging role of mass spectrometry-based proteomics in drug discovery. *Nature Reviews Drug Discovery*, *21*(9), 637–654. https://doi.org/10.1038/s41573-022-00409-3

Michalska, K., & Joachimiak, A. (2021). Structural genomics and the Protein Data Bank. *Journal of Biological Chemistry*, *296*. https://doi.org/10.1016/j.jbc.2021.100747

Mohammadi-Shemirani, P., Sood, T., & Paré, G. (2023). From 'Omics to multi-omics technologies: the discovery of novel causal mediators. *Current Atherosclerosis Reports*, *25*(2), 55–65. https://doi.org/10.1007/s11883-022-01078-8

Moreno, P., Fexova, S., George, N., Manning, J. R., Miao, Z., Mohammed, S., Muñoz-Pomer, A., Fullgrabe, A., Bi, Y., Bush, N., Iqbal, H., Kumbham, U., Solovyev, A., Zhao, L., Prakash, A., García-Seisdedos, D., Kundu, D. J., Wang, S., Walzer, M., … Papatheodorou, I. (2022). Expression Atlas update: gene and protein expression in multiple species. *Nucleic Acids Research*, *50*(D1), D129–D140. https://doi.org/10.1093/NAR/GKAB1030

Moser, K. A., Drábek, E. F., Dwivedi, A., Stucke, E. M., Crabtree, J., Dara, A., Shah, Z., Adams, M., Li, T., Rodrigues, P. T., Koren, S., Phillippy, A. M., Munro, J. B., Ouattara, A., Sparklin, B. C., Dunning Hotopp, J. C., Lyke, K. E., Sadzewicz, L., Tallon, L. J., … Silva, J. C. (2020). Strains used in whole organism Plasmodium falciparum vaccine trials differ in genome structure, sequence, and immunogenic potential. *Genome Medicine*, *12*(1), 1–17. https://doi.org/10.1186/S13073-019-0708-9/FIGURES/6

Mourier, T., de Alvarenga, D. A. M., Kaushik, A., de Pina-Costa, A., Douvropoulou, O., Guan, Q., Guzmán-Vega, F. J., Forrester, S., de Abreu, F. V. S., Júnior, C. B., de Souza Junior, J. C., Moreira, S. B., Hirano, Z. M. B., Pissinatti, A., Ferreira-da-Cruz, M. de F., de Oliveira, R. L., Arold, S. T., Jeffares, D. C., Brasil, P., … Pain, A. (2021). The genome of the zoonotic malaria parasite Plasmodium simium reveals adaptations to host switching. *BMC Biology*, *19*(1), 1–17. https://doi.org/10.1186/S12915-021-01139.

Mthethwa, N. P., Amoah, I. D., Reddy, P., Bux, F., & Kumari, S. (2021). A review on application of next-generation sequencing methods for profiling of protozoan parasites in water: current methodologies, challenges, and perspectives. *Journal of Microbiological Methods*, *187*, 106269. https://doi.org/10.1016/J.MIMET.2021.106269

Muggia, L., Ametrano, C. G., Sterflinger, K., & Tesei, D. (2020). An overview of genomics, phylogenomics and proteomics approaches in ascomycota. *Life*, *10*(12), 356. https://doi.org/10.3390/LIFE10120356

Mutombo, P. N., Man, N. W. Y., Nejsum, P., Ricketson, R., Gordon, C. A., Robertson, G., Clements, A. C. A., Chacón-Fonseca, N., Nissapatorn, V., Webster, J. P., & McLaws, M. L. (2019). Diagnosis and drug resistance of human soil-transmitted helminth infections: A public health perspective. *Advances in Parasitology*, *104*, 247–326. https://doi.org/10.1016/BS.APAR.2019.02.004

Nassar, L. R., Barber, G. P., Benet-Pagès, A., Casper, J., Clawson, H., Diekhans, M., Fischer, C., Gonzalez, J. N., Hinrichs, A. S., Lee, B. T., Lee, C. M., Muthuraman, P., Nguy, B., Pereira, T., Nejad, P., Perez, G., Raney, B. J., Schmelter, D., Speir, M. L., … Kent, W. J. (2023). The UCSC genome browser database: 2023 update. *Nucleic Acids Research*, *51*(D1), D1188–D1195. https://doi.org/10.1093/NAR/GKAC1072

Negi, A., Shukla, A., Jaiswar, A., & Shrinet, J. (2022). Applications and challenges of microarray and RNA-sequencing. *Bioinformatics: Methods and Applications*, 91–103. https://doi.org/10.1016/B978-0-323-89775-4.00016-X

Nussinov, R., Zhang, M., Liu, Y., & Jang, H. (2023). AlphaFold, allosteric, and orthosteric drug discovery: ways forward. *Drug Discovery Today*, *28*(6), 103551. https://doi.org/10.1016/J.DRUDIS.2023.103551

Okombo, J., Kanai, M., Deni, I., & Fidock, D. A. (2021). Genomic and genetic approaches to studying antimalarial drug resistance and plasmodium biology. *Trends in Parasitology*, *37*(6), 476–492. https://doi.org/10.1016/J.PT.2021.02.007

Oli, A. N., Obialor, W. O., Ositadimma, M., Ifeanyichukwu, Odimegwu, D. C., Okoyeh, J. N., Emechebe, G. O., Adejumo, S. A., & Ibeanu, G. C. (2020). Immunoinformatics and vaccine development: an overview. *ImmunoTargets and Therapy*, *9*, 13–30. https://doi .org/10.2147/ITT.S241064

Pal, S., & Dam, S. (2022). CRISPR-Cas9: Taming protozoan parasites with bacterial scissor. *Journal of Parasitic Diseases*, *46*(4), 1204–1212. https://doi.org/10.1007/s12639-022 -01534-x

Paananen, J., & Fortino, V. (2020a). An omics perspective on drug target discovery platforms. *Briefings in Bioinformatics*, *21*(6), 1937–1953. https://doi.org/10.1093/BIB/BBZ122

Paananen, J., & Fortino, V. (2020b). An omics perspective on drug target discovery platforms. *Briefings in Bioinformatics*, *21*(6), 1937–1953. https://doi.org/10.1093/BIB/BBZ122

Pérez-Cobas, A. E., Gomez-Valero, L., & Buchrieser, C. (2020). Metagenomic approaches in microbial ecology: An update on whole-genome and marker gene sequencing analyses. *Microbial Genomics*, *6*(8), 1–22. https://doi.org/10.1099/MGEN.0.000409/CITE/ REFWORKS

Pink, R., Hudson, A., Mouriès, M. A., & Bendig, M. (2005). Opportunities and challenges in antiparasitic drug discovery. *Nature Reviews Drug Discovery*, *4*(9), 727–740. https:// doi.org/10.1038/nrd1824

Piombo, E., Abdelfattah, A., Droby, S., Wisniewski, M., Spadaro, D., & Schena, L. (2021). Metagenomics approaches for the detection and surveillance of emerging and recurrent plant pathogens. *Microorganisms*, *9*(1), 188. https://doi.org/10.3390/MICROORGANI SMS9010188

Pisarski, K. (2019). The global burden of disease of zoonotic parasitic diseases: Top 5 contenders for priority consideration. *Tropical Medicine and Infectious Disease*, *4*(1), 44. https://doi.org/10.3390/TROPICALMED4010044

Rainard, P., Gilbert, F. B., Martins, R. P., Germon, P., & Foucras, G. (2022). Progress towards the elusive mastitis vaccines. *Vaccines*, *10*(2), 296. https://doi.org/10.3390/ VACCINES10020296

Renwick, S., Ganobis, C. M., Elder, R. A., Gianetto-Hill, C., Higgins, G., Robinson, A. V., Vancuren, S. J., Wilde, J., & Allen-Vercoe, E. (2021). Culturing human gut microbiomes in the laboratory. *Annual Review of Microbiology*, *75*, 49–69. https://doi.org/10 .1146/ANNUREV-MICRO-031021-084116

Rocamora, F., & Winzeler, E. A. (2020). Genomic approaches to drug resistance in Malaria. *Annual Review of Microbiology*, *74*, 761–786. https://doi.org/10.1146/ANNUREV -MICRO-012220-064343

Sanchez, C. P., Manson, E. D. T., Moliner Cubel, S., Mandel, L., Weidt, S. K., Barrett, M. P., & Lanzer, M. (2022). The knock-down of the chloroquine resistance transporter PfCRT Is linked to oligopeptide handling in plasmodium falciparum. *Microbiology Spectrum*, *10*(4). https://doi.org/10.1128/SPECTRUM.01101-22/SUPPL_FILE/REVIEWER -COMMENTS.PDF

Satam, H., Joshi, K., Mangrolia, U., Waghoo, S., Zaidi, G., Rawool, S., Thakare, R. P., Banday, S., Mishra, A. K., Das, G., & Malonia, S. K. (2023). Next-generation sequencing technology: current trends and advancements. *Biology*, *12*(7), 997. https://doi.org/10 .3390/BIOLOGY12070997

Sexton, A. E., Doerig, C., Creek, D. J., & Carvalho, T. G. (2019). Post-genomic approaches to understanding malaria parasite biology: linking genes to biological functions. *ACS Infectious Diseases*, *5*(8), 1269–1278. https://doi.org/10.1021/ACSINFECDIS.9B00093/

Shaker, B., Ahmad, S., Lee, J., Jung, C., & Na, D. (2021). In silico methods and tools for drug discovery. *Computers in Biology and Medicine, 137*, 104851. https://doi.org/10.1016/J.COMPBIOMED.2021.104851

Sharpton, T. J., Combrink, L., Arnold, H. K., Gaulke, C. A., & Kent, M. (2020). Harnessing the gut microbiome in the fight against anthelminthic drug resistance. *Current Opinion in Microbiology, 53*, 26–34. https://doi.org/10.1016/J.MIB.2020.01.017

Shi-Kai, Y., Run-Hui, L., Hui-Zi, J., Xin-Ru, L., Ji, Y. E., Lei, S., & Zhang, W.-D. (2015). *"Omics" in pharmaceutical research: overview, applications, challenges, and future perspectives. Chinese Journal of Natural Medicines, 13*(1). https://doi.org/10.3724/SP.J.1009.2015.00003

Singh, S., Sarma, D. K., Verma, V., Nagpal, R., & Kumar, M. (2023). Unveiling the future of metabolic medicine: omics technologies driving personalized solutions for precision treatment of metabolic disorders. *Biochemical and Biophysical Research Communications, 682*, 1–20. https://doi.org/10.1016/J.BBRC.2023.09.064

Stewart, L., Clark, R., & Behnke, C. (2002). High-throughput crystallization and structure determination in drug discovery. *Drug Discovery Today, 7*(3), 187-196. https://doi.org/10.1016/S1359-6446(01)02121-3

Suhre, K., McCarthy, M. I., & Schwenk, J. M. (2020). Genetics meets proteomics: perspectives for large population-based studies. *Nature Reviews Genetics, 22*(1), 19–37. https://doi.org/10.1038/s41576-020-0268-2

Tcheremenskaia, O., Benigni, R., Nikolova, I., Jeliazkova, N., Escher, S. E., Batke, M., Baier, T., Poroikov, V., Lagunin, A., Rautenberg, M., & Hardy, B. (2012). OpenTox predictive toxicology framework: Toxicological ontology and semantic media wiki-based OpenToxipedia. *Journal of Biomedical Semantics, 3*(1), 1–17. https://doi.org/10.1186/2041-1480-3-S1-S7/FIGURES/8

Uppal, K., Salinas, J. L., Monteiro, W. M., Val, F., Cordy, R. J., Liu, K., ... & Jones, D. P. (2017). Plasma metabolomics reveals membrane lipids, aspartate/asparagine and nucleotide metabolism pathway differences associated with chloroquine resistance in Plasmodium vivax malaria. *PLoS One, 12*(8), e0182819. https://doi.org/10.1371/journal.pone.0182819

Van den Kerkhof, M., Sterckx, Y. G. J., Leprohon, P., Maes, L., & Caljon, G. (2020). Experimental strategies to explore drug action and resistance in kinetoplastid parasites. *Microorganisms, 8*(6), 950. https://doi.org/10.3390/MICROORGANISMS8060950

van-Hensbergen, V. P., & Hu, X. (2024). Pattern recognition receptors and the innate immune network. In *Molecular Medical Microbiology*, 3rd edition, 407–441. https://doi.org/10.1016/B978-0-12-818619-0.00131-3

Van Tilbeurgh, M., Lemdani, K., Beignon, A. S., Chapon, C., Tchitchek, N., Cheraitia, L., Lopez, E. M., Pascal, Q., Le Grand, R., Maisonnasse, P., & Manet, C. (2021). Predictive markers of immunogenicity and efficacy for human vaccines. *Vaccines, 9*(6), 579. https://doi.org/10.3390/VACCINES9060579

Varshney, S., Bharti, M., Sundram, S., Malviya, R., & Fuloria, N. K. (2022). The role of bioinformatics tools and technologies in clinical trials. *Bioinformatics Tools and Big Data Analytics for Patient Care*, 1–16. https://doi.org/10.1201/9781003226949-1

Verjee, M. A. (2020). Schistosomiasis: still a cause of significant morbidity and mortality. *Research and Reports in Tropical Medicine, 10*, 153–163. https://doi.org/10.2147/RRTM.S204345

Wijnant, G. J., Dumetz, F., Dirkx, L., Bulté, D., Cuypers, B., Van Bocxlaer, K., & Hendrickx, S. (2022). Tackling drug resistance and other causes of treatment failure in leishmaniasis. *Frontiers in Tropical Diseases, 3*, 837460. https://doi.org/10.3389/FITD.2022.837460/BIBTEX

Wishart, D. S., Feunang, Y. D., Marcu, A., Guo, A. C., Liang, K., Vázquez-Fresno, R., Sajed, T., Johnson, D., Li, C., Karu, N., Sayeeda, Z., Lo, E., Assempour, N., Berjanskii, M., Singhal, S., Arndt, D., Liang, Y., Badran, H., Grant, J., … Scalbert, A. (2018). HMDB 4.0: the human metabolome database for 2018. *Nucleic Acids Research*, *46*(D1), D608–D617. https://doi.org/10.1093/NAR/GKX1089

Wishart, D. S., Knox, C., Guo, A. C., Shrivastava, S., Hassanali, M., Stothard, P., Chang, Z., & Woolsey, J. (2006). DrugBank: a comprehensive resource for in silico drug discovery and exploration. *Nucleic Acids Research*, *34*(Database issue), D668. https://doi.org/10.1093/NAR/GKJ067

Wylezich, C., Belka, A., Hanke, D., Beer, M., Blome, S., & Höper, D. (2019). Metagenomics for broad and improved parasite detection: a proof-of-concept study using swine faecal samples. *International Journal for Parasitology*, *49*(10), 769–777. https://doi.org/10.1016/J.IJPARA.2019.04.007

Yadav, S., & Kapley, A. (2021). Antibiotic resistance: Global health crisis and metagenomics. *Biotechnology Reports*, *29*, e00604. https://doi.org/10.1016/J.BTRE.2021.E00604

Yanai, I., Mellor, J. C., & DeLisi, C. (2002). Identifying functional links between genes using conserved chromosomal proximity. *Trends in genetics*, *18*(4), 176–179. https://doi.org/10.1016/s0168-9525(01)02621-x

Yang, X., Kui, L., Tang, M., Li, D., Wei, K., Chen, W., Miao, J., & Dong, Y. (2020). High-throughput transcriptome profiling in drug and biomarker discovery. *Frontiers in Genetics*, *11*, 505377. https://doi.org/10.3389/FGENE.2020.00019/BIBTEX

Zhang, P., Wu, W., Chen, Q., & Chen, M. (2019). Non-Coding RNAs and their Integrated Networks. *Journal of Integrative Bioinformatics*, *16*(3). https://doi.org/10.1515/JIB-2019-0027

Zhou, M., Varol, A., & Efferth, T. (2021). Multi-omics approaches to improve malaria therapy. *Pharmacological Research*, *167*, 105570. https://doi.org/10.1016/J.PHRS.2021.105570

9 Bioinformatics and Data Analysis in Veterinary Parasitology

Syed Awais Attique[1]*, Qurat Ul Ain[2,3]**,
Mourad Ben Said[4,5], and Muhammad Sohail Sajid[6]

[1]School of Interdisciplinary Engineering & Science (SINES),
National University of Sciences & Technology (NUST),
Islamabad, Pakistan

[2]Department of Forensic Science, Faculty of Medicine and
Allied Health Sciences, The Islamia University of
Bahawalpur, Bahawalpur, Punjab, Pakistan

[3]Center for Advanced Interdisciplinary Science
and Biomedicine of IHM, Division of Life
Sciences and Medicine, University of Science and
Technology of China, Hefei, Anhui, China

[4]Department of Basic Sciences, Higher Institute of
Biotechnology of Sidi Thabet, University of Manouba,
Manouba, Tunisia

[5]Laboratory of Microbiology National School
of Veterinary Medicine of Sidi Thabet,
University of Manouba, Manouba, Tunisia

[6]Department of Parasitology, Faculty of Veterinary
Science, University of Agriculture, Faisalabad, Pakistan
*Corresponding Authors

9.1 INTRODUCTION

Veterinary parasitic diseases encompass a broad spectrum of conditions resulting from infections caused by protozoa, helminths, and arthropods in animals. These diseases not only impact the health and well-being of animals but also wield significant economic consequences within the livestock industry (Grønvold et al., 1996).

The economic ramifications arise from various factors, including reduced productivity, treatment costs, and mortality rates among infected animals. Livestock owners and the industry as a whole face substantial losses, making the effective

DOI: 10.1201/9781032651071-9

management and control of these parasitic diseases imperative for sustaining a thriving livestock sector (Mackenzie et al., 2013).

Furthermore, veterinary parasitic diseases pose a considerable threat to human health through zoonotic infections. Zoonoses are diseases that can be transmitted from animals to humans, and parasitic diseases constitute a significant category within this framework. This dual impact on both animal and human health underscores the intricate interplay between veterinary and public health (Nading, 2013).

Adding to the complexity, the life cycles of these parasites are often intricate and involve multiple stages, hosts, and environmental factors (Poulin & Morand, 2000). This complexity not only challenges the accurate diagnosis of parasitic infections, but also complicates the development of effective treatment strategies (Wobeser, 2013).

Moreover, the emergence of drug resistance among parasites adds another layer of complexity to the management of these diseases (Poulin & Morand, 2000). Conventional treatments may become less effective over time, necessitating the exploration of innovative approaches to combat drug-resistant strains (Sharma et al., 2018).

Veterinary parasitic diseases form a significant category of illnesses affecting a wide spectrum of animals, including livestock, pets, and wildlife. These diseases are induced by various parasitic organisms and are classified into distinct groups with diverse impacts on animal health (Taylor et al., 2015).

Helminths, comprising roundworms, tapeworms, and flukes, are prevalent in the gastrointestinal tract but can also affect other organs and tissues (Mehlhorn, 2016). Diseases caused by helminths, termed helminthiases, can lead to severe consequences such as malnutrition, anaemia, and organ damage. For example, heartworm disease, caused by the helminth *Dirofilaria immitis*, poses a serious and potentially fatal threat to dogs and cats (Santoro et al., 2019).

Protozoa, single-celled organisms, contribute to diseases like toxoplasmosis, giardiasis, and coccidiosis (Lucius & Roberts, 2017). These parasites may reside intracellularly or extracellularly within their hosts, resulting in a broad range of clinical symptoms, from mild diarrhoea to severe systemic infections (Stark et al., 2009).

Ectoparasites, including ticks, fleas, mites, and lice, inflict direct damage by feeding on the host's blood or skin and can act as vectors for various pathogenic microorganisms (Lehmann, 1993). Lyme disease, transmitted by ticks, serves as a prime example of a vector-borne disease with substantial health implications for both animals and humans (Hussain et al., 2021).

Arthropods, besides acting as ectoparasites, can also function as intermediate hosts for various parasitic diseases (Wall & Shearer, 1997). Mosquitoes, for instance, serve as vectors for heartworm disease, transmitting larvae from one host to another (McCall et al., 2008)

The conventional methods employed for controlling veterinary parasitic diseases, including regular deworming, pesticide usage, and management practices aimed at minimising parasite exposure, encounter significant challenges (Waller, 2003). These challenges include the rise of drug-resistant parasites, diagnostic difficulties due to nonspecific clinical signs, environmental and economic concerns associated with widespread drug use, and the global impact of movements and climate change (Waller, 2003).

Drug resistance has become increasingly prevalent among parasites, necessitating the exploration of new and more effective treatment options. The accurate diagnosis of parasitic diseases faces hurdles due to nonspecific clinical signs and limitations in available diagnostic tools (van-der-Ree & Mutapi, 2015). Additionally, the widespread use of anti-parasitic drugs raises concerns about environmental contamination and imposes a substantial economic burden (Konopka et al., 2022).

The global movement of people and goods, coupled with changing weather patterns, has facilitated the spread of parasitic diseases to new regions previously unaffected (Caminade et al., 2019). In response to these challenges, bioinformatics has emerged as an indispensable tool for advancing our understanding of veterinary parasitic diseases (Raszek et al., 2016). By harnessing data from genomic, transcriptomic, and proteomic studies, researchers can uncover the molecular intricacies of parasite biology, host–parasite interactions, and the pathways through which parasites develop drug resistance and evade host immune responses (Merillon & Ramawat, 2020). This wealth of information is crucial for the development of innovative diagnostics, therapeutics, and vaccines to control and prevent parasitic diseases in animals (Suminda et al., 2022).

The advent of bioinformatics has revolutionised veterinary parasitology, enabling the analysis of complex biological data (Baxevanis et al., 2020). Applications in bioinformatics facilitate the identification of new drug targets, the development of vaccines, and the understanding of parasite-host interactions at the molecular level (Yusof, 2022). Data analysis in veterinary parasitic diseases involves the use of statistical methods and computational algorithms to interpret large datasets derived from omics technologies, contributing to more informed decision-making in control strategies (Ezanno et al., 2021).

This chapter provides a comprehensive overview of the tools, resources, methodologies, and applications of bioinformatics and data analysis in the study of veterinary parasitic diseases. It establishes the foundations of data collection and management, delves into omics studies, and explores the future landscape of gene editing, sequencing technologies, and predictive modelling in veterinary research.

9.2 BIOINFORMATICS TOOLS AND RESOURCES

9.2.1 OVERVIEW OF BIOINFORMATICS AND ITS ROLE IN VETERINARY PARASITIC DISEASES

Bioinformatics is an interdisciplinary field that combines biology, computer science, mathematics, and statistics to analyse and interpret biological data (Baxevanis et al., 2020). It encompasses the development and application of computational tools and methods for understanding biological processes (Cantacessi et al., 2012). In the specific context of veterinary parasitic diseases (Cantacessi et al., 2012), bioinformatics plays a pivotal role in various areas, including gene identification, drug target discovery, and vaccine development.

Bioinformatics serves as a crucial ally in tackling the unique challenges posed by veterinary parasitology. These challenges include: a) genomic variability of parasites, b) complex life cycles involving multiple hosts, c) resistance to anti-parasitic drugs, and d) lack of comprehensive data on parasite biology (Yusof, 2022)

Bioinformatics tools are instrumental in overcoming these challenges. They enable the prediction of parasite protein functions, identification of potential antigens for vaccine development, comprehension of drug resistance mechanisms, and the discovery of new diagnostic markers (Cantacessi et al., 2012). By leveraging computational approaches, bioinformatics provides valuable insights that contribute to a deeper understanding of the intricate dynamics of veterinary parasitic diseases, fostering advancements in diagnostics, therapeutics, and preventive strategies (Wong et al., 2023).

9.2.2 Essential Bioinformatics Tools and Databases for Data Analysis

Several databases play a crucial role in providing essential data for research into veterinary parasitic diseases. Here are some key databases:

i) GenBank: GenBank: GenBank is a comprehensive public database that houses nucleotide sequences along with supporting bibliographic and biological annotation (Benson et al., 2018). Researchers can access this database through the National Center for Biotechnology Information (NCBI) webpage using the GenBank database link (https://www.ncbi.nlm.nih.gov/genbank/). GenBank serves as a foundational resource for genetic information, facilitating the exploration of the molecular basis of veterinary parasitic diseases (Benson et al., 2018).

ii) UniProt: UniProt is a high-quality, freely accessible database that compiles protein sequences and functional information (Consortium, 2015). Researchers can access UniProt's wealth of data without charge through the internet at http://www.uniprot.org/. UniProt is an invaluable resource for studying the proteomic aspects of veterinary parasitic diseases, aiding in the identification of proteins relevant to pathogenesis, drug targets, and vaccine development (Consortium, 2019).

iii) VectorBase: VectorBase (Lawson et al., 2009) stands as a bioinformatics resource centre funded by the National Institute of Allergy and Infectious Diseases (NIAID). It focusses primarily on invertebrate vectors that transmit infections to humans. The VectorBase website can be accessed at http://www.vectorbase.org. This platform is dedicated to the annotation and curation of vector genomes, providing a comprehensive online resource for the scientific research community (Megy et al., 2012). Currently, VectorBase includes genomic data for three distinct species of mosquitoes: *Aedes aegypti*, *Anopheles gambiae*, and *Culex quinquefasciatus* (Giraldo-Calderón et al., 2015). This database is instrumental in understanding the genetic makeup of vectors and their role in the transmission of parasitic diseases (Megy et al., 2012)

These databases collectively contribute to the foundation of bioinformatics in veterinary parasitology, offering researchers valuable tools and resources for data analysis, interpretation, and the advancement of knowledge in this critical field (Korhonen et al., 2016).

Commonly used tools for the analysis of parasitic disease data include: i) BLAST (Basic Local Alignment Search Tool), ii) ClustalW, and iii) Bioconductor.

BLAST is a fundamental tool for finding regions of local similarity between sequences, aiding in the inference of functional and evolutionary relationships (Madden, 2002). Widely used in contemporary genomic research, the BLAST algorithm, accessible through the National Center for Biotechnology Information (NCBI) website and various online platforms, allows for the quick alignment and comparison of a query DNA sequence with an extensive library of sequences. It is freely accessible online at https://blast.ncbi.nlm.nih.gov/Blast.cgi#. The ClustalW is a tool designed for multiple sequence alignment, facilitating the alignment of numerous sequences (Lobo, 2008) and enhancing the understanding of evolutionary connections among parasitic organisms. It is used for aligning sequences to identify similarities and differences, aiding in the interpretation of genetic relationships (Goater et al., 2014).

ClustalW alignment tool is accessible at https://www.genome.jp/tools-bin/clustalw. Bioconductor is an open-source software project that provides a suite of tools for the analysis and comprehension of high-throughput genomic data (Gentleman et al., 2005). Specifically designed for the analysis of genomic data, Bioconductor offers a wide range of packages and tools for tasks such as data preprocessing, statistical analysis, and visualisation (Pavlopoulos et al., 2010). As an open-source project, Bioconductor can be freely accessed and utilised for various bioinformatics analyses.

These tools collectively empower researchers in the field of veterinary parasitology to perform intricate analyses, allowing for the extraction of meaningful insights from diverse datasets. Their accessibility and functionalities contribute significantly to the advancement of understanding and addressing challenges posed by parasitic diseases.

9.2.3 Sequence Alignment and Homology Searching

Sequence alignment is a fundamental method used to arrange sequences of DNA, RNA, or proteins to identify regions of similarity (Frith et al., 2004). The detailed process involves the following steps: (i) pairwise alignment (initially, sequences are aligned in pairs to identify matching regions or gaps), (ii) multiple sequence alignment (in cases involving more than two sequences, multiple sequence alignment is performed to highlight conserved regions and variations), (iii) scoring system (a scoring system is employed to assign values to matched or mismatched nucleotides or amino acids, along with gap penalties), (iv) algorithm execution (algorithms, such as dynamic programming algorithms (e.g. Needleman–Wunsch, Smith–Waterman) or heuristic algorithms (e.g. BLAST), are applied to optimise the alignment based on the scoring system), (v) result evaluation (the alignment results are evaluated to identify significant similarities, conserved domains, and potential evolutionary relationships), and (iv) annotation and interpretation (the aligned sequences provide valuable information for annotating unknown sequences, understanding functional genomics, and inferring evolutionary relationships).

Bioinformatics applications in sequence alignment and homology searching have yielded significant outcomes in the identification of genetic markers for parasitic diseases (Mehmood et al., 2014). Sequence alignment has been crucial in identifying genetic markers associated with equine piroplasmosis. These markers contribute to the development of precise diagnostic tests for detecting and monitoring the disease in horses (Tirosh-Levy et al., 2020). Homology searching techniques have been employed to identify genetic markers related to canine heartworms. These markers play a pivotal role in the development of effective treatments and diagnostic tools for managing heartworm infections in dogs (Godel, 2012). Sequence alignment has been instrumental in identifying genetic markers for bovine babesiosis. These markers serve as essential targets for the development of accurate diagnostic tests and therapeutic interventions for cattle (Maan et al., 2018).

The use of bioinformatics tools in sequence alignment not only enhances our understanding of the evolutionary relationships and functional genomics of parasitic diseases but also contributes directly to the development of advanced diagnostic methods and effective treatments.

9.2.4 Phylogenetic Analysis and Evolutionary Studies

Phylogenetic tree construction is a pivotal aspect of phylogenetic analysis, illustrating the evolutionary trajectories and genetic interconnections among species or individual genes (Avise, 1989). This process employs diverse computational algorithms to compare genetic (Kapli et al., 2020), molecular (Patwardhan et al., 2014), or morphological data (Mishler, 1994), culminating in the creation of informative and visually impactful trees. The Table 9.1 compares different bioinformatics tools and databases. This comparative overview offers insight into the tailored utilisation of tools and databases to address the unique challenges posed by veterinary parasitic diseases. Researchers strategically choose these resources, aligning them with the particular demands of their studies, encompassing factors like the type of sequence data, required analytical functions, and the scope of their research inquiries.

9.3   DATA COLLECTION AND MANAGEMENT

9.3.1 Sources of Data for Veterinary Parasitic Diseases

Data for the study of veterinary parasitic diseases can be derived from a diverse array of sources, each offering its own relevance and applications. These sources encompass: (i) laboratory experiments (controlled settings where specific hypotheses related to parasitic diseases are systematically tested, often yielding high-quality and controlled data), (ii) field surveys (collections of data from natural or farm settings,

TABLE 9.1
Bioinformatics Tools and Databases Comparison and Their Functionality

Feature/Tool	BLAST	ClustalW	Bioconductor	GenBank	UniProt	VectorBase
Primary Use	Sequence alignment and comparison	Multiple sequence alignment	Genomic data analysis	Nucleotide sequence database	Protein sequence and function	Invertebrate vector genomics
Accessibility	Free	Free	Free with R statistical software	Free	Free	Free
Data Type	Nucleotide and protein sequences	Nucleotide and protein sequences	Genomic, epigenomic, transcriptomic data	Nucleotide sequences and annotations	Protein sequences, annotations, and functional data	Genomic data of disease vectors

Source: Author's own table

offering valuable insights into the epidemiology and real-world impact of parasitic diseases. Field surveys provide a broader understanding of how these diseases manifest in different environments), and iii) clinical reports (data gathered from veterinary practices, including comprehensive case reports, treatment outcomes, and prevalence data. Clinical reports provide practical, real-world information on the occurrence, diagnosis, and management of parasitic diseases in veterinary settings).

9.3.2   DATA COLLECTION TECHNIQUES AND METHODOLOGIES

In the realm of veterinary parasitic diseases, precise data collection is indispensable for accurate diagnosis, comprehending disease epidemiology, and devising effective treatments (VanderWaal et al., 2017). The integration of bioinformatics and data analysis becomes pivotal with the following techniques:

Polymerase chain reaction (PCR): The PCR, a cornerstone technique in molecular biology, holds equal significance in parasitology research and diagnosis (Zarlenga & Higgins, 2001). In the realm of bioinformatics, a crucial role is played in the design of PCR primers—short DNA sequences initiating the PCR process (Panjkovich & Melo, 2005). Precision in primer design, specific to the parasitic DNA sequences of interest, is paramount for accurate amplification. Bioinformatics databases housing genomic sequences of parasites prove essential in identifying suitable primer sequences (Thaenkham et al., 2022).

Sequencing: Sequencing techniques, especially Next-Generation Sequencing (NGS), generate extensive data on parasite genomes (Greenwood et al., 2016). Bioinformatics is extensively utilised for the handling, storage, and analysis of sequence data. This encompasses tasks like assembling sequences for genome reconstruction and identifying variations and mutations within a parasite population. The execution of these analyses demands sophisticated software and algorithms, often crafted through bioinformatics research (Vashisht et al., 2023).

Immunoassays: In the realm of immunoassays detecting parasitic antigens, bioinformatics plays a pivotal role in antibody selection and design (Kumar et al., 2021). Through the analysis of sequences and prediction of epitopes—the specific binding part of the antigen—bioinformatics tools contribute to enhancing the specificity and sensitivity of immunoassays (Waury et al., 2022).

These methodologies showcase the synergy between traditional laboratory techniques and advanced computational approaches, underscoring the indispensable role of bioinformatics in refining and optimising data collection processes for a comprehensive understanding of veterinary parasitic diseases.

9.3.3   DATA QUALITY CONTROL AND PREPROCESSING

In bioinformatics analyses, the integrity of data holds paramount importance, as the accuracy of drawn conclusions is inherently tied to the quality of the data (Bellazzi et al., 2011). In the domain of data quality control and preprocessing:

Error checking: Bioinformatics relies on a spectrum of software tools to execute thorough quality control checks on raw data. This includes the identification of sequencing errors or contamination through pattern recognition and comparative analysis against reference databases, ensuring the reliability of the dataset (Bao et al., 2014).

Normalisation: Bioinformatics techniques are deployed for the normalisation of data from high-throughput experiments, guaranteeing the validity of comparisons between samples. This process may encompass adjustments for sequencing depth in RNA-seq data or the correction of background signals in microarray data, enhancing the accuracy of subsequent analyses (Hardcastle, 2016).

Data transformation: The transformation of data into a format suitable for analysis is a common practice utilising bioinformatics tools. For instance, raw sequence data might undergo conversion into a count of reads aligned to each gene in the genome. Similarly, expression data might be subjected to log transformation to stabilise variance across a spectrum of values, facilitating more robust analyses (Veselkov et al., 2018).

These steps in data quality control and preprocessing underscore the rigorous standards maintained in bioinformatics analyses, ensuring that the resulting datasets are accurate, standardised, and conducive to deriving meaningful insights in the study of veterinary parasitic diseases.

9.3.4 Data Management Strategies and Tools

In the expansive realm of bioinformatics, effective data management stands as a crucial element, ensuring the integrity, accessibility, and security of research data. Key strategies and tools include:

Laboratory information management systems (LIMS): The LIMS serves as a pivotal tool for orchestrating the flow of samples and associated data throughout the laboratory processing lifecycle (Famili & Cleary, 2022). In parasitology, this involves meticulous tracking of parasite samples from collection through various diagnostic assays. Bioinformatics principles are integrally applied in the design of LIMS, aiming for user-friendly interfaces coupled with comprehensive data handling capabilities (Mehmood et al., 2014).

Bioinformatics pipelines: Bioinformatics pipelines, comprising automated data processing steps, play a pivotal role in parasitology research. These pipelines encompass tasks such as cleaning and analysing sequence data, predicting gene function, and identifying SNP variants linked to drug resistance (Davis-Turak et al., 2017). Created using scripting languages, these pipelines can seamlessly integrate diverse software tools, including those tailored for statistical analysis (Wratten et al., 2021).

These sophisticated data management strategies and tools exemplify the commitment within bioinformatics to streamline processes, enhance accessibility, and fortify the robustness of data in the exploration of veterinary parasitic diseases. Refer to Figure 9.1 for a visual representation of data flow in veterinary parasitic disease research.

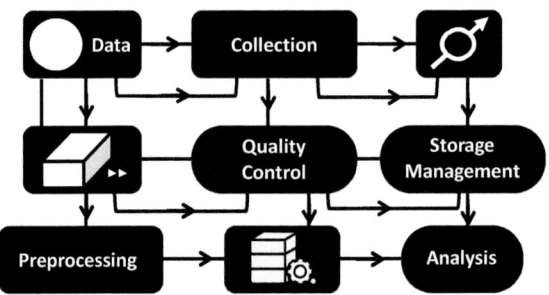

FIGURE 9.1 Parasitic data flow and analysis (Author's own figure).

9.4 STRUCTURAL BIOINFORMATICS

Structural bioinformatics, a sub-discipline of bioinformatics, focusses on analysing and predicting the three-dimensional structures of biological macromolecules. Combining molecular biology, biochemistry, and computer science, this field develops methods for predicting and analysing the structure, function, and interactions of proteins and nucleic acids (Gu & Bourne, 2009). In the context of veterinary parasitic diseases, structural bioinformatics plays a pivotal role in drug discovery and vaccine development (María et al., 2017). The primary objective of structural bioinformatics in drug discovery is understanding the interaction between drugs and their targets (Xia, 2017). Through data analysis and computational modelling, researchers can pinpoint the active or binding sites of proteins expressed by parasites (Crowther et al., 2010). Researchers utilise experimental data from X-ray crystallography, NMR spectroscopy, or Cryo-Electron microscopy to elucidate the structure of parasitic proteins (Merino & Raunser, 2017). In cases where experimental data is lacking, computational techniques like homology modelling predict structures based on related known proteins (Muhammed & Aki-Yalcin, 2019).

Interaction analysis involves analysing geometric and chemical characteristics of potential drug-binding sites. Molecular docking simulations predict how small molecules interact with these sites, including binding affinity and specificity (Henrich et al., 2010). Employing molecular dynamics simulations allows researchers to study the behaviour of a protein–ligand complex over time. This provides insights into the stability of potential drug compounds when bound to their targets (Mortier et al., 2015). Structural bioinformatics aids in refining the selectivity and potency of drug candidates by allowing researchers to visualise and optimise interactions between drugs and parasitic proteins at the atomic level. This reduces the risk of side effects by ensuring drugs target only parasitic proteins without affecting those of the host.

Vaccines function by presenting an antigen to the immune system, eliciting an immune response without causing disease (Storni et al., 2005). Structural bioinformatics plays a crucial role in vaccine development through: (i) Antigen identification (selecting potential antigens based on their structure and surface characteristics, and predicting which parasitic proteins are likely to provoke an immune response), (ii) Epitope mapping (identifying specific parts of an antigen recognised by antibodies (epitopes). Computational tools analyse antigen structures to predict B-cell and T-cell epitope regions, which could serve as vaccine candidates), (iii) Vaccine optimisation (utilising structural data to enhance vaccine design, such as stabilising the conformation of protein antigens to ensure they maintain their shape during vaccine formulation and delivery), and (iv) Evaluating vaccine efficacy (after the design phase, bioinformatics tools assist in interpreting experimental data to assess vaccine efficacy. Simulation of the immune response using structural data offers early insights into the potential success of vaccine candidates before advancing to *in vivo* testing).

9.5   PHYLOGENY ANALYSIS TO MAP THE EVOLUTION OF DIFFERENT PARASITES

Phylogenetic analysis is a method utilised to infer the evolutionary relationships among different species, strains, or taxonomic groups (Hershkovitz & Leipe, 1998). By scrutinising the genetic material of various organisms, scientists construct a "phylogenetic tree," a diagrammatic hypothesis illustrating evolutionary connections and divergence pathways from common ancestors. Understanding parasite evolution is crucial for predicting the emergence and spread of parasitic diseases, designing control measures by identifying transmission origins and vectors, and informing vaccine development by discerning how parasites evolve resistance to treatments (Gutierrez et al., 2015).

Molecular phylogenetics employs DNA, RNA, or protein sequences to construct phylogenetic trees. Comparing these sequences across different organisms facilitates the determination of evolutionary relationships (Page & Holmes, 2009). Several software tools are employed for analysing phylogenetic data. Molecular evolutionary genetics analysis (MEGA) integrates diverse analytical techniques and resources for phylogenomics and phylomedicine (Kumar et al., 2018). Phylogenetic analysis using parsimony (PAUP) is a computational tool designed for phylogenetic analysis utilising parsimony, maximum likelihood, and distance approaches (Swofford, 1998). It offers a range of analysis methods and model selections for various data sources including DNA, RNA, protein, and general data (Page & Holmes, 2009).The PAUP is accessible freely at paup.phylosolutions.com. Bayesian evolutionary analysis by sampling trees (BEAST) is a versatile software tool for investigating evolutionary parameter estimates and hypothesis testing. Its component-based architecture allows for a wide array of evolutionary models, posing challenges in summarisation (Drummond & Rambaut, 2007). Under active development, upcoming improvements include birth-death priors for tree form, codon-based substitution models, structured coalescent framework, continuous character development models, and relaxed clock models (Drummond & Rambaut, 2007). These tools empower researchers to unravel the intricate evolutionary histories of parasites, offering insights crucial for disease management, control, and vaccine development.

Phylogenetic trees serve as fundamental tools in tracing the evolution of parasites, elucidating how current parasitic forms evolved from their ancestors and showcasing the divergence of various parasitic species over time. These trees are pivotal

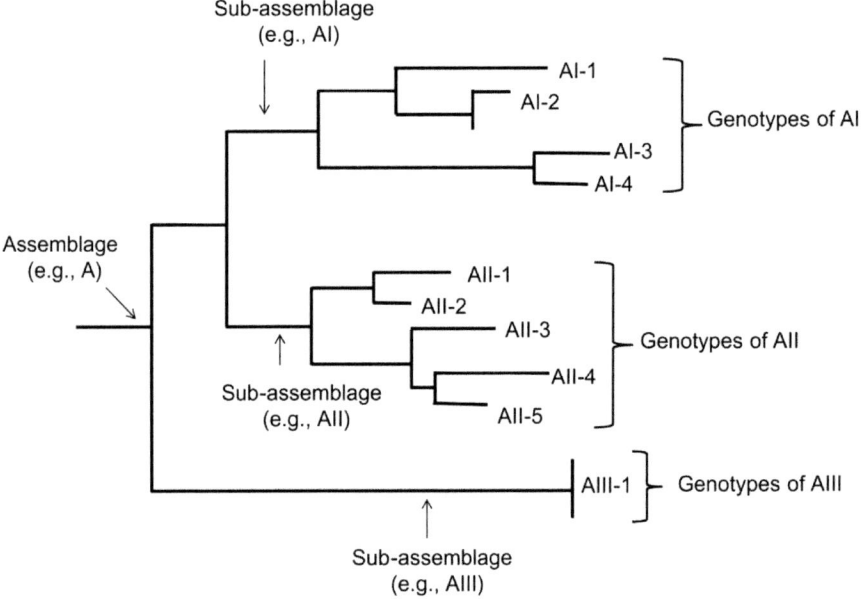

FIGURE 9.2   The sub-assemblages and genotypes present within *Giardia duodenalis*.

in evolutionary biology studies, aiding researchers in comprehending the development of specific traits such as host specificity and resistance to anti-parasitic drugs (Schmid-Hempel, 2021). Research on the phylogenetic tree of the parasite *Giardia* has provided insights into its zoonotic potential—the ability to transfer from animals to humans. The sub-assemblages and genotypes present within *Giardia duodenalis* are given in Figure 9.2. Assemblage A has been identified by the use of a multi-locus typing approach (Ryan & Cacciò, 2013). Similarly, studies on *Trypanosoma* have shed light on its various life cycle stages and how it adapts to different insect vectors and mammalian hosts (Butter et al., 2013). Through these case studies and more, phylogenetic analyses offer invaluable insights into the evolutionary dynamics of parasites, enabling a deeper understanding of their biology, transmission patterns, and potential for host shifts (Figure 9.2).

9.6   COMPARATIVE GENOMICS AND GENOME MAPPING

Bioinformatics empowers researchers to compare complete genome sequences from different parasites and host species. In the realm of veterinary parasitic diseases, bioinformatics tools facilitate the analysis and interpretation of vast genomic datasets generated by sequencing technologies (Norling, 2014). These analyses unveil the intricate biology of parasites, including the identification of genes crucial for infection, survival, host–parasite interactions, and drug resistance (Zheng et al., 2023). Comparative genomics via bioinformatics unveils the impact of evolutionary pressures on parasites (Cai et al., 2012). Bioinformatics analyses of genomic data uncover gene mutations favoured by selective pressures from host immune systems or pharmaceutical treatments (Sironi et al., 2015). Moreover, they assess genetic diversity among parasite populations, crucial for predicting disease patterns and understanding the emergence of drug resistance (Wilson et al., 2016).

Bioinformatics techniques are indispensable for assembling genomes from short reads produced by NGS platforms. Software tools align, merge, and analyse sequencing data to construct complete genomic maps, identifying SNPs, indels, and structural variants (Pereira et al., 2020). Bioinformatics transforms raw data into interpretable genomic maps, facilitating a deeper understanding of parasite biology (Lamichhane et al., 2018).Bioinformatics applications offer dynamic visualisation tools to examine and present genomic synteny and variation. Genome browsers and mapping software depict gene order across different species, enabling comparative analyses and hypotheses on gene function and evolution (Miller et al., 2004). Through bioinformatics, researchers gain insights into the genomic architecture of parasites, enhancing our understanding of their biology and evolution (Korhonen et al., 2016).

Bioinformatics techniques analyse genomic sequences to uncover virulence factors and understand their function (Wren, 2000). Similarly, genomic variations contributing to drug resistance are studied using bioinformatics tools, pinpointing mutations associated with these traits. This insight is crucial for designing new antiparasitic drugs or vaccines (Kwok et al., 2021). Comparative genomics, facilitated by bioinformatics, accelerates the development of new diagnostic tools (Wang et al., 2016). It enables the design of assays targeting specific genomic sequences unique to the parasite. For therapeutics, bioinformatics aids in identifying potential drug targets by highlighting parasitic genes essential for survival but absent in the host (Britton et al., 2014; Swann et al., 2015; Wang et al., 2016).

Specialised software in bioinformatics visualises genomic information, constructing genome maps. These tools provide an intuitive understanding of complex genomic datasets and facilitate the identification of target genes for further study (Nusrat et al., 2019). Bioinformatics visualisation tools interpret synteny blocks and genomic variations effectively. They generate diagrams illustrating the genetic architecture of parasites, crucial for elucidating evolutionary relationships or functional genomics (Korhonen et al., 2016).

9.7 DIFFERENT TECHNIQUES AND ROLE OF BIOINFORMATICS

CRISPR-Cas9 is a revolutionary gene-editing technology applicable to organisms, including parasites (Gupta et al., 2019). Bioinformatics aids in designing guide RNA sequences targeting specific genes within a parasite's genome, predicting off-target effects, and analysing gene-editing outcomes (Qureshi & Connolly, 2022). Bioinformatics analysis is essential in developing gene drive strategies using CRISPR-Cas9. These strategies spread genetic modifications through parasite populations, controlling disease vectors or reducing parasitic virulence (Raban et al., 2022). Ethical considerations and bioinformatics risk assessment models are crucial for evaluating potential consequences (Afshari et al., 2011). The use of

CRISPR-Cas9 raises concerns about unintended ecological impacts and off-target effects. Bioinformatics assists in risk assessment by predicting off-target interactions and simulating gene drive dynamics, addressing ethical considerations associated with gene editing in wild populations (Taning et al., 2017).

Bioinformatics plays a pivotal role in harnessing NGS technologies, which have transformed parasite genome studies by enabling rapid, high-throughput sequencing of DNA and RNA samples. NGS is indispensable for identifying gene expression changes in parasites under different conditions (Cantacessi et al., 2012). The bioinformatics workflow for NGS encompasses sample preparation, sequencing, data cleaning, alignment to reference genomes, assembly, and annotation. Each step is crucial and relies on sophisticated data analysis software to manage the large data volumes efficiently (Sezerman et al., 2019). Bioinformatics applications in NGS include identifying parasite strains, drug resistance markers, and host responses to infection (Maljkovic-Berry et al., 2020). Targeted gene screening aids in discovering new drugs and vaccine candidates by identifying essential genes for parasite survival and virulence (Peraman et al., 2021).

In silico analysis employs computational methods to simulate and predict the behaviour of metabolic and signaing pathways. Utilising databases like KEGG, bioinformatics tools map known and predicted enzyme reactions and pathways in parasites (Hung, 2014). These simulations can pinpoint potential drug targets by revealing critical pathways for parasite survival (Siqueira-Neto et al., 2023). Integrating diverse datasets (genomic, transcriptomic, proteomic, metabolomic) provides a comprehensive view of parasite biology. Bioinformatics methods are used for data integration, which is crucial for understanding complex biological interactions and disease mechanisms (Gligorijević & Pržulj, 2015). Bioinformatics tools like Cytoscape or Gephi create network models visualising biological pathways and interactions, illustrating relationships between molecular entities within a parasite or between the parasite and its host (Smoot et al., 2011).

Machine learning algorithms analyse large and complex datasets to predict disease outbreaks, hotspots for transmission, and the emergence of drug resistance emergence. Bioinformatics is integral to training and validating these models (Kim et al., 2022). Prediction models forecast disease dynamics based on climate models, predict resistance spread using genetic markers, and assess new drug efficacy. Bioinformatics aids in representing these models, summarising predictive performance, and feature sets used (Cao et al., 2020).

9.8   CONCLUSIONS AND FUTURE DIRECTIONS

Bioinformatics has significantly advanced our understanding and control of veterinary parasitic diseases, bridging data resources with clinical insights across various domains. From phylogenetic analysis to predictive modelling, its integration enhances diagnostics, treatment development, and disease prevention. Bioinformatics has facilitated the collection, storage, and analysis of vast amounts of parasitic genomic data. It aids in identifying genetic factors associated with parasite transmission, host specificity, and drug resistance. Bioinformatics tools are instrumental in developing diagnostic assays based on genetic markers, enhancing the accuracy and speed of detecting parasitic infections. This is vital for timely treatment and control measures.

Advancements in CRISPR-Cas9 and gene-editing technologies may lead to novel parasite elimination methods. Decreasing sequencing costs will enable comprehensive multi-omics studies, providing systems biology insights. Machine learning and artificial intelligence will offer more accurate models for disease dynamics, enhancing public health responses. In-silico modelling will predict new drug targets, accelerating therapeutic development. Collaborations between computational scientists, biologists, veterinarians, and epidemiologists will tackle complex parasitic disease issues. Worldwide collaboration and data sharing will improve surveillance and strategic control efforts. Bioinformatics will inform evidence-based public and veterinary health policies and practices, enhancing disease management. In essence, bioinformatics remains pivotal in advancing veterinary parasitology, driving precision medicine and innovative solutions to combat parasitic diseases. Future research directions will focus on leveraging data-intensive analyses to improve livestock health and human well-being globally.

REFERENCES

Afshari, C. A., Hamadeh, H. K., and Bushel, P. R. 2011. The evolution of bioinformatics in toxicology: Advancing toxicogenomics. *Toxicological Sciences*, 120(suppl_1), S225–S237.

Avise, J. C. 1989. Gene trees and organismal histories: A phylogenetic approach to population biology. *Evolution*, 43(6), 1192–1208.

Bao, R., Huang, L., Andrade, J., Tan, W., Kibbe, W. A., Jiang, H., and Feng, G. 2014. Review of current methods, applications, and data management for the bioinformatics analysis of whole exome sequencing. *Cancer Informatics*, 13, CIN. S13779.

Baxevanis, A. D., Bader, G. D., and Wishart, D. S. 2020. *Bioinformatics*. John Wiley & Sons.

Bellazzi, R., Diomidous, M., Sarkar, I. N., Takabayashi, K., Ziegler, A., and McCray, A. T. 2011. Data analysis and data mining: Current issues in biomedical informatics. *Methods of Information in Medicine*, 50(06), 536–544.

Benson, D. A., Cavanaugh, M., Clark, K., Karsch-Mizrachi, I., Ostell, J., Pruitt, K. D., and Sayers, E. W. 2018. GenBank. *Nucleic Acids Research*, 46(Database issue), D41.

Britton, C., Winter, A. D., Gillan, V., and Devaney, E. 2014. microRNAs of parasitic helminths–Identification, characterization and potential as drug targets. *International Journal for Parasitology: Drugs and Drug Resistance*, 4(2), 85–94.

Butter, F., Bucerius, F., Michel, M., Cicova, Z., Mann, M., and Janzen, C. J. 2013. Comparative proteomics of two life cycle stages of stable isotope-labeled Trypanosoma brucei reveals novel components of the parasite's host adaptation machinery. *Molecular & Cellular Proteomics*, 12(1), 172–179.

Cai, H., Zhou, Z., Gu, J., and Wang, Y. 2012. Comparative genomics and systems biology of malaria parasites Plasmodium. *Current Bioinformatics*, 7(4), 478–489.

Caminade, C., McIntyre, K. M., and Jones, A. E. 2019. Impact of recent and future climate change on vector-borne diseases. *Annals of the New York Academy of Sciences*, 1436(1), 157–173.

Cantacessi, C., Campbell, B., Jex, A., Young, N., Hall, R., Ranganathan, S., and Gasser, R. (2012). Bioinformatics meets parasitology. *Parasite Immunology*, 34(5), 265–275.

Cao, Y., Geddes, T. A., Yang, J. Y. H., and Yang, P. 2020. Ensemble deep learning in bioinformatics. *Nature Machine Intelligence*, 2(9), 500–508.

Consortium, U. (2015). UniProt: A hub for protein information. *Nucleic Acids Research*, 43(D1), D204–D212.

Consortium, U. (2019). UniProt: A worldwide hub of protein knowledge. *Nucleic Acids Research*, 47(D1), D506–D515.

Crowther, G. J., Shanmugam, D., Carmona, S. J., Doyle, M. A., Hertz-Fowler, C., Berriman, M., Nwaka, S., Ralph, S. A., Roos, D. S., and Van Voorhis, W. C. 2010. Identification of attractive drug targets in neglected-disease pathogens using an in silico approach. *PLoS Neglected Tropical Diseases*, 4(8), e804.

Davis-Turak, J., Courtney, S. M., Hazard, E. S., Glen Jr, W. B., da Silveira, W. A., Wesselman, T., Harbin, L. P., Wolf, B. J., Chung, D., and Hardiman, G. (2017). Genomics pipelines and data integration: Challenges and opportunities in the research setting. *Expert Review of Molecular Diagnostics*, 17(3), 225–237.

Drummond, A. J., and Rambaut, A. 2007. BEAST: Bayesian evolutionary analysis by sampling trees. *BMC Evolutionary Biology*, 7(1), 1–8.

Ezanno, P., Picault, S., Beaunée, G., Bailly, X., Muñoz, F., Duboz, R., Monod, H., and Guégan, J.-F. 2021. Research perspectives on animal health in the era of artificial intelligence. *Veterinary Research*, 52, 1–15.

Famili, P., and Cleary, S. 2022. Laboratory Information Management System (LIMS) and Electronic Data. In: Huynh-Ba, K. (ed.) *Analytical testing for the pharmaceutical GMP laboratory*. John Wiley & Sons. pp. 345–373.

Frith, M. C., Hansen, U., Spouge, J. L., and Weng, Z. 2004. Finding functional sequence elements by multiple local alignment. *Nucleic Acids Research*, 32(1), 189–200.

Gentleman, R., Carey, V., Huber, W., Irizarry, R., and Dudoit, S. 2005. *Bioinformatics and computational biology solutions using R and Bioconductor*. Springer Science & Business Media.

Giraldo-Calderón, G. I., Emrich, S. J., MacCallum, R. M., Maslen, G., Dialynas, E., Topalis, P., Ho, N., Gesing, S., Consortium, V., and Madey, G. 2015. VectorBase: an updated bioinformatics resource for invertebrate vectors and other organisms related with human diseases. *Nucleic Acids Research*, 43(D1), D707–D713.

Gligorijević, V., and Pržulj, N. 2015. Methods for biological data integration: Perspectives and challenges. *Journal of the Royal Society Interface*, 12(112), 20150571.

Goater, T. M., Goater, C. P., and Esch, G. W. (2014). *Parasitism: The diversity and ecology of animal parasites*. Cambridge University Press.

Godel, C. (2012). *Drug targets of the heartworm," Dirofilaria immitis"*. University_of_Basel.

Greenwood, J. M., Ezquerra, A. L., Behrens, S., Branca, A., & Mallet, L. (2016). Current analysis of host–parasite interactions with a focus on next generation sequencing data. *Zoology*, 119(4), 298–306.

Grønvold, J., Henriksen, S. A., Larsen, M., Nansen, P., and Wolstrup, J. 1996. Biological control aspects of biological control—with special reference to arthropods, protozoans and helminths of domesticated animals. *Veterinary Parasitology*, 64(1–2), 47–64.

Gu, J., and Bourne, P. E. 2009. *Structural bioinformatics* (Vol. 44). John Wiley & Sons.

Gupta, D., Bhattacharjee, O., Mandal, D., Sen, M. K., Dey, D., Dasgupta, A., Kazi, T. A., Gupta, R., Sinharoy, S., and Acharya, K. 2019. CRISPR-Cas9 system: A new-fangled dawn in gene editing. *Life Sciences*, 232, 116636.

Gutierrez, J. B., Galinski, M. R., Cantrell, S., and Voit, E. O. 2015. From within host dynamics to the epidemiology of infectious disease: Scientific overview and challenges. *Mathematical Biosciences*, 270, 143–155.

Hardcastle, T. J. 2016. Generalized empirical Bayesian methods for discovery of differential data in high-throughput biology. *Bioinformatics*, 32(2), 195–202.

Henrich, S., Salo-Ahen, O. M., Huang, B., Rippmann, F. F., Cruciani, G., and Wade, R. C. 2010. Computational approaches to identifying and characterizing protein binding sites for ligand design. *Journal of Molecular Recognition: An Interdisciplinary Journal*, 23(2), 209–219.

Hershkovitz, M. A., and Leipe, D. D. 1998. Phylogenetic analysis. In: Baxevanis, A. D. and Ouellette, B. F. F. (eds.) *Bioinformatics: A practical guide to the analysis of genes and proteins.* John Wiley & Sons, pp. 189–230.

Hung, S. S. 2014. *Metabolic network analysis of apicomplexan parasites to identify novel drug targets.* University of Toronto (Canada).

Hussain, S., Hussain, A., Aziz, U., Song, B., Zeb, J., George, D., Li, J., and Sparagano, O. 2021. The role of ticks in the emergence of Borrelia burgdorferi as a zoonotic pathogen and its vector control: A global systemic review. *Microorganisms*, 9(12), 2412.

Kapli, P., Yang, Z., and Telford, M. J. 2020. Phylogenetic tree building in the genomic age. *Nature Reviews Genetics*, 21(7), 428–444.

Kim, J. I., Maguire, F., Tsang, K. K., Gouliouris, T., Peacock, S. J., McAllister, T. A., McArthur, A. G., and Beiko, R. G. 2022. Machine learning for antimicrobial resistance prediction: Current practice, limitations, and clinical perspective. *Clinical Microbiology Reviews*, 35(3), e00179–00121.

Konopka, J. K., Chatterjee, P., LaMontagne, C., and Brown, J. (2022). Environmental impacts of mass drug administration programs: Exposures, risks, and mitigation of antimicrobial resistance. *Infectious Diseases of Poverty*, 11(1), 1–14.

Korhonen, P. K., Young, N. D., and Gasser, R. B. 2016. Making sense of genomes of parasitic worms: Tackling bioinformatic challenges. *Biotechnology Advances*, 34(5), 663–686.

Kumar, S., Gupta, S., Mohmad, A., Fular, A., Parthasarathi, B., and Chaubey, A. K. 2021. Molecular tools-advances, opportunities and prospects for the control of parasites of veterinary importance. *International Journal of Tropical Insect Science*, 41, 33–42.

Kumar, S., Stecher, G., Li, M., Knyaz, C., and Tamura, K. 2018. MEGA X: Molecular evolutionary genetics analysis across computing platforms. *Molecular Biology and Evolution*, 35(6), 1547.

Kwok, A. J., Mentzer, A., and Knight, J. C. 2021. Host genetics and infectious disease: New tools, insights and translational opportunities. *Nature Reviews Genetics*, 22(3), 137–153.

Lamichhane, S., Sen, P., Dickens, A. M., Hyötyläinen, T., and Orešič, M. 2018. An overview of metabolomics data analysis: Current tools and future perspectives. *Comprehensive Analytical Chemistry*, 82, 387–413.

Lawson, D., Arensburger, P., Atkinson, P., Besansky, N. J., Bruggner, R. V., Butler, R., Campbell, K. S., Christophides, G. K., Christley, S., and Dialynas, E. 2009. VectorBase: A data resource for invertebrate vector genomics. *Nucleic Acids Research*, 37(suppl_1), D583–D587.

Lehmann, T. 1993. Ectoparasites: Direct impact on host fitness. *Parasitology Today*, 9(1), 8–13.

Lobo, I. 2008. Basic local alignment search tool (BLAST). *Nature Education*, 1(1), 215.

Lucius, R., and Roberts, C. W. 2017. Biology of parasitic Protozoa. In: Lucius, R., Loos-Frank, B., Lane, R. P., Poulin, R., Roberts, C., Grencis, R. K., Shankland, R., and Roy, R. F. (eds.) *The biology of parasites.* Wiley-Blackwell, pp. 95–224.

Maan, S., Dalal, S., Kumar, A., Dalal, A., Bansal, N., Chaudhary, D., Gupta, A., and Maan, N. S. 2018. Novel molecular diagnostics and therapeutic tools for livestock diseases. *Advances in Animal Biotechnology and its Applications*, 26, 229–245.

Mackenzie, J. S., Jeggo, M., Daszak, P., and Richt, J. A. 2013. *One Health: The human-animal-environment interfaces in emerging infectious diseases* (Vol. 366). Springer.

Madden, T. L. 2002. The BLAST sequence analysis tool. In: McEntyre, J. (eds.) *The NCBI handbook* (Vol. 2), National Library of Medicine (US), National Center for Biotechnology Information, Bethesda, MD. pp. 425–436.

Maljkovic-Berry, I., Melendrez, M. C., Bishop-Lilly, K. A., Rutvisuttinunt, W., Pollett, S., Talundzic, E., Morton, L., and Jarman, R. G. 2020. Next generation sequencing and bioinformatics methodologies for infectious disease research and public health: Approaches, applications, and considerations for development of laboratory capacity. *The Journal of Infectious Diseases*, 221(Supplement_3), S292–S307.

María, R., Arturo, C., Alicia, J. A., Paulina, M., and Gerardo, A. O. 2017. The impact of bioinformatics on vaccine design and development. *Vaccines*, 2, 3–6.

McCall, J. W., Genchi, C., Kramer, L. H., Guerrero, J., and Venco, L. 2008. Heartworm disease in animals and humans. *Advances in Parasitology*, 66, 193–285.

Megy, K., Emrich, S. J., Lawson, D., Campbell, D., Dialynas, E., Hughes, D. S., Koscielny, G., Louis, C., MacCallum, R. M., and Redmond, S. N. 2012. VectorBase: Improvements to a bioinformatics resource for invertebrate vector genomics. *Nucleic Acids Research*, 40(D1), D729–D734.

Mehlhorn, H. 2016. Worms (Helminths). In: Mehlhorn, H. (ed.) *Animal parasites: Diagnosis, treatment, prevention.* Springer, pp. 251–498.

Mehmood, M. A., Sehar, U., and Ahmad, N. 2014. Use of bioinformatics tools in different spheres of life sciences. *Journal of Data Mining in Genomics & Proteomics*, 5(2), 1.

Merillon, J.-M., and Ramawat, K. G. 2020. *Co-evolution of secondary metabolites.* Springer.

Merino, F., and Raunser, S. 2017. Electron cryo-microscopy as a tool for structure-based drug development. *Angewandte Chemie International Edition*, 56(11), 2846–2860.

Miller, W., Makova, K. D., Nekrutenko, A., and Hardison, R. C. 2004. Comparative genomics. *Annual Review of Genomics and Human Genetics*, 5, 15–56.

Mishler, B. D. 1994. Cladistic analysis of molecular and morphological data. *American Journal of Physical Anthropology*, 94(1), 143–156.

Mortier, J., Rakers, C., Bermudez, M., Murgueitio, M. S., Riniker, S., and Wolber, G. 2015. The impact of molecular dynamics on drug design: Applications for the characterization of ligand–macromolecule complexes. *Drug Discovery Today*, 20(6), 686–702.

Muhammed, M. T., and Aki-Yalcin, E. 2019. Homology modeling in drug discovery: Overview, current applications, and future perspectives. *Chemical Biology & Drug Design*, 93(1), 12–20.

Nading, A. M. 2013. Humans, animals, and health. *Environment and Society: Advances in Research*, 4, 60–78.

Norling, M. 2014. *Bioinformatic methods for metagenomics and comparative genetics in veterinary medicine.* Doctoral Thesis, Department of Animal Breeding and Genetics, Swedish University of Agricultural Sciences, Uppsala, Sweden.

Nusrat, S., Harbig, T., and Gehlenborg, N. 2019. Tasks, techniques, and tools for genomic data visualization. *Computer Graphics Forum*, 38(3), 781–805.

Page, R. D., and Holmes, E. C. 2009. *Molecular evolution: A phylogenetic approach.* John Wiley & Sons.

Panjkovich, A., and Melo, F. 2005. Comparison of different melting temperature calculation methods for short DNA sequences. *Bioinformatics*, 21(6), 711–722.

Patwardhan, A., Ray, S., and Roy, A. 2014. Molecular markers in phylogenetic studies-a review. *Journal of Phylogenetics & Evolutionary Biology*, 2(2), 131.

Pavlopoulos, G. A., Soldatos, T. G., Barbosa-Silva, A., and Schneider, R. 2010. A reference guide for tree analysis and visualization. *BioData Mining*, 3, 1–24.

Peraman, R., Sure, S. K., Dusthackeer, V. A., Chilamakuru, N. B., Yiragamreddy, P. R., Pokuri, C., Kutagulla, V. K., and Chinni, S. 2021. Insights on recent approaches in drug discovery strategies and untapped drug targets against drug resistance. *Future Journal of Pharmaceutical Sciences*, 7, 1–25.

Pereira, R., Oliveira, J., and Sousa, M. 2020. Bioinformatics and computational tools for next-generation sequencing analysis in clinical genetics. *Journal of Clinical Medicine*, 9(1), 132.

Poulin, R., and Morand, S. 2000. The diversity of parasites. *The Quarterly Review of Biology*, 75(3), 277–293.

Qureshi, A., and Connolly, J. B. 2022. Bioinformatic and literature assessment of toxicity and allergenicity of a CRISPR-Cas9 engineered gene drive to control the human malaria mosquito vector Anopheles gambiae. *Malaria Journal*, 22(1), 234

Raban, R., Gendron, W. A., and Akbari, O. S. 2022. A perspective on the expansion of the genetic technologies to support the control of neglected vector-borne diseases and conservation. *Frontiers in Tropical Diseases*, 3, 999273.

Raszek, M. M., Guan, L. L., and Plastow, G. S. 2016. Use of genomic tools to improve cattle health in the context of infectious diseases. *Frontiers in Genetics*, 7, 30.

Ryan, U., and Cacciò, S. M. 2013. Zoonotic potential of *Giardia*. *International Journal for Parasitology*, 43(12–13), 943–956.

Santoro, M., Miletti, G., Vangone, L., Spadari, L., Reccia, S., and Fusco, G. 2019. Heartworm disease (*Dirofilaria immitis*) in two roaming dogs from the urban area of Castel Volturno, Southern Italy. *Frontiers in Veterinary Science*, 6, 270.

Schmid-Hempel, P. 2021. *Evolutionary parasitology: The integrated study of infections, immunology, ecology, and genetics*. Oxford University Press.

Sezerman, O. U., Ulgen, E., Seymen, N., and Durasi, I. M. 2019. Bioinformatics workflows for genomic variant discovery, interpretation and prioritization. In: Samadikuchaksaraei, A., and Seifi, M. (eds.) *Bioinformatics tools for detection and clinical interpretation of genomic variations*. IntechOpen, p. 15.

Sharma, C., Rokana, N., Chandra, M., Singh, B. P., Gulhane, R. D., Gill, J. P. S., Ray, P., Puniya, A. K., and Panwar, H. 2018. Antimicrobial resistance: Its surveillance, impact, and alternative management strategies in dairy animals. *Frontiers in Veterinary Science*, 4, 237.

Siqueira-Neto, J. L., Wicht, K. J., Chibale, K., Burrows, J. N., Fidock, D. A., and Winzeler, E. A. 2023. Antimalarial drug discovery: Progress and approaches. *Nature Reviews Drug Discovery*, 22(10), 807–826.

Sironi, M., Cagliani, R., Forni, D., and Clerici, M. 2015. Evolutionary insights into host–pathogen interactions from mammalian sequence data. *Nature Reviews Genetics*, 16(4), 224–236.

Smoot, M. E., Ono, K., Ruscheinski, J., Wang, P.-L., and Ideker, T. 2011. Cytoscape 2.8: New features for data integration and network visualization. *Bioinformatics*, 27(3), 431–432.

Stark, D., Barratt, J., Van Hal, S., Marriott, D., Harkness, J., and Ellis, J. 2009. Clinical significance of enteric protozoa in the immunosuppressed human population. *Clinical Microbiology Reviews*, 22(4), 634–650.

Storni, T., Kündig, T. M., Senti, G., and Johansen, P. 2005. Immunity in response to particulate antigen-delivery systems. *Advanced Drug Delivery Reviews*, 57(3), 333–355.

Suminda, G. G. D., Bhandari, S., Won, Y., Goutam, U., Pulicherla, K. K., Son, Y.-O., and Ghosh, M. 2022. High-throughput sequencing technologies in the detection of livestock pathogens, diagnosis, and zoonotic surveillance. *Computational and Structural Biotechnology Journal*, 20, 5378–5392.

Swann, J., Jamshidi, N., Lewis, N. E., and Winzeler, E. A. 2015. Systems analysis of host–parasite interactions. *Wiley Interdisciplinary Reviews: Systems Biology and Medicine*, 7(6), 381–400.

Swofford, D. L. 1998. *Phylogenetic analysis using parsimony. version 4.0.* Sinauer.

Taning, C. N. T., Van Eynde, B., Yu, N., Ma, S., and Smagghe, G. 2017. CRISPR/Cas9 in insects: Applications, best practices and biosafety concerns. *Journal of Insect Physiology*, 98, 245–257.

Taylor, M. A., Coop, R. L., and Wall, R. L. 2015. *Veterinary parasitology*. John Wiley & Sons.

Thaenkham, U., Chaisiri, K., and Hui En Chan, A. 2022. PCR and DNA sequencing: Guidelines for PCR, primer design, and sequencing for molecular systematics and identification. In: Thaenkham, U., Chaisiri, K., and Hui En Chan (eds.) *Molecular systematics of parasitic helminths*. Springer, pp. 183–199.

Tirosh-Levy, S., Gottlieb, Y., Fry, L. M., Knowles, D. P., and Steinman, A. 2020. Twenty years of equine piroplasmosis research: Global distribution, molecular diagnosis, and phylogeny. *Pathogens*, 9(11), 926.

van-der-Ree, A. M., and Mutapi, F. 2015. The helminth parasite proteome at the host–parasite interface–Informing diagnosis and control. *Experimental Parasitology*, 157, 48–58.

VanderWaal, K., Morrison, R. B., Neuhauser, C., Vilalta, C., and Perez, A. M. 2017. Translating big data into smart data for veterinary epidemiology. *Frontiers in Veterinary Science*, 4, 110.

Vashisht, V., Vashisht, A., Mondal, A. K., Farmaha, J., Alptekin, A., Singh, H., Ahluwalia, P., Srinivas, A., and Kolhe, R. 2023. Genomics for emerging pathogen identification and monitoring: Prospects and obstacles. *BioMedInformatics*, 3(4), 1145–1177.

Veselkov, K., Sleeman, J., Claude, E., Vissers, J. P., Galea, D., Mroz, A., Laponogov, I., Towers, M., Tonge, R., and Mirnezami, R. 2018. BASIS: High-performance bioinformatics platform for processing of large-scale mass spectrometry imaging data in chemically augmented histology. *Scientific Reports*, 8(1), 4053.

Wall, R., and Shearer, D. 1997. *Veterinary entomology: Arthropod ectoparasites of veterinary importance*. Springer Science & Business Media.

Waller, P. J. 2003. Global perspectives on nematode parasite control in ruminant livestock: The need to adopt alternatives to chemotherapy, with emphasis on biological control. *Animal Health Research Reviews*, 4(1), 35–44.

Wang, S., Wang, S., Luo, Y., Xiao, L., Luo, X., Gao, S., Dou, Y., Zhang, H., Guo, A., and Meng, Q. 2016. Comparative genomics reveals adaptive evolution of Asian tapeworm in switching to a new intermediate host. *Nature Communications*, 7(1), 12845.

Waury, K., Willemse, E. A., Vanmechelen, E., Zetterberg, H., Teunissen, C. E., and Abeln, S. 2022. Bioinformatics tools and data resources for assay development of fluid protein biomarkers. *Biomarker Research*, 10(1), 83.

Wilson, B. A., Garud, N. R., Feder, A. F., Assaf, Z. J., and Pennings, P. S. 2016. The population genetics of drug resistance evolution in natural populations of viral, bacterial and eukaryotic pathogens. *Molecular Ecology*, 25(1), 42–66.

Wobeser, G. A. 2013. *Essentials of disease in wild animals*. John Wiley & Sons.

Wong, F., de la Fuente-Nunez, C., and Collins, J. J. 2023. Leveraging artificial intelligence in the fight against infectious diseases. *Science*, 381(6654), 164–170.

Wratten, L., Wilm, A., and Göke, J. 2021. Reproducible, scalable, and shareable analysis pipelines with bioinformatics workflow managers. *Nature Methods*, 18(10), 1161–1168.

Wren, B. W. 2000. Microbial genome analysis: Insights into virulence, host adaptation and evolution. *Nature Reviews Genetics*, 1(1), 30–39.

Xia, X. 2017. Bioinformatics and drug discovery. *Current Topics in Medicinal Chemistry*, 17(15), 1709–1726.

Yusof, A. M. 2022. Bioinformatics applications on cryptosporidium research: A review. *Bangladesh Journal of Medical Science*, 21(1), 8.

Zarlenga, D. S., and Higgins, J. 2001. PCR as a diagnostic and quantitative technique in veterinary parasitology. *Veterinary Parasitology*, 101(3–4), 215–230.

Zheng, Y., Young, N. D., Song, J., and Gasser, R. B. 2023. Genome-wide analysis of *Haemonchus contortus* proteases and protease inhibitors using advanced informatics provides insights into parasite biology and host–parasite interactions. *International Journal of Molecular Sciences*, 24(15), 12320.

Index